PENGUIN BOOKS
THE PENGUIN DICTIONARY OF ALTERNATIVE MEDICINE

T.V. Sairam holds a doctorate in alternative medicine and has published about 400 articles in reputed journals on an assortment of subjects. He is the author of *Home Remedies* (in four volumes), hand books of herbal cures for common ailments.

The Penguin Dictionary of Alternative Medicine

T.V. Sairam

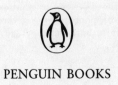

PENGUIN BOOKS

PENGUIN BOOKS
Published by the Penguin Group
Penguin Books India Pvt Ltd, 11 Community Centre, Panchsheel Park, New Delhi 110 017, India
Penguin Group (USA) Inc., 375 Hudson Street, New York, NY 10014, USA
Penguin Group (Canada), 90 Eglinton Avenue East, Suite 700, Toronto, Ontario, M4P 2Y3, Canada (a division of Pearson Penguin Canada Inc.)
Penguin Books Ltd, 80 Strand, London WC2R 0RL, England
Penguin Ireland, 25 St Stephen's Green, Dublin 2, Ireland (a division of Penguin Books Ltd)
Penguin Group (Australia), 250 Camberwell Road, Camberwell, Victoria 3124, Australia (a division of Pearson Australia Group Pty Ltd)
Penguin Group (NZ), 67 Apollo Drive, Rosedale, North Shore 0632, New Zealand (a division of Pearson New Zealand Ltd)
Penguin Group (South Africa) (Pty) Ltd, 24 Sturdee Avenue, Rosebank, Johannesburg 2196, South Africa
Penguin Books Ltd, Registered Offices: 80 Strand, London WC2R 0RL, England

First published by Penguin Books India 2007
Copyright © T.V. Sairam 2007

ISBN 10: 0-14306-307-3   ISBN 13: 978-0-14306-307-0

Typeset in ITC Stone by InoSoft Systems, Noida
Printed at Thomson Press, Noida

For my late wife, Radha

Introduction

Alternative medicine is the core of the health-care system of 80 per cent of the world's population and is one of the fastest growing sectors of healthcare. Herbs and supplements are not largely regulated by consumer-protection agencies, but studies show there is a huge surge in the demand for these alternative remedies. Between 1991 and 1997, the use of herbal medicines in the US grew by 380 per cent and, according to a 2001 study, nearly 70 per cent Americans have used as least one form of alternative treatment in their lifetime.

While conventional medicine is preferred in the treatment of trauma and emergencies (although homoeopathy can provide very effective first-aid), alternative medicine is most subscribed to in the treatment of chronic diseases. It lends gentle long-term support to release the body's own innate powers of healing with dietary modifications, herbal medicines, homoeopathy, acupuncture, hydrotherapy, massage and lifestyle counselling. Alternative medicine systems believe that the body is suffused by a network of channels that carry a subtle form of life energy and generally prefers that the patient take an active part in both prevention and treatment. Conventional medicine, on the other hand, sees the body as a mechanical system and believes most disorders can be traced to chemical imbalances best treated with powerful drugs.

Alternative medicine encompasses an array of different systems and therapies and places equal emphasis on the mind, body and spirit, with a personalized approach to bring an individual to a state of health where he or she is in harmony with their environment. It encompasses alternative medical systems including Traditional Chinese Medicine (which focusses on the balance of qi, or vital energy and incorporates the use of acupuncture, herbal medicine, massage, and qigong) and ayurveda (India's traditional healthcare system which places equal emphasis on body, mind, and spirit and strives to restore the inner harmony of the individual through diet, exercise, meditation, herbs, massage, exposure to sunlight and controlled breathing). It also includes homoeopathic medicine (based on the principle 'like cures like' i.e., the same substance that in large doses produces the symptom of an illness, in very minuscule doses may cure it) and naturopathic medicine (which emphasises health restoration rather than the treatment of disease and incorporates diet, clinical nutrition, herbal medicine, hydrotherapy, spinal and soft-tissue manipulation electric current, ultrasound and light therapies), biological medicine (which uses herbs, food and vitamins found in nature), energy medicine (which involves the use of energy fields, including qigong, reiki and systems which involve the use of electromagnetic fields such as electroacupuncture, manual medicine which is based on manipulation and/or movement of parts of the body, including osteopathy, massage, chiropractic, Feldenkrais and reflexology), and mind–body medicine (which uses techniques to help enhance the mind's ability to influence body functions and includes biofeedback, guided imagery, hypnotherapy, meditation, prayer, tai chi, qigong and yoga). Traditional medical systems are also practised by

Native American, Aboriginal Australian, African, Middle-Eastern, Tibetan and Central and South American cultures.

To physicians trained in allopathic medicine, alternative medicine is just not taught in medical schools and one they know little about. But nearly half the doctors who responded to an American survey subscribed to alternative therapies themselves. The practice of conventional medicine is also intimately linked in the medico–pharmaceutical–industrial complex whose first priority is to make profit, but more and more insurance plans covering treatments such as acupuncture and chiropractic.

Ayurvedic medicine is as applicable today as it was 5000 years ago; the powder made from the beans of *Mucuna pruriens*, commonly called velvet beans or cowitch (from the Hindi kiwatch) was used to treat Parkinson's disease for centuries in India (the disease was called kampavata in India, before it acquired its present name from James Parkinson who described it in 1817 AD), is now receiving attention in conventional medicine for the high amount of l-dopa, a precursor to dopamine, a neurotransmitter required by the central nervous system and lacking in patients of Parkinson's.

Similarly, gingko biloba, made from an extract of the leaf of the gingko tree, is now the most prescribed drug in Germany and found effective in preventing and treating Alzheimer's disease. Also in Germany, the herb saw palmetto is now prescribed in 90 per cent of all cases of enlarged prostate.

St. John's wort (*Hypericum perforatum*) has a history of medicinal use going back to ancient Greece where it was thought to treat several illnesses, including nervous conditions. It is now one of the most commonly purchased herbal products in the US where it is researched to treat alcoholism, bacterial infections, ear infections, AIDS, premenstrual syndrome, Seasonal Affective Disorder, wounds, minor burns and haemorrhoids.

Valerian, native to the Americas, Asia and Europe has been used to ease insomnia, stress-related anxiety and nervous restlessness for thousands of years and modern-day research has now confirmed the scientific validity of its historical uses. It may additionally ease menstrual and stomach cramps, Irritable Bowel syndrome, migraine symptoms and some of the restlessness that accompanies ADHD. Its most well-researched use, however, is to help people sleep.

Traditional Chinese Medicine , practised for over 3000 years in China, has one or more of its therapies used by over a quarter of the world's population. TCM, which combines the use of medicinal herbs, acupuncture and therapeutic exercises such as qigong, proved in efficacy in many chronic diseases including cancer, allergies, heart disease and AIDS. Like Ayurveda, TCM also focusses on the individual and looks for and corrects underlying causes of imbalance and patterns of disharmony.

The dictionary is a compilation of terms, ideas and concepts commonly used across the world in alternative systems healing so as to make them available in one book. A list of abbreviations used to indicate medicinal systems to which an entry belongs (in brackets against the entry) has been included at the beginning of the book. Cross references to entries are indicated through words in small capitals. There are also illustrations for the reader to refer to, although this is not specifically an illustrated dictionary. Several sources have referred to including various materia medicas, pharmacopoeias, encyclopaedias, books on various systems of medicines and websites.

Alternative medicine is a large canvass, including several techniques and healing traditions, and while every effort has been made to ensure accuracy and authenticity, there may be errors and omissions. I take complete responsibility for the material in this book, and would welcome suggestions for improvement in future editions.

T.V. Sairam

Abbreviations

Abbreviations, representing medicinal systems, used in this book are:

Afr.	African folk practices/traditions
Am. Ind.	American Indian folk practices/traditions
Arab.	Arabic/Islamic folk practices/traditions
Aus.	Australian folk practices/traditions
Cos.	Cosmetic and beauty care practices/traditions
Chi.	Chinese folk practices/traditions
Egy.	Egyptian folk practices/traditions
Eur.	European folk practices/traditions
Flo.	Flower remedies and Aromatherapy
Gem.	Therapeutic gems and crystals traditions
Grk	Greek folk practices/traditions
Haw.	Hawaiian folk practices/traditions
Heb.	Hebrew folk practices/traditions
Hom.	Homoeopathy
Ind.	Indian folk practices/traditions (Ayurveda, Siddha and Unani)
Jap.	Japanese folk practices/traditions
Kor.	Korean folk practices/traditions
Mod.	Modern medicine
Misc.	Miscellaneous
Nat.	Naturopathy and nature cure practices—traditional and modern
Num.	Numerology/Astrology
New Age	New Age concepts and practices
Occ.	Occult practices—traditional and modern
Per.	Persian folk practices/traditions
Rom.	Roman folk practices/traditions
Spa	Health treatments in Spa
Sufi	Sufi healing practices/traditions
Tib.	Ancient Tibetan and Buddhist tradition
Turk.	Turkish folk practices/traditions
Vib.	Vibrational/energy medicine
Yoga	Traditions in Yoga

abdominal breathing (Nat.) A technique of BREATHING wherein by contracting and lowering the diaphragm, the abdomen expands, facilitating optimal inhalation of oxygen. Subsequently, the abdomen is contracted by relaxing the diaphragm and letting it rise so that maximum air is expunged. A noteworthy feature of this technique is that it involves no motion of the chest or shoulders. This exercise helps not only in toning up abdominal muscles, but also in expunging the extra fat accumulation in the abdominal region.

abdominal touch diagnosis (Jap.) A traditional Japanese diagnostic method wherein pressure is applied to different areas around the abdomen, each linked to a specific organ of the body. Touch diagnosis is a specialized method in several ancient medical schools around the world, including AYURVEDA and SIDDHA.

abhava yoga (Yoga) The yoga of non-being; a higher yogic practice, involving focussing one's AWARENESS on one's CONSCIOUSNESS. There is no object or MANTRA upon which a person meditates; one's own self is meditated on as a void and without qualities, unlike in MAHA YOGA. Every action which is self-determined and ruled from within is considered in yoga philosophy as an act of Universal Oneness.

abhaya See HARITAKI.

Abhinaya Darpana (Ind.) An ancient treatise on kinesics, dealing with ABHINAYA, non-verbal communicative gestures, employing the fingers, palm, hands, legs, head, elbows, wrist, face and body. Traditional dance in India, like its architecture, music, poetry and sculpture, seeks to communicate impersonal, universal emotions, through the medium of the human anatomy, which create movement in a composition of form, both sensuous and spiritual. Dance movements and gestures were based on the alignment of the body, mind and spirit, advocated in the esoteric philosophy of YOGA.

abhiru See SATAVARI.

abhukta (Ind.) The administration of medicine on an empty stomach. An empty stomach is often regarded as an ideal setting for increasing the efficacy of medication. There has been a tradition of FASTING which itself is used as a method to fight common ailments such as headaches and fevers.

abhyanga (Ind.) The daily application of medicated oils, intended to remove dryness of the skin, besides neutralizing the aggravation of VATA, one of the three humoral defaults. Medicated oils are prepared by cooking the herbs with oil, usually in earthenware pots. Vata shamaka oil is one such oil, used to counter vata aggravation.

abhyantara kumbhaka (Yoga) An ancient technique for breath-retention (KUMBHAKA), performed with the deep-breathing exercise (PRANAYAMA). The practice is aimed at increasing one's longevity by boosting one's spiritual force, vigour and vitality.

abhyantara snehana (Ind.) The internal administration of medicated oils, intended to liquefy and dislodge toxins. In

AYURVEDA, medicated oils are applied through the mouth, eyes, nostrils, ears and anus as preventive and therapeutic measures.

abhichaara (Occ.) The employing of spells, believed to cause physical and mental harm to those they are used against. The spell components consist of certain special words, gestures, a magical object such as a wand, or a combination of the three. Once an abhichaara is cast, it has a one-time magical effect and cannot be cast again until the spell-caster re-prepares it.

abjad (Ind.) A domain of NUMEROLOGY, which is an integral part of SUFI HEALING.

abourk (Egy.) An Egyptian system of healing, based on ENERGY BALANCING.

abracadabra (Heb.) A Kabbalistic charm, derived from the initials of the Hebraic words *Ab, Ben* and *ruach a Cadesch* (Father, Son and the Holy Ghost).

Abrams, Albert (1863–1924) (New Age) A pathologist from Stanford University, Abrams was the inventor of RADIONICS, which he referred to as radio therapy. He was greatly influenced by Herman von Helmholts, a famous medical scientist, physical scientist and philosopher under whom he studied at Heidelberg University. His interest in exploring the connection between the theories of biology and physics led to the discovery of radionics.

absent healing (Vib.) Also, absentee healing. A traditional concept of healing according to which it is not essential that the healer be in close physical proximity with his patient for a diagnosis or prophylaxis. A healer, irrespective of his location, can transmit the healing energy and vibrations through his prayers to a patient *in absentia*. Saints and sages from the past are believed to continue to serve the sick and suffering with their healing energy and vibrations.

acceptance acupressure method (New Age) A system of ACUPUNCTURE which recognizes the attitude of acceptance or non-judgement as fundamental to coping with problems.

achara (Ind.) Conduct; an overall approach to a healthy lifestyle.

acid foods (Nat.) FOOD items which enhance acidity in the stomach, e.g., vegetable oils, starchy food, flour, cooked and canned vegetables, meat, fowl and fish, preserves, processed milk, pickles, butter and cheese.

aconite (Ind./Hom.) *Aconitum ferox.* Also, monkhood. A diluted non-toxic extract of the poisonous herb aconite is used in homoeopathy to treat symptoms similar to those which ingesting the poison causes; it is used to treat anxiety, fear and restlessness.

acquired knowledge (Mod.) Empirical knowledge of the material world, as distinguished from intuitive knowledge.

acro-sage (New Age) A form of Inversion Therapy in which a person is suspended upside down. By reversing the 'damaging effects' of gravity, this treatment is believed to strengthen the immune and nervous system. Developed by Benjamin Maratz, a former circus clown, in the 1990s, it is a combination of MASSAGE YOGA and gymnastics.

acu-ball pressure (New Age) A system of ACUPRESSURE, using soft balls of solid rubber to help activate the flow of CHI energy.

acu-diet (New Age) A diet leading to weight loss, usually designed to suppress hunger, regulate the appetite and reduce the stress involved in dieting. German Frank R. Bahr popularized this method in his book *Acu-diet: Weight Loss at your Fingertips*, published in 1978. According to the acu-diet theory, the 'compulsive eating centre' in the brain can be influenced favourably by massaging specific ACUPOINTS.

acuPath (Mod.) A modern motion analysis device used by ergonomists and safety engineers to prevent work-related back injuries. A similar product is also under development for use in clinical applications for patients who have sustained lower- back injuries.

acupoints (Chi.) Also, acupuncture points. ACUPUNCTURE points located along the MERIDIANS.

acupoint bloodletting (Chi.) A system of ACUPUNCTURE, characterized by puncturing ACUPOINTS with needles. The technique is designed to activate blood flow and clear the channels (MERIDIANS) of accumulated toxins.

acupoint therapy (Mod./New Age) A modern therapeutic approach, designed by Mitchell J. Rabin, a stress-management consultant. The system is based on psychological counselling and ACUPUNCTURE theory.

acupowder (New Age) Powdered herbs, applied over ACUPOINTS for activating energy flow in the region.

acupressure (Chi.) A traditional Chinese system of healing aimed at activating the flow of CHI by using finger pressure at ACUPOINTS; any treatment involving the surface stimulation of acupuncture points either with the hands or with hand-held tools. The word may also refer to SHIATSU.

acupressure facial (Cos./New Age) A facial massage which manipulates fifty energy points in the face muscles and skin to relieve stress, and ease and prevent wrinkles.

acupressure touch (Chi.) A system of ACUPRESSURE, characterized by gentle touch.

acupuncture (Chi.) A traditional Chinese system of HEALING, in which tiny needles are inserted at ACUPOINTS, aimed at activating the flow of CHI. Acupuncture may be effective in the treatment of addiction, asthma, carpal tunnel syndrome, fibromyalgia, headache, low-back pain, menstrual cramps, myofascial pain, nausea and vomiting, osteo-arthritis, post-operative dental pain, stroke rehabilitation and tennis elbow.

acupuncture analgesia (New Age) See ACUPUNCTURE ANAESTHESIA.

acupuncture anaesthesia (New Age) The application of the technique of ACUPUNCTURE in pain management, first used in China in 1958.

acupuncture-assisted anaesthesia (New Age) See ACUPUNCTURE ANAESTHESIA.

acupuncture cupping (New Age) A technique which integrates ACUPUNCTURE and CUPPING. Cupping is a technique that is used in the treatment of stagnation of CHI energy in the channels (MERIDIANS) or stagnation in blood-flow. It is normally performed as an alternative to acupuncture.

acupuncture imaging (New Age) The use of modern imaging techniques to explore connections between ACUPOINTS and the brain. Aimed at body–mind integration, the technique involves the practitioner's palpating the acupuncture zone, and simultaneously describing it to the client in inspirational terms.

acupuncture needles (Chi.) Tiny, sterile, hair-thin needles used in ACUPUNCTURE.

acupuncture points See ACUPOINTS.

acupuncture therapy (Chi.) Any treatment aimed at the subcutaneous stimulation of ACUPOINTS, enabling direct influence on the flow of CHI energy. See ZHENJIU.

ACUSCEN (Mod./New Age) The acronym of Adaptive Compact Universal Self-Correcting Electro Neuro-Stimulator, an electro-stimulator with biofeedback, used in pain or stress management. It delivers bi-polar electrical pulses, which resemble the natural pulses of neural cells every few milli-seconds.

acuscope (Mod./New Age) Also electro-acuscope. A computerized device designed to balance the body's electrical current. It monitors electrical activity in the body and indicates the mode of treatment, based on the information fed into its computers. The instrument is employed for promoting the healing of wounds and injuries.

acuscope therapy (Mod./New Age) Also electro-acuscope therapy. The therapeutic application of ACUSCOPE.

acuscope myopulse therapy (Mod./New Age) The therapeutic application of ACUSCOPE, designed for measuring a wide range of neuro-muscular conditions.

acu therapy (New Age) Gentle touching of specific areas of the body, designed to remove pain by relieving tension and muscle spasms. Acutherapy uses the body's reflex system and energy flows. This PAIN-management technique was developed in recent years by Jim Foster, an anatomist at the Myotherapy Institute Research Center at Salt Lake City, Utah.

acu-vision (New Age) A software conceived for practitioners of Traditional Chinese Medicine (TCM) and offering a ready database from Chinese traditional texts, along with a diagnostic module. By selecting a symptom, a diagnostic method established in terms of acu-points or plant formulae can be retrieved. It is also possible to transfer data on the response from the patient to the software, which in turn works like an authentic source of reference for subsequent applications.

adhama pranayama (Yoga) A system of PRANAYAMA wherein inhalation is fixed at twelve matras. As the normal ratio followed is 1:4:2, the duration for retention (KUMBHAKA) and exhalation (RECHAKA) becomes forty-eight and twenty-four matras respectively.

adhara prasadhanam (Ind.) A traditional Indian cosmetic preparation, made of tropical herbs, applied to cracked, peeling or chafed lips.

adhatoda See VASAKA.

adhisthana (Ind.) The location and virulence of a DISEASE.

adhobhukta (Ind.) The administration of medicines after eating.

adhyatma yoga (Yoga) An approach to self-realization derived from the Upanishads, and meaning the unifying discipline of the inner self. It refers to the method of realizing BRAHMAN, achieved more by being than by knowing. It also refers to an expansion of consciousness from an individual plane to the Universal plane, avoiding intellectual or emotional interferences.

adjuration (Eur./Occ.) A prayer formula used in conjuring or exorcising evil spirits and negative energies. Water, oil and salt are exorcised and these in turn are used in personal exorcism and to bless or consecrate places or objects used for worship. God is sought to endow supernatural power on these material elements to protect those who use them against evil influences.

advanced energy healing (New Age) A system of HEALING which integrates AURA ANALYSIS, AWARENESS RELEASE TECHNIQUE, CLAIRVOYANT DIAGNOSIS, MAGNETIC HEALING, SOUL MERGING and THIRD-EYE AWAKENING. It was developed by Robert Jaffe, a contemporary medical doctor and energy healer from California.

aeromancy (Eur./Occ.) From the Greek *aero*, meaning air, and *manteia*, meaning divination; one of the oldest forms of DIVI-

NATION, it is a means of foretelling events by observing atmospheric conditions such as storms, wind currents, cloud formations, comets and falling stars. The types of divination that can be included in aeromancy are AUSTROMANCY, divination by observing wind direction and intensity; NEPHOMANCY, divination by observing cloud formations and movements; ceraunoscopy, the interpretation of thunder and lightning; CHAOMANCY, aerial vision; cometomancy, interpreting the appearance of comet tails; and meteormancy, interpretation based on observing shooting stars and meteors. Ancient Hindus, Etruscans and Babylonians found portents in the sky of great interest and this was reflected in the gods worshipped by them. In medieval times, aeromancy involved summoning ghosts to project images of approaching events onto clouds. Modern aeromancy is more introspective, almost a meditative process. See also AUROMANCY.

aetites (Eur./Grk.) Also aquilaeus, eagle stone and rattlestone. A purple-coloured concretion of mostly iron oxide, filled with loose sand that rattles when shaken. Said to be imbued with magical powers, it was believed to have been found in the neck or stomach of an eagle and that eagles transported this stone to facilitate the laying of their eggs. It is traditionally worn bound to the arm, as a protection against miscarriage, to prevent impending sickness and to prevent untimely births. It is also said to heal epilepsy and prevent premature births, and to aid in childbirth when worn on the thigh.

affirmation (New Age) Expressions conceived in the belief of investing the SELF with power; often written down, spelt or chanted repeatedly, with the conviction that the utterance can alter an actual situation. While formulating affirmation, positive statements of immediacy (e.g., 'I am perfectly all right now.') are found to be more effective than the ones that affirm a future event (e.g., 'I'll be all right.').

affusion therapy (Nat./Spa) The application of WATER of varying temperatures to achieve specific therapeutic effects such as enhancement in circulation. The technique is employed extensively in HEALTH spas in Europe.

African holistic health (Afr./New Age) An African version of NATUROPATHY, as developed by Llaila O. Afrika, a contemporary herbalist and a massage therapist who devised certain biochemical diagnostic tests using saliva and urine specimens. See AFRICAN HOLISTIC HEALTH.

agada tantra (Ind.) Toxicology; a branch of AYURVEDA which deals with various methods for eliminating toxins from the body.

agape (Grk.) A Greek word meaning unconditional love; it is also the New Testament word for love and was used by early Christians to refer to the self-sacrificing love they believed each should have for the other, and returned evil with good. Greek philosophers contemporary to Plato used the word in a way that suggested love for that which was below you, rather than *philia*, love between equals, and *eros*, love for that which is above you. *Eros* was seen as the highest, and *agape* as the lowest.

agape eros-being centre (Grk.) One of the four dynamic-being centres which the embodied soul is divided into. It consists of the upper frontal portion of the body which is believed to mediate feelings of openness towards others. The other three centres are the hara-being centre (the abdominal portion of the body, supposedly permitting self-love), the logos-being centre (the upper dorsal portion of the body, possessing limitless intuitive faculties) and the phallic–spiritual warrior-being centre (the lower back and the limbs enabling resoluteness and perseverance).

agape quest programme (New Age) An integrated approach to KINESIOLOGY, including ACUPRESSURE and BACH FLOWER REMEDIES.

agar See AGURU.

agarbha pranayama (Yoga) One of the two types of PRANAYAMA. It excludes JAPA or MEDITATION unlike SAGARBHA PRANAYAMA, which is accompanied by JAPA or MANTRA. Many yoga teachers encourage only sagarbha pranayama.

agarwood tree See AGURU.

agate (Gem) A naturally striped chalcedony quartz, named after a river in Sicily, and widely used in the system of talismans. There are two forms of agate: the dark-green moss agate, also called gardener's stone, said to strengthen the heart chakra, bring peace and balance and enable its wearer to remain close to nature; and the green-and-white tree agate, believed to enhance its wearer's introspection and broaden his outlook.

agati (Ind.) *Sesbania grandiflora*. A folk remedy; the bark, leaves, gum and flowers of this plant are used in the treatment of bruises, catarrh, dysentery, fevers, headaches, anaemia, bronchitis, pain, sores, sore throats and stomatitis.

> 'One who consumes agati avoids aggravation of pitta.'
>
> —Sage Agastya

agathodemon (Egy.) A good spirit, worshipped by ancient Egyptians, depicted as a serpent with a human head.

age of Aquarius See NEW AGE.

age regression (New Age) A system of HYPNOTHERAPY based on the belief that all forms of diseases are linked to events in one's past.

ageing (Misc.) The accumulation of free radicals, oxidants, which can appropriate electrons from other molecules, is believed to be the cause of ageing. Recent clinical trials have reportedly shown that the daily intake of natural antioxidants can delay the process of ageing. Current concepts of ageing believe that this phenomenon is not the result of a single mechanism but represents several phenomena—all orchestrated. Physiological theories of ageing focus on organ systems and their interrelationships: wrinkling of the skin, shrinking of the body and limbs, fading eyesight, and loss of enthusiasm, memory and strength are some symptoms of ageing. While ageing is not a state of disease, some diseases are caused due to ageing.

agni (Ind./Yoga) Fire; in the context of living organisms, agni represents the heat energy responsible for digestion and other metabolic activities. The active element in the digestive processes taking place in the stomach and gastrointestinal tract is called JATHARAGNI. BHUTAGNI works at nourishing and DHATUAGNI enables the formation of DHATUS in the body. Agni is also one of FIVE ELEMENTS of AYURVEDA. The four different body states of the fire element in AYURVEDA are indicated in the following table:

Agni

Type of digestive fire or agni	Associated digestive conditions/symptoms
Vishamagni, as influenced by VAYU	Upward movement of gas in the stomach, causing noise and heaviness, resulting in constipation or dysentery, distension of abdomen and/or colic pain
Tikshnagni, as influenced by PITTA	Burning sensation and heat, resulting in parched lips, palate and throat, quick digestion, coupled with enormous appetite
Mandagni, as influenced by KAPHA	Difficulties in digestion, causing heaviness in abdomen and also in the head, dyspnoea, salivation and fatigue
Samagni, as influenced by an equilibrium state of the three DOSHAs	Normal digestion, paving way for good health

agni anushasan mudra (Yoga) A MUDRA, formed by touching of tips of thumbs and projecting the index fingers downwards and keeping the remaining three fingers closed. This mudra is believed to work on the lower abdomen and intestines and is recommended as an aid for digestion.

agni-karmal See MOXIBUSTION.

agnimantha (Ind.) *Premna integrifolia.* One of the ten celebrated roots, or DASAMULA, in AYURVEDA. The bark of the tree is used in the treatment of abdominal diseases, fevers, flatulence, liver complaints, neuralgic disorders and rheumatism. (The other nine roots widely used in ayurveda are *Aegle marmelos, Ailanthus excelsa, Stereospermum suaveolens, Phaseolus trilobus, Teramnus labialis, Tick trefoil, Uraria picta, Solanum indicum* and *Solanum xanthocarpum*).

agni mushti mudra (Yoga) A MUDRA formed by touching the tips of both the thumbs and closing all other fingers. As this mudra is believed to produce heat in the body, it is considered an aid for digestion.

Agni Yoga (Yoga) Inspired by Vedic traditions, Buddhism and Theosophy, and also called the Teaching of Living Ethics, Agni Yoga was founded by Russian painter Nicholas Roerich and his wife Helena. The word 'agni' refers to a spiritual fire within the heart or psychic energy, seen as the core on which life is based. Agni Yoga is just not a path of physical exercises, meditation and asceticism, but also of conscious altruism. In the early 1920s, the Roerichs attracted a following in New York City, where they built a museum, and also in India where they retired.

agrimony (Chi./Flo.) *Agrimonia eupatoria.* A perennial herb indigenous to the swamps in Europe and North America and used in folk remedies to heal ulcers and wounds. The ancient Greeks used it to treat eye conditions. In traditional Chinese medicine, agrimony is used to eliminate tape worms and treat digestive conditions. When the plant flowers, the entire plant is cut above the root, then chopped, dried and stored for use in folk medicine.

agudagandha See ASAFOETIDA.

aguru (Ind.) *Aquilaria agalloch.* Also, agar, agarwood tree. The tree, now endangered, grows in the foothills of Assam, Burma, Vietnam and Papua New Guinea. It produces a valuable aromatic resin, in great demand for its use in incense and medicine. The wood of this tree is used to remove wrinkles and flabbiness from the face and in the treatment of nausea and diarrhoea.

'Aguru rejuvenates the body shattered by ageing.'

—A Tamil Siddha song

ahamkara (Yoga) Ego, one of the three factors constituting CHITTA or consciousness.

ahara (Ind.) Food.

ahara rasa (Ind.) The essence of food.

ahara shakti (Ind.) An assessment of the capacity of a patient to ingest, digest, and assimilate food. The duration between consuming a meal and the next one is a measure of *agnibala*, or the strength of the digestive fire. An optimal ahara shakti, indicates a quicker expected recovery from disease and imbalance. The capacity of consumption of food and its digestion is thus taken as an indicator of health or morbidity.

ahimsa (Ind./Yoga) Non-violence, in the Hindu, Jain and Buddhist traditions. In its wider sense, it encompasses an abstinence from causing harm to any living creature, by thought, word or deed. It involves the development of a mental attitude in which hatred is replaced by love.

aikido (Jap.) A Japanese martial art which focusses on using the opponents' energy to gain control over them. It is not a static art, but places great emphasis on motion and the dynamics of movement. Although the idea of a martial discipline striving for peace and harmony may seem paradoxical, at least to the uninitiated, aikido also refers to spiritual enlightenment, physical health and peace of mind.

air-ion therapy See NEGATIVE ION THERAPY.

air-pumping cupping method (New Age) A form of CUPPING that requires a suction device, such as an air-pumping cup.

air therapy (New Age) Exposure to the air in natural surroundings, such as beaches, caves, groves, mountains, rivers, springs, waterfalls and wells, for their high concentration of NEGATIVE IONS. Research suggests that while some allergy-provoking substances, such as dust and pollen, exhibit a positive electrical charge, they can be counteracted with negative ions which are believed to be curative for their beneficial effects on respiration.

ajamoda See AJWAIN.

ajapa japa (Yoga) Ceaseless awareness; the practice of JAPA without the mental effort normally needed to repeat a MANTRA; the automatic repetition of mantras.

ajasrika (Ind./Yoga) Activities that promote positive health and wellbeing such as yoga, PRANAYAMA, regulated food intake, an attitude of gratitude and unconditional love for all God's creations.

ajirna (Ind.) Dyspepsia. Often, dyspepsia is caused by a stomach ulcer or acid reflux disease. In the latter, stomach acid finds its way back into the oesophagus, the tube leading from the mouth to the stomach, and causes pain in the chest. Antacids, which neutralize the acidity in the stomach, are prescribed when such symptoms occur.

ajna chakra (Yoga) Located at the point of the THIRD EYE, which is the conscience, the ajna chakra reveals insight. It is one of the fourteen CHAKRAS.

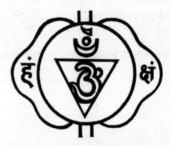

Ajna Chakra

ajna's tube (Yoga) A psychic passageway that runs from the AJNA CHAKRA to the back of the head.

ajwain (Ind.) *Trachispermum ammi*. Also, ammi bishop's weed. The fruit, often inaccurately referred to as a seed, is used as an antispasmodic, stimulant, tonic and carminative and to ease asthma and indigestion and treat diarrhoea and flatulence.

Ajwain alone helps in digesting a hundred varieties of food.

—A Sanskrit saying

akasha (Ind./Yoga) Sky, ether; the all-pervading space in the universe; the first of the five elements (PANCHABHUTAS) of which the physical universe is made. Also used to designate 'inner' space, that is the space of CONSCIOUSNESS (called cid-akasha).

akasha mudra (Yoga) A MUDRA, made by conjoining tips of the thumb and index finger (or, sometimes, the middle finger). It is believed to increase the composition of ether in the body.

akshara mushtika (Yoga) The art of communicating syllables or ideas by fingers.

akshaya See VIBHITAKI.

akriti (Ind.) A term for physical shape; external shape.

Alastor (Grk.) The avenging god. In Greek mythology, Alastor is the avenging demon, associated with blood feuds between families, and is the term for an avenging power that visits the sins of the fathers on their children.

Albucasis See AL-ZAHRAWI.

alchemical bodywork (New Age) An approach to EMOTIONAL RELEASE, using BODYWORK and HYPNOSIS.

alchemical hypnotherapy (New Age) An approach to healing, which combines the use of insight, EMOTIONAL RELEASE, and emotional clearing. Developed in the 1970s by David Quigley, a hypnotist and psychotherapist, the method is said to help a patient find and transform any imagery that affects him adversely.

alectorius (Gem) A real or supposed animal concretion, thought to come from a cock's throat. Known from ancient times, it was believed to make its wearer invincible and wealthy, help regain lost kingdoms, and even find new ones. It was also used as an antidote for poison.

alectromancy (Eur./Occ.) A method of DIVINATION, using a cock or a hen.

aleuromancy (Eur./Occ.) A method of DIVINATION, using flour.

Alexander, Gerda See EUTONY.

Alexander technique (Mod.) A method for improving ease and freedom of movement, balance, support and coordination, as formulated by Frederick Matthias Alexander (1869–1955), a Shakespearean actor from Australia. Optimum bodily movements are believed to flow from one basic movement, the maximum lengthening of the spine, which Alexander called the 'primary' control. Though the technique is more a re-education process than a prophylactic treatment, it is found to improve neuro-muscular coordination.

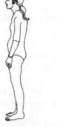
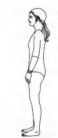

The wrong way   The correct way
of standing   of standing

Alexander Technique

alextoromantia (Occ.) A DIVINATION method based on the direction in which a rooster immediately turns when let loose in a circle. The circle made indicates all the eight directions to facilitate the observer's identifying the direction instantly.

Alextryomancy (Occ.) A DIVINATION method in which random configurations assumed by grains of wheat scattered on the ground are studied to infer divine logic and plan one's future course of action.

alfalfa (Chi./Ind.) *Medicago sativa.* A herb native to the Mediterranean region. The dried leaves and seeds of this plant have long been used in folk medicine, especially in India and China. Alfafa saponins has anti-fungal properties, reported to act on the cardiovascular, nervous and digestive systems. The leaves contain eight essential amino acids and are rich in calcium, magnesium, potassium and carotene. It is also a folk remedy for joint stress and is considered a galactogogue.

algotherapy (Cos./Mod./Spa) A form of THALASSOTHERAPY; also known as seaweed bath. Algotherapy uses seaweeds in facials, body wraps, and baths for detoxification and rejuvenation. Treatment with seaweeds are found useful in stress management, muscle and skin restoration and weight control.

alkaline food (Mod.) A high intake of foods that alkalize, viz., agar, alfalfa, dried ginger, almonds, dried coconut, peanuts, fruits and raw vegetables, buttermilk, yoghurt and raw milk, is recommended for the upkeep of health. Allergic reactions and other forms of stress tend to produce acid in the stomach; eating alkalizing food counters acidity.

alliance method (New Age) The Usui system of REIKI; a form of reiki training as developed by Chujiro Hayashi, a retired naval officer and a successor to Sensei Usui. Hayashi made changes in the reiki system and introduced the twelve hand positions currently used in reiki. The Usui system of reiki generates energy for personal and family healing, as a gentle complementary therapy.

> 'This power (reiki) is unfathomable, immeasurable, and being a universal life force, it is incomprehensible to man. Yet, every single living being is receiving its blessings daily, awake and asleep.'
>
> —Hawayo Takata

allium cepa (Mod.) Also, red onion. The diluted extract of the red onion is used to treat symptoms similar to those caused by the red onion, e.g. burning and watering eyes.

allopathy (Mod.) Conventional medicine. The term was coined by Samuel Hahnemann, the founder of homoeopathy with which it is often contrasted. Allopathy treats a disease with drugs having the opposite effect to the existing symptoms. This formidable body of knowledge is the most organized and widely used system of medicine; each finding is based on extensive research, has helped alleviate pain and suffering and increased life spans. As the system emphasizes the symptomatic cure of a disease, as opposed to viewing the patient as a whole, the need for specialists for specific organs and diseases has arisen.

allspice (Am.Ind.) *Pimenta dioica*. The dried, unripe berry of this evergreen tree tastes like a blend of cinnamon, cloves and nutmeg, hence its name. The tree is a native to south Mexico and the Caribbean. The berries are used in folk medicine for relief from indigestion.

almond (Ind.) *Prunus amygdalus*. Also, badam. The tree is a native of south-west Asia. The parts of this tree are used variously in different parts of the globe: leaves, bark and fruit fight dysentery (south-east Asia) and are used as dressings for rheumatic joints (Indonesia); the bark is used to treat diarrhoea (Samoa), dysentery and fever (Brazil); leaves are used to treat scabies (India and Pakistan), colic (South America), liver diseases (Taiwan), control bleeding during teeth extraction (Mexico) and intestinal parasites (Philippines); the fruit is used in the treatment of nausea and asthma (Mexico), leprosy and headaches (India) and coughs (Samoa).

> 'Almond renders beauty.'
>
> —*Atanga Samgraham*

alochak pitta (Ind.) One of the five types of PITTA, alochak pitta is believed to reside in the eyes and at the THIRD EYE, the point between the two eyebrows. According to AYURVEDA, it transforms the reflection of an object on the retina into an image and thus initiates vision, both sensory and spiritual. See also DOSHA.

aloe (Chi./Grk./Ind./Sufi.) Also kumari, aloe vera. Native to the Cape Verde islands, off the West African coast, the plant, known for its healing qualities, is now grown in many parts of the world. About 2,000 years ago, the Greek historian Dioscorides and Roman naturalist Pliny recommended aloe vera as an effective household remedy for burns, bruises, cuts, scrapes,

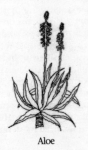

Aloe

constipation and skin irritation. Aloe was also an important part of famed Egyptian queen Cleopatra's toilette.

> 'Aloe vera contains the greatest number of active substances of any plant I've looked at.'
>
> —Dr Robert H. Davis

alomancy (Eur./Occ.) A method of DIVINATION, using salt.

alpha calm therapy (New Age) An integrated approach to healing, which combines VISUALIZATION and ERIKSONIAN HYPNOSIS.

alpha waves (Mod./New Age) A type of BRAINWAVES, with a range of frequencies between 8 and 12 Hz, believed to be the gateway to meditation, and providing a bridge between the conscious and the unconscious mind. Characterized by a relaxed state of mind with enough room for VISUALIZATION and CREATIVITY, a concentration of alpha waves is often associated with a liberating sense of peace, pleasure and well-being. In BIOFEEDBACK, alpha-centred programmes are often recommended for addressing stress and stress-related disorders.

alphitomancy (Eur./Occ.) A form of DIVINATION using barley cakes or loaves of barley bread, chiefly employed in ancient times to prove the innocence or guilt of suspected people. Suspects would be fed barley cakes or slices; those who got indigestion were held as guilty and the rest innocent.

Al-Razi, Abu Bakr Mohammad Ibn Zakariya (841–926) Persian physician, philosopher and scholar who made enduring contributions to medicine, alchemy and philosophy. Although he was initially inclined towards music, he later learnt medicine, mathematics, astronomy, chemistry and philosophy. His was the first treatise on smallpox and chickenpox, and he was the first to draw a distinction between them. He was also an expert surgeon, and introduced the use of opium in anaesthesia. A notable feature of his medical system was that he favoured cure through correct and regulated food and emphasized the importance of psychological factors on health. His contribution greatly influenced the development of medicine.

> 'An intelligent physician cannot heal all diseases since that is simply not possible.'
>
> —Al-Razi

alternate hot and cold hand bath (Nat.) A simple form of treatment in WATER THERAPY. The hands are plunged first in hot water (for, say, three minutes), followed by cold water (for say, half a minute). The process is repeated thrice and ends with cold-water immersion. This treatment, ideal for cold hands, is aimed at improving blood circulation in the wrists and hands.

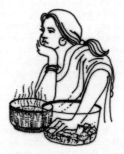

Alternate hot and cold hand bath

alternate hot and cold leg bath (Nat.) A simple form of treatment in water therapy, in which the legs (up to the calves) are plunged first in hot water (for, say, three minutes) and then in COLD WATER (for, say, half a minute). The process, repeated thrice, ends with cold-water immersion. This treatment is often recommended for congestion of lungs, insomnia, pelvic pain, painful periods and suppressed menstruation.

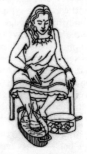

Alternate hot and cold leg bath

alternate nostril breathing method See ANULOMA VILOMA.

alternative childbirth (Nat.) The natural approach to childbirth as administered by midwives in traditional societies.

alternative medicine (Mod.) Methods of healing used in place of conventional medical treatment, ALLOPATHY. It is distinct from complementary medicine which is used in conjunction with, rather than instead of, allopathy.

alternative nutrition (New Age) An approach to nutrition which falls outside the scope of dietary systems as recognized by modern medicine.

Altman, Nathaniel See SCIENTIFIC PALMISTRY.

Al-Zahrawi, Abu al-Qasim Khalaf bin Abbas (AD 936–1013) A famous Arab surgeon and physician for the king of Spain, Al-Zahrawi was known to the West by his Latin name Albucasis. He invented several surgical instruments, including instruments for the internal examination of the ear and for removing foreign bodies from the throat. He also wrote an encyclopaedia on surgery.

ama (Ind.) The accumulation of toxic undigested food and waste products in the body.

ama deus (Am. Ind./Occ.) Literally 'to love God'. A 6,000-year-old system of DIVINATION, HEALING and MAGIC, developed by the Guarani Indians of the Amazon Rain Forest, ama deus uses BREATHING, symbols and vibrational energy to accelerate the healing process in the body.

amantilla See TAGARA.

amla See AMALAKI.

amalaki (Ind.) *Emblica officinale*. Also, amla, emblic myrobalan, Indian gooseberry. It grows all over the Indian subcontinent, from Myanmar to Afghanistan and from the Himalayas in the north to the Deccan in the south.

The fruit contains natural antioxidants and is the richest natural source of vitamin C. It is cooling and laxative. The dried fruit is used traditionally in the treatment of diarrhoea, dysentery and haemorrhage.

Amalaki is one of the three myrobalans, which combine together to form the popular rejuvenating formula, TRIPHALA.

> 'Amalaki is the best among all the rejuvenating herbs.'
>
> —*Charaka Samhita*

amanae (New Age) Bodywork aimed at releasing emotional blockages, generally comprising bitter, old memories and traumatizing experiences. A typical amanae session involves a brief discussion with the client, encouraging him or her to go deep into his or her being, and assisting in releasing emotional blockages that surface and separate the patient from his original self. Proper breathing and other physical techniques are also employed to achieve this goal. The deep emotional shifting is said to result in the liberation of energy which has often been locked up for years in emotional blockages, thus enhancing one's wellbeing.

amandinus (Gem) A variously coloured gemstone, believed to enable its wearer to overcome bad dreams.

amaragandhiharidra See MANGO-GINGER.

amaroli See AUTOURINE THERAPY.

ambahava See GUGGULU.

amber (Gem) A fossilized resin, believed to stimulate friendship and happiness. In folk remedies, it is prescribed in the treatment of ailments connected with the stomach, liver and kidneys. Amber beads are also traditionally worn to insulate the wearer from ailments such as headaches, jaundice, rheumatism, rickets and toothaches.

America, herbal medicine in The term herbal medicine generally refers in the US to a system of medicine that uses European or North American plants. The traditional use of medicinal plants in North America traces its origin to the coming together of both European settlers and Native Americans during the eighteenth and nineteenth centuries. The practice of medicine is, however, restricted to professionals who have a license. There are no restrictions on teaching people how to take better care of themselves. Most herbalists, therefore, call themselves teachers, healers or counsellors, rather than medical practitioners.

amethyst (Gem) A transparent, purple quartz, the birth stone for people born in February. It is traditionally worn in rings, bracelets and necklaces to soothe the pain of migraine, arthritis and gout. Amethyst is also believed to keep its wearer calm and in control of his various emotional levels. It is kept under pillows to bring pleasant dreams.

'Amethyst can dissipate all evil thoughts and quicken the intelligence.'

—Leonardo da Vinci

AMI (Mod./New Age) See APPARATUS FOR MEASURING THE FUNCTIONAL CONDITIONS OF MERIDIANS AND THEIR CORRESPONDING INTERNAL ORGANS.

amiante (Gem) A fireproof stone, traditionally considered to counter the charms of magic.

amla See AMALAKI.

amlika See AMALAKI.

amplification (New Age) Elaboration and clarification, especially of dream images, by ideas associated with it or by drawing parallels from mythology, folklore and ethnology.

amplified-energy therapy (New Age) A contemporary form of ENERGY HEALING, popularized by Richard Gordon, and based on the principle that one can manoeuvre one's own life-energy for healing by following the body's innate intelligence.

amra (Ind.) *Mangifera indica.* Also, mango. This popular fruit tree is also used in traditional Indian medicine. The leaf decoction is taken as a remedy for diarrhoea, fever, chest complaints, diabetes and hypertension, its dried flowers are used in the treatment of diarrhoea and chronic dysentery, the bark in rheumatic conditions and diphtheria, and the resinous gum from the tree trunk to treat cracks in the skin of the feet, scabies and syphilitic sores.

'A year in which I don't eat my mangoes should be deleted from my lifespan.'

—Rabindranath Tagore

amritalata See GUDUCHI.

amritavalli See GUDUCHI.

amritavallari See GUDUCHI.

amritpan (Yoga) 'The quaffing of nectar'. A DHARANA practice, involving the control of BREATHING, focussing AWARENESS on CHAKRAS and the VISUALIZATION of drawing up nectar from the MANIPURA to the VISHUDDHI through the spinal pathway with the help of the suction pressure in one's BREATH.

amulet (Eur./Occ.) An object, image, inscription or drawing which is imbued with magical properties, worn to ward off disease and the evil eye. Semi-precious stones, metals such as iron, copper or silver, fruit and vegetables are commonly used as amulets.

Ana Be'ko'ach (Eur./Occ.) An ancient practice of MEDITATION and PRAYER, built around a sequence of forty-two letters from the *Book of Genesis.*

anacard See BHALLATAKA.

anaesthetic acupuncture (New Age) See ACUPUNCTURE ANAESTHESIA.

anahata chakra (Yoga) 1. Heart chakra; one of the fourteen CHAKRAS representing cognition, compassion and what is called the 'I-love attitude'; 2. a sound without boundaries; the inner sound.

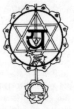

Anahata Chakra

'The Great Instrument is uncompleted. The Great Tone has an inaudible sound.'

—Lao Tzu

analytical psychology (Mod.) A school of depth psychology, based on the movement started by Carl Gustav Jung. It includes a comprehensive view of the human psyche, in both its conscious and unconscious aspects, and primordial images deriving from the deepest layers of the unconscious psyche ('archetypes of the collective unconscious'). Jung described striking parallels between the unconscious images produced by individuals in dreams and visions and the universal motifs found in the religions and mythologies of all ages.

anandamaya kosha (Yoga) The innermost of the five sheaths (PANCHAKOSHA) which constitute the body–mind–spirit complex in Indian philosophy, this sheath represents perennial bliss. The other four sheaths are the annamaya kosha, the sheath of food, pranamaya kosha, the sheath of life, manomaya kosha, the sheath of the mind, and vijnanamaya kosha, the sheath of knowledge.

Ananda Yoga (New Age/Yoga) A version of HATHA YOGA, with a much gentler approach towards exercises. Besides the physical exercises (asana), breathing exercises (PRANAYAMA) and mental exercises (DHYANA), Ananda Yoga also makes use of silent affirmations which contribute to its uniqueness. The system was developed by Swami Kriyananda, a disciple of Paramahamsa Yogananda, a practitioner of Kriya Yoga, who recorded his spiritual journey in *An Autobiography of Yogi*.

anapana sati (Yoga) Meditation on breathing as expounded by the Buddha in his Great Discourse on the Foundations of Mindfulness. It is considered the gateway to enlightenment and the very basis of Buddhahood.

androdamas (Gem) A mystical stone, resembling a diamond, found in squares in the sands of the Red Sea. It is believed to restrain anger and alleviate lunacy.

anemoscopy (Eur./Occ.) A form of DIVINATION which takes into account aspects of wind, such as its intensity, direction and sound. It also includes the observation of objects such as dust or smoke carried by the wind. A method in anemoscopy involves asking a question and then tossing a handful of dirt, sand or seeds into the air and observing the answer from the pattern of the resulting dust clouds. Another, the pendulum method, involves holding a pendulum over a circle lined with runes or other symbols and, after formulating the question to be asked, observing how the wind moves the pendulum.

angel chiropractic care (New Age) A holistic approach for healing, which includes APPLIED KINESIOLOGY, BACH FLOWER REMEDIES, BIOMAGNETISM, CHIROPRACTIC, CRANIOSACRAL THERAPY, NUTRITIONAL COUNSELLING, REFLEXOLOGY and VIBRATIONAL MEDICINE.

angelic healing (New Age) A holistic method of HEALING, consisting of PRAYER, MEDITATION and VISUALIZATION, based on the belief that angels guide, protect and heal people invisibly.

angelica root (Chi.) *Angelica sinensis*. Also, Chinese angelica, dong quai, female ginseng, tang-kuei. A multi-purpose root, widely used in China to treat gynaecological disorders, fatigue and mild anaemia. It is also used as an aphrodisiac.

anima (Yoga) One of the eight SIDDHIS, it enables one to perceive oneself as minute as an atom.

Anima mundi (Eur./New Age) 'Soul of the world'; the divine essence that envelopes the universe; a concept that the world as such represents a whole, living entity.

animal electricity (Mod.) Accidentally discovered by Italian physician Luigi Galvani in the eighteenth century, it led to the foundation of a new science, electrophysiology, the study of the electrical properties of biological cells and tissues. It involves measurements of voltage change or electrical current flow on a wide variety of scales from single-ion channel proteins to whole tissues like the heart.

animal magnetism (New Age) An organic magnetism, similar to physical magnetism; a vital force that can be transmitted from one person to another without physical contact, and believed to enhance healing. The existence of such a force and its therapeutic role was asserted by an Austrian physician, Franz Anton MESMER (1734–1815). He reasoned that his own body acted as a type of magnet, reinforcing the fluid in the bodies of his patients. He considered all ailments as caused by an obstacle to the flow of this body-fluid and was of the view that the same can be overcome by correcting the flow. His theories and methods came to be known as MESMERISM. Although several of his contemporaries regarded Mesmer's practice as quackery, his theory of animal magnetism laid the foundation for modern hypnosis and suggestion therapy.

animal psi (Eur.) Also, anspsi. The term animal psi, coined by J.B. Rhine, refers to paranormal abilities as may be exhibited by some animals. PSI talents such as CLAIRVOYANCE, PRECOGNITION, and TELEPATHY are believed to exist in some animals and birds. Pet dogs, for instance, have been found to behave uncharacteristically to exhibit their forecasting an adverse event in the family.

animism (Eur./Occ.) The term refers to the belief that supernatural beings, endowed with intelligence, inhabit even inanimate objects, such as stones, groves, lakes and rivers, i.e., that everything possesses a soul or consciousness. Animists can be found today in significant numbers in several countries around the globe, including Congo, Ethiopia, Gabon, India, Indonesia, Japan, Laos, Myanmar, Papua New Guinea, the Philippines, Russia, Sweden, Thailand, the US and Zambia.

anjali mudra (Yoga) A MUDRA in which the two palms are brought together at the chest level. This posture is considered a yogic process of the unification of all universal forces to achieve balance and harmony. It is also a common Asian form of salutation.

anma (Jap.) Also, anma, pu tong an mo. *An* means press, *mo* means rub, and *an mo* means massage. A general form of Chinese QIGONG massage, which recognizes 361 'energy points' (TSUBOS) in the body. The massage is aimed at improving blood circulation and relaxation. See also, ANMA THERAPY.

anma therapy (New Age) A BODYWORK programme employing techniques and treatment procedures borrowed both from traditional Oriental medicine and the Western school of medicine. Anma therapy helps in restoring and maintaining the optimum by addressing the physical body, bio-energy and emotions. This copyrighted treatment programme, as developed in recent times by Korean-born Tina Sohn, includes the use of dietary therapy, herbs, nutritional supplements and the external application of herbal preparations.

anna (Ind.) Food, diet.

anise (Eur./Ind.) *Pimpinella anisum*. The herb, native to Asia Minor, was widely cultivated in ancient Egypt. It is used to treat dry coughs, where expectoration is difficult. Its stimulant and carminative properties also make it useful in flatulence and colic. Its volatile oil, obtained from the seeds, is mixed with spirits of wine and made into a liqueur (anisette) which is useful in bronchial problems. The oil is also a good antiseptic.

antimonium tartaricum (Hom.) Also, ant-t; ant. tart, tart emetic. Though it is highly poisonous, ant. tart. in homeopathic dosages assists in the healing of measles, chicken pox, whooping cough, pneumonia, bronchitis, nausea and vomiting.

anspsi (Eur.) See ANIMAL PSI.

antaranga kumbhaka (Yoga) The suspension of breath after full inhalation during PRANAYAMA. The retention of breath inside the body is believed to enhance the value of respiration.

antaranga sadhana (Yoga) Literally, the mental practice. The term also refers to emotional and mental disciplining (say, through PRANAYAMA) and mental detachment (as brought about by practising, say, PRATYAHARA). The ancient system of yoga recognizes the inherent, untapped power of emotions and, through various practices, aims at harnessing and channelizing it for the benefit of individuals as well as society.

> 'The aim of yoga is to calm down the chaos of conflicting impulses.'
>
> —Sage Patanjali

antaranga trataka (Yoga) A form of TRATAKA involving intense VISUALIZATION of a CHAKRA or a presiding deity. This yoga system is oriented towards tapping the inherent, hidden, unmanifested and untapped energy within an individual's body–mind complex.

antaratma sadhana (Yoga) The quest for the soul through meditative practices, viz., DHARANA, DHYANA and SAMADHI. These three practices relate to the higher realms of the eight-fold yoga system, codified by PATANJALI.

anthotherapy (New Age) Therapeutic spa treatments, provided either in dry conditions or in hot and humid caves filled with vapours. The high humidity and absence of pollen in caves makes them an ideal setting to treat people with allergies and ailments of the respiratory system.

anthropomancy (Eur./Occ.) A method of DIVINATION, using the entrails of a dead or dying person. Although this barbaric practice has long been outlawed, there are instances of this method being practised in recent history.

anthropometry (Mod.) A system of measurement of the various body segments and their proportions. In AYURVEDA, the height, length and breadth of the various limbs are measured in terms of the breadth of a person's own finger.

anthroposophical medicine (Eur.) The remedies of ANTHROPOSOPHY. While analytical medicine forms the backbone of the Western school, in the Eastern tradition, physicians employ their intuitive skills not only for diagnosis but also for the treatment of ailments.

anthroposophy (New Age/Occ.) Derived from the Greek *anthropo,* meaning human, and *sophia,* meaning wisdom. An esoteric, curative philosophy, aimed at reviving the human ability to use spiritual perceptions for HEALING. Rudolf Steiner, an Australian social philosopher, was the main architect of this philosophy. Anthroposophy to concerned with life with regard to its spiritual reality.

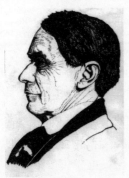

Rudolf Steiner

anti-candida diet (Mod./New Age) A diet which excludes foodstuffs that contrib-

ute to a susceptibility to candida infections. Foods such as sugar in all its forms, yeast-risen breads and bakery products, malted cereals, cheeses, mushroom and fruit are excluded in an anti-candida diet. There is, however, some disagreement about how restrictive the anti-candida diet needs to be with regard to starch, grains, vegetables, and breads. Some dieticians recommend a very low total carbohydrate diet with no yeast-containing products, whereas others recommend the focus on the elimination of fermentable sugars alone.

anti-nutrients (Mod.) Food items which are devoid of minerals and vitamins (such as sugar and white flour) and can cause the severe depletion of critical glucose-metabolizing minerals such as chromium.

antioxidants (Mod.) Molecules that prevent the toxic effects of free radicals by lending electrons to them, without turning into toxic radicals themselves. Vitamin C, Vitamin E and beta-carotenes found in the body are important antioxidants, and are considered essential for rejuvenation.

anuloma viloma (Yoga) Also, alternate-nostril BREATHING method. Inhalation is done through only one nostril and exhalation through the other. Between inhalation and exhalation, the BREATH is retained. Also, see PRANAYAMA.

anunasika (Yoga) A technique of BREATHING aimed at cleansing the respiratory passages and orifices of the sinuses in the skull.

anupana (Ind.) A fluid vehicle for medicine, such as water, milk and honey.

anurasa (Ind.) A secondary taste as, for example, a little sweetness found in an otherwise sour fruit.

Anusara Yoga (New Age/Yoga) A version of HATHA YOGA, developed by John Friend in 1997. The system embodies an uplifting philosophy, 'a celebration of the heart', which aims at looking for the good and positive side in all people, things and events in our lives. This life-affirming vision forms the backbone of the system. It is also rooted in a community of highly trained teachers and fun-loving students.

anushasan mudra (Yoga) A MUDRA formed by holding the index finger straight and folding the other fingers. It is believed to curtail anger, fury and impatience.

anusthana (Yoga) The observance; the resolve to act with total discipline.

anuvasana basti (Ind.) An enema, given with herbal oil. See also, 'BASTI.

anuyoga (Tib.) Also, 'further yoga'. A system of yoga practised by the Tibetan Buddhists. It contains several works designated as SUTRAS.

apamarga (Ind.) *Achyranthes aspera*. Also, chirchita. A common Indian wasteland plant, regarded as the 'divine herb' by CHARAKA. Apamarga is known for its purgative, pungent and digestive qualities. It is also a folk remedy, used to treat inflammation of the internal organs, piles, itch, abdominal enlargements and enlarged cervical glands. The herb is also known for its diuretic properties.

apana (Ind.) One of the five forms of the LIFE FORCE which occupies the lower part of the body, below one's navel. This life-force is said to be responsible for functions connected with the evacuation of bowels, urine, gas, menstrual fluids and semen from the body.

apana mudra (Yoga) A MUDRA or finger-lock formed by touching the base of the thumb with the tip of index finger, while the tips of middle and ring fingers touch the tip of the thumb. This finger-lock is aimed at accelerating the healing process especially in the treatment of abdominal ailments such as diabetes, flatulence, indigestion, jaundice, piles and ulcers.

apana vata (Ind.) The aspect of VATA which controls elimination and reproduction. If unbalanced, the colon becomes dry, and the stool gets hardened, causing constipation. AYURVEDA prescribes demulcent herbs such as LICQURICE to remove dryness in the colon and re-establish its naturally moist and unctuous environment. Eating laxative foods (e.g., stewed fruits like prunes, figs or dates) and lifestyle changes (e.g., eating fibre-rich foods, drinking adequate water and physical work-outs) are other prescriptions.

apana vayu mudra See APANA MUDRA.

aparajita (Ind.) *Clitoria ternatea*. Also, butterfly pea. The juice of the leaf of this plant is used in folk remedy, along with JAIPHAL, to treat migraines and in certain tribal pockets, constipation. In India women insert the roots of this plant into the vagina to avoid unwanted pregnancies.

aparigraha (Yoga) Non-possessiveness. One of the five forms of self-restraint (YAMA) in the Yoga system of PATANJALI.

aphrodisiac (Misc.) A food, drink, medicine, fragrance or tool which is believed to arouse sexual desire. The definition also includes products that improve sexual performance.

The sexual effects of aphrodisiacs are based on folklore. In 1989, the US Food and Drug Administration stated that there was no scientific proof that over-the-counter aphrodisiacs worked to treat sexual dysfunction. Some ancient Chinese recipes of aphrodisiacs, bizarre to the uninitiated, are given in the following table:

aphrodisiac	Traditional recipe
The Hunting Lion	The paws of bears, the horn of the rhino and distilled human urine, simmered over a slow fire
Celestial Thunder	The tongue of peacock spiced with chilli powder and flavoured with the sperm of pubescent boys
Three-day Glory	Soy beans mixed with fresh ginseng, the penis of an ox, and dried human placenta

The moon is nothing
But a circumambulating aphrodisiac
Divinely subsidized to provoke the world
Into a rising birth-rate

—Christopher Fry

apis (Hom.) Also, honeybee. A remedy in HOMOEOPATHY made from the body of the bee, apis is used to treat symptoms similar to those caused by bee stings, i.e., burning stinging pains, blisters with swellings, cystitis, fluid retention and fevers with a lack of thirst.

apitherapy (New Age) Also, bee therapy, bee-sting therapy. The use of products from the bee (usually the European honey bee, *Apis mellifera*) to promote health and healing. BEE POLLEN, BEE VENOM, beeswax, HONEY, PROPOLIS and ROYAL JELLY are considered to be effective against ailments such as arthritis, chronic pain, multiple sclerosis and cancer. This therapy was known by the ancient Chinese, Egyptians and the Greeks. Hippocrates used bee venom in the treatment of arthritic joints, the venom being administered either by needle or by actual bee-stings.

Bee pollen is marketed as a nutritional supplement. An allergic reaction is a possibility with any bee product.

aporrheta (New Age) Esoteric instructions revealed to initiates during rituals in FREEMASONRY.

Apparatus for Measuring the Functional Conditions of Meridians and their Corresponding Internal Organs (Mod./New Age) Also, AMI. An apparatus, designed to measure the initial skin currents as well as steady-state currents, in response to DC voltage externally applied at SEI points. It can be used to teach exercises in health clubs or yoga sessions, apart from more conventional use in hospitals and acupuncture clinics.

apple diet (Mod./New Age) A purification DIET regimen in which food intake is restricted to raw apples. It is recommended for anaemia and weakness.

'An apple a day keeps the doctor away.'
    —An old English saying

applied kinesiology (Mod./New Age) Also, muscle testing. The term was first coined in 1964 by George J. Goodheart Jr, a chiropractor from Detroit, to refer to a method of diagnosis and treatment developed by him. The method is based on the concept that muscle groups share energy pathways with internal organs in the body and that every organ dysfunction is relatable to a particular muscle.

aqua acupuncture (New Age) Also, auricular point injection. A form of ACUPUNCTURE that employs the hypodermic injection of substances such as liquid herbal extracts and vitamin preparations at ACUPOINTS.

aqua aerobics (Mod.) Aerobic exercise performed in a swimming pool where the water provides support and added resistance. The reduced impact to the body makes this a particularly advantageous form of exercise for the overweight, elderly or pregnant exerciser, or in post-medical trauma.

aqua balancing (Mod.) A warm-water treatment done in a shallow pool in which the practitioner, standing in a water cradle, manipulates the floating patient through a series of gentle movements and stretches to induce a state of relaxation.

aquamarine (Gem) A gemstone, in a range of beautiful blue shades, believed to stabilize love and positive energies and create harmony and well-being.

aqua puncture (New Age) See AQUA ACUPUNCTURE.

Aquarian age See NEW AGE.

aquilaeus See AETITES.

Arabic medicine (Arab.) Also, traditional Arabic medicine; TIBB. A system of medicine, with its roots in Islamic tradition, dating back to the fall of the Roman Empire. Greek medical texts were translated into Arabic and along with sophisticated pharmaceutical information available from the East as a consequence of the trade route which existed with India through land and sea, the Arabs improved many Greek and Roman medical, especially ocular, techniques. Many herbs and spices of the orient, like nutmeg, cloves, and mace, were known for their medicinal values. Many Arabic medicinal terms (such as drug, syrup, alcohol and alkali) seeped into European languages and became popular in Western schools.

aravinda See LOTUS.

arcanum (Eur.) From the Latin *arcanus*, meaning secret or hidden. It implies esoteric wisdom, which remains secret or mysterious. The term also refers to a secret known exclusively to members of a small group. It also refers to secrets in nature, the kind sought by the alchemists of the past.

archana (Yoga) Worship in its ritualistic form, traditionally recommended as a cure for mental depression. PRAYER is used as an effective healing method in many cultures around the world.

archetypal psychology (Mod.) A branch of psychology, first named as such by James Hillman (1970). It was affiliated with the arts, culture and the history of ideas, arising as they do from the imagination, rather than with medical and empirical psychologies.

ardha kati chakrasana(Yoga) An ASANA, as illustrated, considered beneficial for the spine.

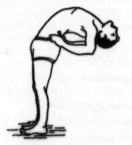

Ardha kati chakrasana

ardha linga chakra mudra (Yoga) A MUDRA formed by locking the fingers and rotating the unlocked thumbs around each other in a clockwise direction. It is recommended as an aid to digestion.

ardha matsyendra asana (Yoga) An ASANA, as illustrated, considered beneficial for diabetics and those with kidney-related ailments.

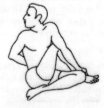

Ardha matsyendra asana

argentum nitricum (Hom.) Also, arg. nit., devil's stone, hellstone, lunar caustic, silver nitrate. Extracted from the mineral ore acanthite which is derived from silver, arg. nit. is prescribed as a remedy for anticipatory anxiety and gastro-intestinal problems such as belching and flatulence. It is believed to suit warm-blooded people who are impulsive and in a hurry to do things.

arhatic yoga (Yoga) A form of yoga aimed at activating and aligning CHAKRAS as developed by Choa Kok Sui, a contemporary Chinese-Filipino scientist.

Arica (Mod./New Age) A contemporary method of enlightenment, which employs biology and psychology in order to clarify human CONSCIOUSNESS with modern knowledge. The Arica School provides a clearly defined map of the human psyche in order for each person to discover the basis of their ego process and to transcend this process into a higher state of consciousness. The school was founded in 1968 by Oscar Ichazo (b. 1931), a Bolivian teacher who specialized in ENNEAGRAM. His followers are often referred to as Aricans. Arica's system and methodology, known as protoanalysis, draws its inspiration from G.I. Gurdjieff's teachings on consciousness. The methodologies of Arica are similar to those from traditions like I-CHING, KABBALAH, SUFISM, TIBETAN BUDDHISM, YOGA and ZEN.

ariolater (Eur.) A person who practises DIVINATION.

arishta See SOAP NUT TREE.

arithmomancy (Eur./Occ.) A method of DIVINATION which involves the interpretation of values in numbers and letters. The method is based on the esoteric principles of Pythagoras who recognized a correspondence between gods, men and numbers. Arithmomancy is a part of the Jewish KABBALAH and is considered a forerunner to NUMEROLOGY.

arjuna (Ind.) *Terminalia arjuna*. Every part of this tall tree, common in India, is considered medicinal. Its grey bark has a long medicinal history as a cardiac tonic. Arjuna is widely used in both AYURVEDA and UNANI, both externally and internally, in the treatment of various ailments including fractures, ulcers, heart diseases, biliousness, urinary discharges, asthma, tumours, leucoderma, anaemia and excessive perspiration.

It is used as an expectorant, aphrodisiac, tonic and diuretic. The tree also is ecologically important and is recommended for the reclamation of saline, alkaline soils and deep ravines.

arkah See ARKH.

arkh (Ind.) *Calotropis gigantea*. Also, ak, madar. This shrub, which grows all over India, especially in wastelands, is used in folk medicine to treat various ailments such as asthma, cold, cough, diarrhoea, eczema, elephantiasis, fevers, indigestion, nausea, rheumatism and vomiting. The leaves are known for their use in the treatment of paralysis, arthralgia, swellings, and intermittent fevers. The Flowers are bitter, digestive astringent and anthelmintic. Calstropis is also a reputed homoeopathic drug.

Arndt-Schultz Law (Mod.) A hypothesis propounded by Arndt Schulz (1853–1932), a German pharmacologist. According to it, weak stimuli on living cells accelerate physiological activities, moderate ones inhibit and the stronger ones stop them. In other words, every stimulus elicits an activity inversely proportional to the intensity of the stimulus.

arnica (Hom.) *Arnica montana*. Also, leopard's bane. In folk medicine, the plant is a popular remedy, rubbed on the skin to soothe and heal chapped lips, bruises and sprains. It is also a homoeopathic anti-inflammatory that may be used for traumatic injury, bruises, stiffness and muscle soreness. It is widely used as a salve or tincture for anti-inflammatory and pain-relieving purposes.

arogya (Ind.) Health.

aroma bath (Mod./New Age/Spa) Bathing in water sprinkled with aromatic oils which contain complex chemicals that act at a psycho-physical level to induce relaxation by stimulating blood and lymph flow. Many oils are also known for their anti-bacterial and antifungal properties. Oils of basil, eucalyptus, jasmine, rosemary and sandalwood are widely used in aroma baths.

aroma genera (New Age) A system of AROMATHERAPY, developed by Valerie Ann Worwood, a British naturopath. It is based on the principle that certain groups of ESSENTIAL OILS correspond with certain personalities and emotional types.

aromapuncture (New Age) Puncturing acupoints with an acupuncture needle, soaked in an ESSENTIAL OILS remedy.

aromatherapy (New Age) Also, aromatic medicine. A term coined in 1928 by Gatter Fosse, a French chemist, to refer to the therapeutic application of ESSENTIAL OILS from plants, flowers, or wood resins, to affect mood or promote health. Treatments include sniffing, ingestion and application on the skin (usually with MASSAGE). The oils are believed to act simultaneously at the physical, emotional, mental and spiritual levels.

aromatology (New Age) A system of AROMATHERAPY, which prescribes the use of ESSENTIAL OILS in compresses, inhalations, diffusers, spritzers, baths, creams and lotions.

aromics (New Age) A healing system, blending AROMATHERAPY and NLP, as popularized in 1993 by Bill McMahan, a healer from California.

arrowroot (Am. Ind.) *Marantha arundinace*. The powdery substance from the root of this plant was used by the Arawaks, natives of the West Indies, to draw out toxins from victims of poisonous arrows. Its English name is derived from this practice. Arrowroot is used in herbal medicine as a soothing demulcent and for easing digestion, and is a nutrient with benefit in convalescence.

arsenicum album (Hom.) Also, ars. alb. A diluted form of arsenic, a metallic poison, used in HOMOEOPATHY to treat symptoms similar to those caused by arsenic poisoning, including dehydration and burning pain.

Art of Living (Mod./New Age) A self-development programme, including the practices of PRANAYAMA and SUDARSHAN KRIYA (sudarshan means right vision, and kriya means purifying action), as popularized by Bangalore-based Sri Sri Ravi Shankar (b. 1956). The practise of Sudarshan Kriya helps in shifting one's awareness beyond one's thoughts and emotions, resulting in a feeling of being more even and natural, and centered in one's self. The practice is said to facilitate physical, mental and emotional renewal, with elevated spirituality.

art of lymphatic system activation
See LYMPHASIZING.

art psychotherapy See ART THERAPY.

art therapy (New Age) The use of art and other visual media in a therapeutic setting.

> 'Without art the crudeness of reality would make the world unbearable.'
>
> —George Bernard Shaw

> 'In morals, always do as others do; in art, never.'
>
> —Jules Renard

artainment (Mod.) A stress reduction programme, based on music.

asafoetida (Ind.) *Ferula asafetida*. Also, devil's dung, giant's funnel, hing. The dried latex obtained from the root of this plant is a herbal medicine, traditionally used to treat asthma, bronchitis, constipation, cough, flatulence, nervousness and palpitation. A favourite of ancient Romans, it was valued for its aroma, more persistent than of garlic. Because of its pungent smell, asafoetida when applied acts as an insect repellent.

asana (Yoga) Also, yogasana. Asana refers to a body posture attained by a person while in harmony with his or her inner CON-SCIOUSNESS, to facilitate meditation. Asanas are generally performed in five steps:

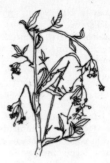

Asafoetida

Step 1: Bodily postures that exercise the organs of action in a voluntary manner, releasing tension, increasing flexibility and the flow of the vital spirit (PRANA).

Step 2: Cognitive action or directing one's awareness within oneself, with a view to creating a rhythmic flow of positive energy.

Step 3: Mental state of pure joy (ANANDA).

Step 4: Intellectual absorption of the mind (DHARANA).

Step 5: Fusion of the individual spirit (microcosm) with the divine or universal spirit (macrocosm).

There are several asanas, each unique in its own way as indicated in the following table:

Asana

Asana	Examples	Possible therapeutic role
Standing	ardha chandrasana, tadasana, utthita parsvakonasana, utthita trikonasana, virabhadrasana	Physical stamina and hence can be useful to police and security personnel, athletes and sportsmen
Forward bending and stretching of the posterior half of the body	paschimottasana, upavisthakonasana	Physical and mental flexibility and hence can be useful to sedentary workers and thinkers
Sitting and supine	baddha kona asana, padmasana, supta baddha kona asana, supta padangusthanasana, simhasana, vajrasana, virasana	A preparatory asana, said to be helpful for those who undertake KRIYAs
Inverted	adho mukha svanasa,	Emotional stability and balance and

	urdhva mukha svanasa	hence can be helpful in recovering from everyday stress
Focussed on the abdominal and lumbar regions	bharadvajasana and marichyasana	Abdominal organs strengthened as the pelvic and lumbar muscles are toned up
Twisting the body	ardha matsyendrasana, jathara parivartanasana	Mental peace as the internal organs are strengthened
Body bending backwards	bhujangasana, matsyasana, ustrasana	Said to be invigorating
Balancing the body	niralamba sarvangasana, salamba sarvangasana, salamba sirsasana	Arms and wrists are strengthened, as the body is made light

The regular practise of asanas is believed to control cholesterol level, reduce weight, normalize blood pressure and improve heart performance. Thus reduction of physical stress enhances one's vitality. It may also be helpful in clearing emotional blockages, thus making the mind strong.

> 'Perfection (in an asana) is achieved when the effort to perform it becomes effortless and the infinite being within it is reached.'
>
> —Sage Patanjali

asana, training in (Yoga) Training in ASANA involves four stages: a) focussing on body movements, flexibility and stability; b) sending awareness to every nook of the body; c) familiarizing mind with body and; d) locking of mind with the body.

> 'While practising an asana, one must focus attention on the inner body, drawing the mind inward to sharpen the intellect.'
>
> —B.K.S. Iyengar

asana therapy (New Age) A form of ancient healing, based on selecting and sequencing ASANAs, taking into consideration the physical and emotional constituents of the patient and nature of ailment.

ASAT CORE counselling (New Age) Promoted by the American Society of Alternative Therapists (ASAT), CORE, an acronym for Consciousness, Ownership, Retrieval/Release and Engage is a healing method based on the belief that there exists unlimited human capacity for the conscious creation of life.

Asclepiades of Bithynia (124–40 BC) (Grk.) A Greek physician who theorized that diseases are caused by the inharmonious flow of corpuscles of the body. In order to restore harmony in the body, he recommended a proper diet, physical work or exercise and bathing and hydrotherapy. He was also an advocate for the humane treatment of the mentally ill.

Asclepius (Grk.) The most important Greek mythical figure, associated with health and healing. His staff, entwined in a serpent's coils, is a symbol of the modern medical profession. Other Greek mythical figures associated with health are Apollo, the god of healing, and Hygieia, the daughter of the god Asclepius who represents the forces of cleanliness.

ashgandh See ASVAGANDHA.

ash gourd (Ind.) *Benincasa hispida*. Also, kushmanda. The fruit of this climber has been used in the Orient as a food and medicine for thousands of years. All its parts are used medicinally: the rind is a diuretic, used in the treatment of urinary dysfunction; the ash of the rind is applied to painful wounds; the seed is used in the treatment of coughs, fevers, excessive thirst and to expel tapeworms.

ashoka (Ind.) *Saraca indica*. Also gandha pushpa. An Indian tree attributed with mystical qualities. It is used to alleviate depression, especially in women. The plant drug also finds its application in the treatment of excessive uterine bleeding and bleeding caused by piles.

Ashtanga Hridaya (Ind.) An ancient text on AYURVEDA, written by Vagabhatta.

Ashtanga Sangraha (Ind.) An ancient text written in the seventh century AD by Buddhist physician Vagabhatta. It discusses the eight branches of Ayurveda: salya tantra (major surgery), salakya tantra (minor surgery), kaya chikitsa (therapeutics), bhuta vidya (demonology), kaumara bhrtya (paediatrics), agada tantra (toxicology), rasayana (elixirs), and vaji karana (aphrodisiacs).

Ashtanga Yoga (Yoga) The 'eight-limbed' system of YOGA, as codified by the sage Patanjali. The system consists of eight stages: the practice of self-restraint, prescribed observances, prescribed body postures, breath-control, withdrawal of mind from the sense-organs, concentration, meditation and, finally, absorption of one's being into one's self. Yoga is more than just a physical discipline; it helps balance physical, mental, emotional and spiritual needs, eliminating the inherent conflicts between each other.

Yoga's guidelines of restraints and observances (See YAMAS and NIYAMAS) are grounded in common sense and help in efficiently managing one's energy towards the goal of self-realization. The system extends the freedom to find one's own truth without mindlessly accepting externally imposed rules. Even the greatest gurus simply indicate direction. It is ultimately for an individual to embark on his or her journey. See YOGA SUTRA.

Ashtoreth (Misc.) The moon goddess of the Phoenicians, representing the passive principles in nature. Many ancient civilizations acknowledged the importance of female principles in nature and symbolized them for worship and adoration. The Phoenicians were the earliest settlers in present-day Lebanon and are believed to have migrated from the Arabian peninsula in 1200 BC.

ashtanga ayurveda (Ind.) From the Sanskrit ashtanga, meaning eight limbs; the eight branches in the science of AYURVEDA, including internal medicine (kaya chikitsa), paediatrics (koumara brtya), psychiatry (bhuta vaidya), toxicology (agadatantra), ENT-cum-ophthalmology (shalakya tantra), surgery (shalya tantra), geriatrics (rasayana) and virilization therapy (vajikarana).

asparsha yoga (Yoga) Also, Intangible Yoga. From the Sanskrit asparsha, meaning free from contact. A yogic concept of non-dualism, introduced by Gaudapada (eighth century AD), referred to as the grand-guru of Shankaracharya, asparsha yoga is a discipline of non-contact. According to some authors, this yoga system refers to asceticism (sanyasa).

ashvagandha (Ind.) *Withania somnifera.* Also, ashgandh; Indian ginseng; wintercherry; Indian ginseng. The leaves, fruit and roots of this plant have been in use in India for the last four millennia. It is believed to impart the fabled sexual energy of the horse; the plant is to Indian medicine what ginseng is to Chinese. In Africa, ashvagandha leave have been used for fighting fevers and inflammatory conditions. Its root has a wide range of application in the treatment of various physiological disorders.

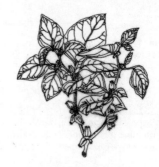

Ashvagandha

ashvattha (Ind.) *Ficus religiosa.* Also, bo, bodhi tree, peepul, sacred fig. A native Indian tree, believed by Hindus to be the abode of Trimurti, the Trinity of Gods, representing Creation (Brahma), Preservation (Vishnu) and Destruction (Shiva). Buddhists believe that Gautama Buddha meditated under this tree and achieved nirvana.

Its bark, roots, fruits, leaves and latex of this tree have been used in native medicines for centuries. In folk medicine, its roots are used in the treatment of gout and lumbago. They are chewed to prevent gum diseases. The leaves are fried in *ghee* (clarified butter) and used as a poultice, applied to swollen glands in mumps. The leaves and bark together are used to relieve diarrhoea and dysentery. Its latex is used externally in haemorrhoids. Unani practitioners blow the powder of the dried bark into the rectum through a pipe to cure anal fistula.

aspen (Flo.) *Populus tremula*. The bark of this tree is anodyne, anti-inflammatory and febrifuge.

assumption of responsibility (Mod./ New Age) A method of BEHAVIOUR THERAPY in which patients are made to accept that it is they who are responsible for their thoughts, feelings and actions. In the case of alternative medicine, the patient is made to take up the responsibility for his cure himself.

Astara's healing science (New Age) A form of SPIRITUAL HEALING as practised by a neo-Christian, interfaith church, founded in 1951. The methods used include ABSENT HEALING, CRYSTALS, VISUALIZATION and PRAYER.

asteya (Yoga) Honesty and non-theft. One of the five forms of self-restraints (YAMA) in the Yoga system of PATANJALI.

asthi (Ind.) The bodily tissue of bones.

asthi-vaha srotas (Ind.) CHANNELS that carry nutrients to the bones.

asthma mudra (Yoga) A MUDRA formed by touching the fingernails of the middle fingers of both the hands, keeping the other fingers straight. It is said to impact the clearance of congestion in the trachea, resulting in easy breathing.

Aston-patterning (Mod.) An approach to healing, combining DEEP-TISSUE, MASSAGE and movement education, as developed by Judith Aston.

astral body (Yoga) The subtle, invisible, luminous and vibrating PSYCHIC body, believed by occultists to survive death and decay of the organism.

astragalomancy (Eur./Occ.) A method of DIVINATION, with dice or bones.

astral flight (Yoga/Occ.) Also, astral projection; astral travel. An out-of-body experience often occurring during sleep or meditation, when the etheric body, separated from the physical body, travels great distances resulting in an altered state of consciousness.

astral projection See ASTRAL FLIGHT.

astral travel See ASTRAL FLIGHT.

astrological counselling (Num.) A form of PSYCHOTHERAPY, based on ASTROLOGY.

astrological diagnosis (Num.) Also, astro diagnosis. The examination of the birth chart of the patient to obtain clues to the emotional reason for an illness. This ancient method is based on the premise that certain personality types, as governed by the astrological signs, are pre-disposed to certain predictable illnesses.

astrologic medicine (Num.) Also, astral healing, astro-medicine; medical astrology. An ancient body of knowledge, based on the principle that specific mental and physical conditions correspond to the relative positions of celestial bodies. Astrological medicine includes astrological-diagnosis, prognosis, selection and timing of treatment and preventive medicine. A trained medical astrologer on analyzing a person's birth chart (horoscope) determines his or her bodily strengths and weaknesses, proneness to various disease states, and possible nutritional inadequacies.

astrology (Num.) A study professing to foretell the future by interpreting the movements of heavenly bodies upon the destiny of an individual or nation. It is also considered to give insights into emotional, professional and health matters.

astromedicine See ASTROLOGIC MEDICINE.

asvini mudra (Yoga) A MUDRA formed by contracting the sphincter muscles of the anus for half a second and then relaxing them for another half a second and repeating the process.

atala (Yoga) One of the fourteen CHAKRAS, situated at the level of hips, which symbolize fear and lust. There are seven chakras, situated below the base of the spine and all of them are known as 'lower chakras'. While meditating on the lower chakras, a practitioner normally focusses his awareness, as if spinning anti-clockwise on his lower parts of the body: hips, thighs, knees, calves, ankles, feet and soles, each representing a chakra, spinning anti-clockwise. The chakras below the base of the spine are given in the following table:

Chakras Below The Base of The Spine

Chakra	Location in the human body	Human characteristic represented
Atala	Hips	Fear and lust
Vitala	Thighs	Rage
Sutala	Knees	Jealousy and vengeance
Talatala	Calves	Confusion
Rasatala	Ankles	Selfishness
Mahatala	Feet	Lack of conscience
Patala	Soles	Malice and murder

atapsevan (Ind.) The application of solar rays for mitigating diseases and symptoms.

atarusa See VASAKA.

Atkins diet (Mod.) A diet prescription which advocates a restricted consumption of carbohydrates with an unlimited quantity of protein in combination with specific nutritional supplements. Devised by Robert Atkins in the late 1960s, the diet won the support of millions of dieters for its efficacy in shedding pounds rapidly in spite of several teams of scientists and nutritionists finding that the Atkins regime could cause several diseases due to nutritional imbalances, which went beyond bad breath, constipation, cramps, culinary boredom and weakness.

atma (Yoga) Soul; spirit; true self.

attenuation (Hom./Occ.) A reduction in the strength of a signal with respect to distance travelled through a medium. In the context of HOMOEOPATHY, it is indicated by a symbol consisting of a number and a letter. The number indicates the number of times the liquid is diluted and the letter, the kind of diluting step used; the letter X, for instance, indicates that the diluting step was ten-fold, D indicates the European version of the ten-fold step, C and K the hundred-fold step. See also, KORSAKOVIAN METHOD OF ATTENUATION, HAHNEMANNIAN METHOD OF ATTENUATION, SUCCUSSION.

attitude of gratitude (New Age) An age-old concept according to which people who feel gratitude have better lives than those who dwell on their disappointments.

A healthy state of emotions is often linked to a good state of physical as well as mental health.

attitudinal healing (New Age) The regulation of physical, mental and spiritual health, by assuming a proper mental attitude or world-view. Systems such as CHRISTIAN SCIENCE, TRANSPERSONAL PSYCHOLOGY and YOGA are oriented towards attitudinal healing.

> The more you praise and celebrate your life, the more there is in life to celebrate.
>
> —Oprah Winfrey

attunement (New Age) A state of being, a spiritual discipline and a way of healing with life energy; a process of opening and expanding the QI-holding capacity and ENERGY BALANCING. It also refers to the ritual or process of the activation of REIKI within a person's palms. Performed by a Master, the process is said to empower the initiate to tap into and direct the energy to the desired person or area of the body.

augur (Eur./Occ.) A diviner or a soothsayer. In ancient Rome, an augur was a priest or official who interpreted the will of gods to the king by referring to various natural phenomena such as the flight of the birds and their behaviour while flying. An augur observed, for instance, the type of birds which fly, the flight formation (whether they are flying in groups or alone), sounds made by them while flying and the direction of flight. Decisions taken by the king on important issues such as war and trading took into consideration the augur's findings.

aum (Yoga) The divine vibration; a sound chanted in meditation; a primordial sound from which all speech and thought in the universe are thought to be derived; a symbol of super-consciousness; a vital tool, a phenomenon and a mystery of the science of yoga; an outcome of the primordial energy, containing latent power; a BIJA MANTRA of AJNA CHAKRA. Aum is comparable with other sacred sounds around the globe: *hum* of the Tibetans, *amin* of the Muslims, and amen of the Christians, Egyptians, Greeks and Romans.

> 'The letter "a" symbolizes the conscious or waking state; the letter "u" the dream state, and the letter "m" the dreamless sleep state of the mind and spirit. The entire symbol stands for the realization of man's divinity within himself.'
>
> —B.K.S. Iyengar

aum healing technique (Yoga) An approach to healing by chanting aum in daily meditation, as popularized by Paramahansa Yogananda in 1920. According to Yogananda, everything in the universe is composed of energy and the apparent difference between solids, liquids, gases, sound and light is merely a difference in their vibratory rates. By chanting aum, the divine vibration, we can increase the body's supply of cosmic energy and even direct it as a healing force to any part of the body, mind and soul.

> 'Aum, the vibration of the Cosmic Motor.'
>
> —Paramahansa Yogananda

aura (Yoga) A subtle, invisible energy field that surrounds matter, both living and non-living. Aura is also defined as an electrophotonic vibration response of an object to certain external stimuli. The aura around a living object (plant, animal or human) is reported to change very quickly. On the other hand, the aura around a non-living object, such as RUDRAKSHA, birthstones, crystals and water, is essentially stable. The aura system is said to be made of seven types of auras: astral, celestial, emotional, etheric, etheric template, mental and ketheric template. It is said that children up to the age of five years have the natural tendency to see auras. Infants are believed to look above a person in front of them and when they don't like the colour of the aura above the head, or if this colour is distinct from their parent's aura, they cry.

The aura around humans is said to be made of electromagnetic radiation. The most exploited characteristic of aura seems to be the fact that it contains information about the object; while the infrared part of the spectrum (body heat) is said to be related to the body functions like circulation and metabolism, the ultraviolet part is attributed to mental work such as thinking, sense of humour and emotions. An aura is said to be visible only to those born with the skill to see it, although it is naturally found in children and some adults have retained this ability.

A visible aura containing various colours can indicate the spiritual and emotional personality of a plant, human, or of even nonconscious matter. An aura can also be felt, heard or sensed through other means.

aura analysis (New Age/Yoga) Also, aura-diagnosis, auric analysis. The examination of AURA with or without equipment (e.g., KIRLIAN PHOTOGRAPHY) so as to ascertain the health of a person. The state of health of a person is said to be revealed by the quality of his or her aura. The colours of aura are often associated with glands, organs, organ systems and psychological states such as anger, frustration and hatred.

aura balancing (Yoga/New Age) Also, aura cleansing, aura clearing, aura healing, auric healing, aura massage. A subtle but profound energy adjustment administered to AURA which is said to catalyze recuperation. By correcting the auric field around the patient's head or body, it is believed that a healthy state can be achieved.

aura brushing (Yoga/New Age) Also, aura cleansing, auric brushing. Grooming one's auric fields by running down one's aura from top to bottom, aimed at releasing blockages or cobwebs in aura. Usually a client stands with legs apart, at shoulder width, arms at his sides, with eyes closed. The practitioner starts with the front of the client's body. With fingers spread wide apart, reaching above the head of the client, and imagining that his fingers are growing several inches longer, the practitioner makes long continuous strokes from above the head down through the body, all the way to the ground. The same procedure is repeated several times around the body of the client till the practitioner finally reaches the place where he commenced.

aura cleansing See AURA BRUSHING.

aura clearing See AURA BALANCING.

aura diagnosis See AURA ANALYSIS.

aura healing See AURA BALANCING.

aura reading See AURA ANALYSIS.

aura–soma therapy (New Age) A non-intrusive therapy as developed by Vicky Wall (1918–91), a chiropodist and apothecary. A variation of AURA-BALANCING, COLOUR THERAPY and CHAKRA-healing. A client is asked to choose 'the most attractive' of four different-coloured bottles out of a selection of NINETY-EIGHT coloured bottles. This method is aimed at identifying areas of the body which crave for attention. This method does not diagnose or treat, but can pinpoint areas of the body, mind and spirit that are in need of attention by the patients themselves.

auric analysis See AURA ANALYSIS.

auric brushing See AURA BRUSHING.

auric healing See AURA BALANCING.

auric massage A form of AURA BALANCING.

auricle (Misc.) The outer portion of ear; the oval-shaped appendage on the lateral surface of the head, whose function is sound localization and its amplification. Professor Park Jae Woo, founder of the Sujok school of acupuncture, was the first to note the affinity between the auricle and the various internal organs through their physical resemblance to one another. According to him, the resemblance of the auricle to the internal organs, especially the heart, lung, spleen, and kidney, indicates a correspondence with the actual organs in the body.

auricular acupuncture (Chi./New Age) The stimulation of acumeridian points in the ear has a long history of success in bringing about health improvements. Chinese in origin, it is considered an important part of an integrative medicine programme. See also, AURICULAR THERAPY.

auricular analgesia (New Age/Mod.) A form of AURICULAR THERAPY, aimed at alleviating pain in fully conscious patients.

auricular magnetic therapy (New Age) A form of auricular therapy, in which magnetic pellets or balls are taped over the auricular ACUPOINTS.

auricular massage (New Age) A form of AURICULAR THERAPY, in which all or part of the ear is pinched, pressed and rotated.

auricular medicine See AURICULAR THERAPY.

auricular moxibustion (New Age) A form of MOXIBUSTION, forming part of AURICULAR THERAPY.

auricular point injection See AQUA-ACUPUNCTURE.

auricular point laser-stimulating method (New Age) Also, auricular needling. A form of AURICULAR THERAPY.

auricular reflexology (Mod./New Age) Developed in 1967 by P.F.M. Nogier, a French medical professional, this form of REFLEXOLOGY works with the ears; it aims at treating health conditions in remote parts of the body through the external stimulation of points in the ear. These stimulations are aimed at not only helping problems connected to the face or head, but also for relieving pathological disorders in the abdomen, chest, feet and lower back. The system was based more on clinical trials and laboratory experiments rather than on metaphysical abstract theories characteristic of Traditional Chinese Medicine. The therapeutic principles were applied according to Western understanding of the human body.

auricular therapy (Chi.) Also, auricular medicine, auriculotherapy, Chinese auricular therapy, Chinese auricular ACUPUNCTURE, traditional Chinese auricular acu-points therapy, traditional Chinese auricular acupuncture, traditional Chinese auricular therapy. An important component of traditional Chinese acupuncture, auricular therapy deals with the AURICLE, which is used to stimulate specific organs and meridians in the body. The auricle represents a foetus in the womb, in an inverted position, and thus represents the whole body. It is based on the idea that energy travels along a unique system of pathways which correspond neither to the vessels nor nerves, but converge at the auricle on which about 100 different ACUPOINTs are identified. The earliest recorded mention of the close relationship between the ear and the body can be seen in the *Silk Book Meridians*, written around 500 BC, which states that the ear meridian originates in the back of the hand and ascends to enter the ear. Auricular diagnostic and therapeutic methods were first documented in *Nei Jing*, the classic of medicine, written in about 200 BC, which stated that the nature and location of various diseases could be determined by inspecting the shape, colour, moistness and collaterals of the ear. It also referred to the use of bloodletting puncturing of the collaterals of the ear to treat headaches and side pain.

Auricular therapy developed further in Europe, particularly in France and Germany, over the last few decades. It is also well-recorded that the ancient Egyptians used certain earrings to treat vision and fertility problems. The Romans learned this technique, through the Mediterranean trading routes, and used it for, for example, cauterizing specific points on the ears for the treatment of sciatica.

The development of modern science has also contributed towards new treatment methods and equipment for this ancient system. At present, auricular therapy can be performed in fifteen different ways including MASSAGE, electric stimulation, needles, MOXA, seeds, magnets and laser. Afflictions treated with Chinese auricular therapy include acne, amenorrhoea, angina pectoris, anorexia, appendicitis, bronchial asthma, bronchitis, cardiac arrhythmia, cataract, common cold, conjunctivitis, coronary heart diseases, diabetes, dysentery, eczema, epilepsy, female infertility, gastric and duodenal ulcers, gastritis, glaucoma, hearing decrement, hypertension, hyperthyroidism, hypertrophy of the female breast, hypotension, impotence, insomnia, leucorrhoea, migraine, musculoskeletal problems, nephritis, obesity, pneumonia, prolapsed uterus, psoriasis, psychosis, respiratory disorders, rheumatic heart diseases, rhinitis, schizophrenia, sciatica, sprain and contusion, tonsillitis, ulcerative colitis, uterine bleeding, vomiting and whooping cough.

auricular magnetic therapy (Chi.) A form of AURICULAR THERAPY in which magnetic pearls are used, especially for the elderly suffering from insomnia. The underlying idea is that the nerves in the specific areas of the external ear correspond to specific parts of the brain, which has a reflex connection to the body. These reflexes are believed to get activated when problems in part of the body induce reflex reactions in the external ear, manifested as changes in tenderness and altered blood circulation. These reflexes are activated when specific points on the ear are stimulated with the help of magnets, resulting in relief in another area of the body.

auriculotherapy See AURICULAR THERAPY.

Aurobindo, Sri See AUROTHERAPY; INTEGRAL YOGA.

aurotherapy (Misc.) A practical therapeutic practice, aimed at growth, transformation and healing, based on Sri Aurobindo's ideas on CONSCIOUSNESS.

aurum met (Hom.) Gold. It is used to lift depression, sadness moodiness and stress.

Australian fever tree (Aus.) See BLUE GUM EUCALYPTUS.

aushadha (Ind.) Drugs.

audhadhi (Ind.) The management of diseases with medicines—herbal or other. Also, one of the three pillars of AYURVEDA.

austromancy (Eur./Occ.) A branch of AEROMANCY, which is DIVINATION through astral phenomena such as thunder and lightening. It is concerned with the observance and interpretation of winds; a method of DIVINATION, using clouds and winds.

autogenic discharge (Mod.) Sensation of muscle movements that accompany the release of stored tensions.

autogenic training (Mod.) Also, autogenic therapy. A system of very specific auto-suggestive formulas to tackle stress and tension and to alleviate PSYCHOSOMATIC ILLNESS such as constipation, hypertension, insomnia, obesity and skin problems as developed in the 1930s by Johannes Schultz, a German therapist. The system involves the creation of resolutions which can help sort out problems.

autoimmune disorders (Mod.) Disorders which occur in the body and result in the destruction of one or more types of body tissues, abnormal growth of an organ, or changes in organ function. The disorder may either affect an organ or tissue type or multiple organs and tissues. Organs and tissues commonly affected by autoimmune disorders include blood components like red blood cells, blood vessels, connective tissues, endocrine glands such as the thyroid or pancreas, muscles, joints and skin. A patient may have more than one autoimmune disorder at a time. Examples of autoimmune (or autoimmune-related) disorders include Addisons' disease, dermatomyostitis, Grave's disease, lupus, multiple sclerosis, myasthenia gravis, pernicious anaemia, Reiter's syndrome and rheumatoid arthritis.

Automated Computerized Treatment System (ACTS) (Mod.) An electronic database, developed by Major Gordon Smith, a British radionics pioneer. It contains 260,000 treatments which include ACUPUNCTURE, COLOUR THERAPY, FLOWER REMEDIES, GEM THERAPY, LIGHT THERAPY and SOUND THERAPY. Aimed at evaluating the scientific measurements of the effectiveness of RADIONICS, the system is based on clients' self-reported improvement ratings for over 200 common ailments, some of which were professionally diagnosed. With less than 100 patients for each illness, such 'data' do not meet the requirements for calculating common measures of statistical reliability used in standard experimental studies, such as mean, variance, and z-scores. However, a large database of anecdotal evidence suggests that radionic machines can produce positive healing effects on people, animals and plants. The database can be useful in assessing the need of the right dose of treatment at the right time.

automatic writing (New Age) A surrealist technique, which comprises both the process and the product of writing or scribbling, which is believed not to have originated from the conscious thoughts of the writer, but by his putting himself in a 'receptive' frame of mind. In other words, the writer is said to be unaware of what he or she is writing as it is often done in trance. What is crucial here is the unpremeditated mind, free of thoughts.

autonomic reflex testing (New Age) A non-invasive test based on the energy changes (that precede the biochemical changes that lead to diseases) for assessing and treating imbalances in the body's energy fields.

autopoiesis (Mod./New Age) (from the Greek *auto*, meaning self, and *poiesis*, meaning creation) A phenomenon which manifests in self-maintaining systems. It represents a network of processes of production, transformation and destruction of components which through their continuous interactions regenerate and realize the network of processes (relations) that produced them. The space defined by an autopoietic system is self-contained and cannot be described by using dimensions that define another space. The concept implies a fundamental complementarity between structure and functions. The term was introduced in 1973 by Francisco Varela, a Chilean biologist, and Humberto Matuana.

From this very general point of view, the notion of autopoiesis is often associated with that of self-organization. The phenomenon represents any entity which metabolizes, maintains and perpetuates its identity, despite constant environmental disturbances.

autosuggestion therapy (New Age) An approach to healing, in which one repeats affirmations and positive suggestions, till the body and mind begin to act accordingly.

autourine injections (New Age) The use of one's own urine as injectable medicine has been practised in recent years. The procedure helps sidestep the revulsion generally associated with drinking it, to prevent and treat degenerative diseases. See also AUTOURINE THERAPY.

autourine therapy (Ind./Chi./Egy./Nat./New Age) Also amaroli, auto-urotherapy, manav mutra, shivambu, uropathy, urine therapy, urotherapy, water of life therapy. The use of one's own urine as medicine, especially in degenerative diseases, is an ancient method of healing. Urine therapy has its roots in ancient Egypt, ancient China and ancient India.

Urine is considered anti-bacterial, anti-fungal and anti-viral. It is used in AIDS, cancer, fatigue, anaemia, urinary disease, for weight loss, colds and flu, candida, diabetes, digestive problems and jaundice.

Most toxins in the food are filtered out of the blood, through the liver and kidneys. Toxic matter which finds its way into the urine is said to be highly diluted. Urine is therefore believed to be actually less toxic and more alive than much of the food and drink that actually goes into the body. According to Martha Christy, the author of *Your Own Perfect Medicine*, the re-introduction of urine into one's own body boosts the body's immune defence and accelerates the process of healing. John Armstrong, a British naturopath who did pioneering research on urine in the early-twentieth century, recommends its use as an effective mouthwash, aftershave lotion, antiseptic, and to fight obesity. Armstrong also recommends urine massage for all types of skin infections. (See also AUTOURINE INJECTIONS).

> 'If you believe in me, you will never thirst... Rivers of living water shall flow from your bellies.'
>
> —Jesus (in John 7:38)

autourotherapy See AUTOURINE THERAPY.

avalamban kapha (Ind.) An aspect of KAPHA situated in the chest and thoracic areas, supporting the functions of the heart and lungs by protecting them from wear and tear.

avapidana nasya (Ind.) Herbal mixtures, crushed and squeezed into the nostrils.

avastha (Ind.) The condition or state of one's health.

aversion conditioning (Mod.) A technique of behaviour therapy in which a stimulus which is attractive to the patient, but would lead to undesirable results, is paired with an unpleasant event in order to break the pattern.

aversion therapy (Mod.) A form of behaviour modification, which employs unpleasant or painful stimuli in an effort to help a patient overcome his or her socially unacceptable or harmful behavior. Aversion therapy was used first in 1930 for the treatment of alcoholism. By 1950s and 1960s the therapy became a popular method in the treatment of sexual deviation. By gradually increasing familiarity with the detested objects or events, the therapy aims at the elimination of undesirable responses.

Avicenna (Per.) (AD 980-1037) Also, Ibn Sina. The Latinized version of the name Ibn Sina, the greatest of the medieval Persian physicians. He is also known as the 'prince' of physicians. Of the 450-odd books written by him on medicine and its philosophy, his principal work, *The Canon of Medicine,* is rated as a classic. Another of his books, *The Book of Healing,* is also popular. He is considered by many as the father of modern medicine, as he made fundamental contributions to medicine and European reawakening.

avidya (Ind.) Ignorance; a state of mind, unawareness of reality. Buddhism believes that it is avidya that mistakes the illusory phenomena of this world (maya) for reality. Oriental medicine is developed on the premise that ill-health is due to fundamental spiritual disharmony resulting from avidya.

avupattikara churna (Ind.) A popular formulation used in hyperacidity.

awareness (Misc.) The recognition of a condition that calls for attention. To be spiritual is to be aware of what one thinks, speaks or does at a given moment of time. Expanding awareness is said to lead one to true spirituality.

> 'Discipline and focussed awareness... contribute to the act of creation.'
>
> —John Poppy

> 'Fate is non-awareness.'
>
> —Jan Kott

awareness through movement See FELDENKRAIS THERAPY.

axinomancy (Eur./Occ.) One of the several obscure methods involved in DIVINATION in which an axe is used. The method may involve throwing an axe into the ground, or swinging it into a tree and interpreting the direction of the handle or the quivering of the blade. This form of divination was used in predicting the ruin of Jerusalem.

ayurveda (Ind.) Literally, the science of life. Considered the oldest health-care system known to mankind, and the fifth Veda, dating from 3000 to 1000 BC, ayurveda is more than a system of medicine. It refers broadly to a way of healthy and contented living with a four-fold purpose of life; virtue, wealth, enjoyment and salvation. The philosophy and practise of Ayurveda emphasizes the use of one's physical and mental abilities to achieve harmony with the environment. Ayurveda is considered to be a supplement to *Atharva Veda*.

ayurveda, the eight branches of (Ind.) According to CHARAKA, the eight branches of Ayurveda are: general medicine, surgery, ear, diseases of the nose, throat, eye and mouth, psychiatry, midwifery and paediatrics, toxicology, rejuvenation and aphrodisiacs.

ayurvedic (Ind.) Of, or pertaining to, AYURVEDA.

ayurvedic acupuncture (Ind.) A form of KALARI CHIKITSA, based on *Suchi Veda*, a 3000-year-old Vedic text which in the system of AYURVEDA is considered the science of acupuncture.

ayurvedic aromatherapy (Ind.) See GANDHACHIKITSA.

ayurvedic facial (Ind.) A therapeutic skin-care treatment, employing DOSHA-specific products and facial massage, focussing on MARMA points.

ayurvedic nutrition (Ind.) A concept based on the doctrine that one should select one's food according to the individual constitution and the season, and one should lessen one's intake of foods that aggravate the ascendant DOSHA.

babul (Ind.) *Acacia arabica, Acacia nilotica* Also, gum arabic; wattle bark. The bark of This tree, native to India and Africa, has been traditionally used in a strong decoction as a gargle to treat coughs and sore throats and as a mouthwash for spongy gums. The gum of the tree is also medicinal. It is used as a douche in gonorrhoea, cystitis, vaginitis, leucorrhoea, piles and in anal prolapse. The bark of the tree is also used for tanning and dyeing to various shades of brown.

baby BEST (Eur./New Age/Vib.) A version of Bio-Energetic Synchronization Technique, meant only for infants. This nonforceful, self-healing procedure, employing the hands, is aimed at energy-balancing in the infant's body to re-establish its natural healing abilities.

baby massage (Ind./Vib.) Also, Indian infant-massage, infant massage. A daily massage, based on gentle strokes for promoting general health in infants. The baby is laid on his stomach on his mother's outstretched legs and bath oil is applied while slowly stretching his body parts. The massage usually ends with a hot-water shower. After drying, the baby's body is fumigated with burning incense. The massage prolongs sleep and is also said to be helpful in stimulating the organs responsible for respiration, circulation and digestion. It also prevents gas and colic, the most common complaints in infants. According to some reports, the precocious motor development of many Indian babies can be attributed to baby massages. It is also recommended for children with special needs, as human touch is therapeutic for them.

Infant massage as a childcare practice is not unknown in other parts of Asia and in Africa and is being researched in Europe. In the US, massage therapy schools train young mothers and mothers-to-be in baby massage.

Bach, Edward (1886–1936) (Flo.) The British pathologist who was the pioneer in developing a healing system based on floral essence. The system is rooted on classical homoeopathic concepts. See BACH FLOWER REMEDIES.

> 'Disease will never be cured or eradicated by present materialistic methods, for the simple reason that disease in its origin is not material . . . Disease is in essence the result of conflict between the Soul and Mind and will never be eradicated except by spiritual and mental effort.'
>
> —Edward Bach

Bach Flower Remedies (Flo.) A healing system, based on floral essence, as developed in the 1920s by Edward Bach, a British pathologist. Some of these flower remedies are used in the treatment of common ailments as indicated:

Bach flower remedies	Ailments
Agrimony, aspen, crab apple, red chestnut	Anxiety
Agrimony	Suppressed feelings and emotions
Aspen	Fear of the unknown
Beech, impatiens	Intolerance, irritability
Centaury	Exhaustion
Cerato, larch	Lack of confidence
Cherry plum	Irrational behaviour, lack of confidence, persecution complex
Chestnut bud	Lack of concentration, repetition of faults
Chicory	Depression, narcissism, possessive and over-protective tendencies
Clematis	Absent-mindedness, day-dreaming, dementia
Crab apple	Feeling unclean or polluted
Elm	Feeling of inadequacy
Gentian	Doubt and despondency
Gorse	Feeling of hopelessness, pessimistic outlook
Heather	Over-talkative and self-obsessed nature
Holly	Feelings of anger, hatred, jealousy and suspicion
Honeysuckle	Living in the past, nostalgia
Hornbeam	Feeling tired and withdrawn
Impatiens	Impatience and irritability
Larch	Lack of confidence and feeling worthless
Mustard	Depression
Mimulus	Fear psychosis
Oak	Fighting nature that exhausts
Olive	Exhaustion
Pine	Self-reproach and guilt
Red chestnut	Over-anxious nature
Rock rose	Panic, shock, trauma
Rock water	Rigid approach, being hard on oneself, always demanding perfection
Scleranthus	Indecision
Star of Bethlehem	Trauma due to accident, loss, etc.
Sweet chestnut	Depression and hopelessness
Vervain	Restlessness
Vine	Aggressiveness, bullying, tyranny
Walnut	Habituation (to facilitate change)
Water Violet	Aloofness, reserved nature
White chestnut	Over-active mind, full of unwanted patterns of thoughts, stress, worrying nature
Wild oat	Directionlessness
Wild rose	Lack of interest or initiative, fatalism
Willow	Self-pity, resentment
Rescue remedies	Accident, crisis or trauma

badara (Ayur./Chi.) *Zizyphus jujube* Also, Chinese date, sour date, jujube, suanzaoren, zaoren, zizyphus. This plant is native to China where it is regarded as one of the 'five great fruits'. The Vitamin C-rich fruit of this tree has a long history of medicinal use. According to an ancient Chinese text written in AD 100, zizyphus is sour and 'balanced' (i.e. it is both warming and cooling). It is used mainly in the treatment of abdominal ailments and pains in the limbs. The protracted use of zizyphus is believed to make one's body light and promote longevity.

> 'Jujube imparts taste to the tongue.'
>
> —*Raja Nighantu*

baddha kona asana (Yoga) An asana considered good for the kidneys and prostate gland and useful in relieving sciatic pain, pain in the testicles and vaginal irritation.

bael (Ind.) *Aegle marmelos*. Also, stone apple, Bengal quince. A woody tree, native to India, known for the medicinal use of its leaves and fruits. Its leaves are believed to be Lord Shiva's favourite, hence the tree is sacred to Hindus. Bael also grows in Sri Lanka, Pakistan, Bangladesh, Myanmar, Thailand and most south-east Asian countries. It is used in several indigenous systems of medicine in India, China, Burma and Sri Lanka, particularly for its hypoglycaemic quality and in the treatment of diabetes mellitus.

> 'Plant a bael and please Shiva!'
>
> —*Padma Purana*

bagua (Chi.) From the Chinese for eight symbols. Also, pa kua. An ancient Chinese philosophical concept, symbolized by an octagonal diagram with one trigram on each side, representing the interaction between YIN and YANG. Each direction on the

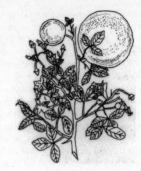

Bael

octagon (north, north-east, west, south-west and so on) is associated with certain significant aspects believed to affect one's life. By mapping the ba gua onto a home, for example, guidelines on correct orientation can be deduced. In FENG SHUI, particularly, the bagua octagon (see illustration) is placed, with its bottom downwards, at the front door to help harmonize domestic activities, associated with the prescribed directions.

The table below indicates the nature of QI emanating from different directions, as understood in the Chinese tradition:

Direction	Nature	Symbol	Remarks
qi from the north	nourishing and mystic	black tortoise, an animal of winter; Moon	intuitive, compliant and diplomatic
qi from the south	energizing and lucky	red phoenix, a summer bird that heralds good fortune; Sun	energetic, restless and dynamic
qi from the east	protecting and kind	golden dragon, the green animal of spring; thunderbolt	growing, warm and generous
qi from the west	disruptive and unpredictable	white tiger, an animal of autumn; lake	forceful, unyielding self-reliant

An example of the application of the ba gua is avoiding the construction of a kitchen in the northern part of a house because the hearth or stove could be dampened by the water element associated with the north. According to Chinese philosophy, each kind of qi seeks to achieve balance and harmony by coveting its opposite. As the hot qi of the south seeks the cool qi of the north, the wise qi of the east seeks novelty from the unpredictabe qi of the west. At the centre lies the earth, a 'home' for all directions, seeking to harmonize them with its patience, prudence and stability.

bagua map (Chi.) A map, drawn on the basis of *I-CHING*, the ancient Chinese book on DIVINATION. The map incorporates eight fundamental aspects which are considered essential in human existence: love, wealth, reputation, health, creativity, knowledge, career and friends/well-wishers. The map finds its application in FENG SHUI consultations, to decide on the location of a building on land and for allotting various functional areas in an auspicious manner.

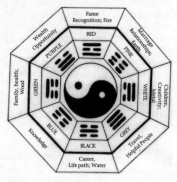

Bagua map

baguazhang (New Age) Also, circle walking. A holistic healing practice aimed at improving QI energy as developed by Dong Hai-Chuan, a Chinese practitioner in the mid-1800s. It comprises walking in a circle in a variety of postures, referred to variously as the chicken step, elephant step, snake step, mud-walking step, etc. Its practise is said to improve VITAL FORCE.

bahiranga kumbhaka (Yoga) Also, bahya kumbhaka. From bahiranga, meaning outside. Bahiranga kumbhaka is an important stage in the regulation of breath (PRANAYAMA). In this stage, the breath is held outside the body after exhalation, and is distinct from the practice of holding the breath inside the body, ANTARANGA KUMBHAKA. See also, KUMBHAKA.

bahiranga trataka (Yoga) Also, outer gaze (bahiranga means outside). The esoteric practice of gazing steadily at objects, the commonly used ones including candle flames, a full moon, or a rising or setting sun. This practice is said to correct, over time, eye disorders, besides developing concentration skills. Steady gazing is one of the six cleansing methods specified in HATHA YOGA, a branch of yoga which treats the body and its physiology as the perfect instrument for SELF-REALIZATION. See also, KRIYA.

Bahr, Frank R. (Mod./New Age) An acutherapist who combined a special diet regimen with acupressure, aimed at reducing obesity. Dr Bahr's book on ACU-DIET prescribes a ten-second-a-day acupressure, along with diet regulations, for weight reduction.

bahupatra See BHUMYAMALAKI.

bahya kumbhaka (Yoga) See BAHIRANGA KUMBHAKA.

bahya snehana (Ind.) The external application of medicated oil; one of the procedures prescribed in PURVAKARMA. The application is often carried out by two therapists who stand on either side of the patient, who lies on a special wooden bed, and vigorously massage the body in synchronicity.

bai zhi (Chi.) *Angelica dahurica.* Also, Chinese angelica. A herb known in Chinese folklore for its anti-inflammatory properties. It is also used in the treatment of allergies and colds, as it helps clear congestion by opening up nasal passages.

bai shao (Chi./Jap.) *Paeonia lactiflora.* Also, Chinese peony, white peony root. An attractive ornamental plant, known for its medicinal use for over 3,000 years in China. The root of the white peony is known for its regulatory action on liver QI. Along with LIQUORICE, bai shao is used in China and Japan in the formulation shakuyaku-kanzo.

bai zhu (Chi./Jap.) *Angelica sinensis.* A fragrant, medicinal herb grown in China, Japan and Korea, traditionally used in ailments connected with the bowels, heart, lungs and liver. A tonic prepared from this herb is also administered to women to regulate their menstrual cycles.

bakuchi (Ind./Chi.) *Psoralea corylifolia.*

Also, babchi, bemchi. A medicinal herb, celebrated both in the Chinese and Indian folklores since ancient times. The herb is usually used in topical preparations for the treatment of alopoaecia and vitiligo.

> 'Destroyer of leprosy.'
> —a Sanskrit name for bakuchi

bakula (Ind.) *Mimusops elengi*. Also, simha-kesara, vakula, Spanish cherry. An ornamental garden tree, with white fragrant flowers, common in India, Malaysia, Myanmar, Sri Lanka, Thailand and Vietnam. Its roots, fruit and seeds are known for their astringent properties and are also used in the treatment of gonorrhoea. Chewing the unripe fruit is said to prevent the falling of loose teeth. An extract of its bark is used as a mouthwash in severe gum ailments. Its dried and powdered flowers are used as a snuff to induce copious defluxion from the nose, to relieve congestion in the head.

bala (Ind.) *Sida rhombifolia* and *Sida orientalis*. Also, mahabala. A weed which grows in the Indian subcontinent. Its stem, rich in mucilage, is employed internally in combination with pepper as an emollient, diuretic and febrifuge. The roots are anthelminthic.

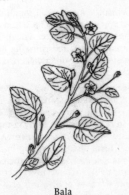

Bala

balaka (Ind.) See TAGARA.

balance breathing (Mod./New Age) A general health practice, which trains a person to assess the condition of his or her personal energy. It is based on the belief that by applying appropriate breath interventions, one can bring one's personal energy into balance.

balance therapies (Mod.) A holistic approach to healing, which employs herbs, HOMOEOPATHY and KYO-JITSU. The method is attributed to Arcadi Beliavtsev, who also developed FACE MODELLING.

balneotherapy (Nat.) A holistic approach in which baths are recommended for curing various disease, particularly afflictions of the skin. Baths and sulphur springs have been known for their therapeutic use from ancient times; the remains of ancient baths can still be seen in Europe and Britain. The pre-Aryan Great Bath of Mohenjodaro existed in the Indian subcontinent almost 5,000 years ago.

Water is known to enhance the immune mechanism in the body by improving the circulation of blood and lymph. In Japan, repeated immersion in hot-water springs is practised and in Europe bathing in hot water loaded with minerals is considered therapeutic. Hot water also reduces pain and stress. See also, HOT BATHS, HYDROPATHY, HYDROTHERAPY.

balsam apple See BITTER GOURD.

ban xia (Chi.) *Pinellia ternata*. Also, banha. A toxic plant, rich in calcium oxalate which is destroyed by thoroughly cooking or drying. The medicinal root is known in folk medicine for its use in strengthening the spleen and in removing gall-stones. It is also used in the treatment of coughs and in controlling nausea and vomiting, and there have been few reported cases of it being used in the treatment of cancer as well.

band music, therapeutic role of (New Age) Band music, employing brass instruments, cymbals, drums and trumpets, is characterized by loud and activating tunes and sounds and considered therapeutic for children, adolescents and adults. The appropriate rhythm can bring cheer which may help overcome depression and can also be useful in the treatment of addictions. Military band music is also known for boosting the morale of the armed forces and inspiring movement and lightness. See also, MOZART EFFECT, MUSIC THERAPY.

> 'After silence, that which comes nearest to expressing the inexpressible is music.'
>
> —Aldous Huxley

bandha (Yoga) Energy lock. An exercise, prescribed in YOGA, involving the contraction and relaxation of specific muscles in the body. The exercise is aimed at harnessing PRANA, the life-force, which is, after it is harnessed, believed to get distributed to the areas in the body which thirst for it.

The table below gives information on the three bandhas:

Bandha	Location	Methodology	Probable role
Uddiyana bandha	Navel	Performed at the end of breath retention (KUMBHAKA) and at the commencement of inhalation (RECHAKA)	Prevention and cure of stomach-related disorders
Jalandhara bandha	Neck	Performed by bending the head downwards so that the chin touches the chest, thereby contracting the neck. Practised at the end of puraka	Facilitation of the shift of prana into the whole of sushumna
Mula bandha	Anus	Performed while sitting in padmasana, and by pressing the perineum with the left heel, keeping the right heel above the genital organs and contracting the anal muscles. Mula bandha can be done during puraka, kumbhaka, rechaka and also while meditating and doing japa	Prevention and cure of all mind-related illness and mental tension

> 'The regular practise of the three bandhas ensures perfect health.'
>
> —Adi Sankaracharya

banha See BAN XIA.

baoding balls (Chi.) Also, Chinese health balls. Smooth-surfaced, hand-held balls, in use in China for over a millennium to alleviate arthritis in the hands and fingers.

baptisia (Am. Ind./Hom.) *Baptisia tinctoria*. Also, wild indigo, baptis. An acrid, bitter herb, popular with North American Indians for its medicinal use. A decoction of the root has antiseptic properties and is used especially for washing wounds and skin ulcers. When used as a mouthwash, it serves as a remedy for gum infections and sore throats. Modern research has confirmed its anti-bacterial role. It is also recognized as a stimulant for the immune system.

The fresh root and bark are used to make homoeopathic medicine. Though it has a limited range of action, it finds its use especially in the treatment of certain types of flu. Confused or impaired thinking and delirium are some of the indications of this medicine.

barberry (Chi./Hom./Ind.) *Berberis vulgaris, B. aristata*. Also, daru haridra. A plant known since ancient times for its medicinal value in rheumatic and gouty complaints and diseases of the urinary organs. Ancient medical texts of China dating back over 3,000 years, acknowledge its medicinal role. Due to its ability to correct liver function and promote the flow of bile, it is also a liver cleanser. In homoeopathy, barberry is used in the treatment of gallstones, gout and urinary tract infections.

> 'Daru haridra, one of the ten drugs that reduce corpulence.'
>
> —*Charaka Samhita*

barefoot shiatsu (Jap.) A Japanese approach to heal the body through massage; a form of SHIATSU in which CHANNELS are pressed with hands, feet, elbows or knees. The therapist walks barefoot on the back of the patient to remove tension. Though the word shiatsu refers to finger pressure, Shizuku Yamamoto, a contemporary expert, incorporated foot and toe pressure for a deeper massage which, according to him, enables the freer flow of QI energy in the body.

Barhydt, Elizabeth and Hamilton (Mod./New Age) The Barhydts innovated simple but profound self-help techniques to relieve chronic pain, learning disability and stress. They are founders of a non-profit organization, Loving Life, which follows Ken Keyes' concepts of personal growth through love and sharing. The organization aims at teaching people how to relieve stress and overcome pain while increasing one's energy level and quality of life. See also, SELF-HELP FOR STRESS AND PAIN.

barley (Eur.) *Hordeum vulgare*. Also, common barley. The decorticated seed of this plant is known commercially as pearl barley and is used in soups and stews. Malt, obtained from the roasted sprouts of whole seeds, is used in breweries, and the seeds are used for their digestive and nutritive properties. Barley water, an infusion of the germinated seeds in water, has long been prescribed for babies and invalids. It is also a folk remedy to reduce excessive lactation. Barley has also been in use as a poultice for burns and wounds. The plant also has a folk history of anti-tumour activity. Modern research has shown that barley may be of aid in the treatment of hepatitis, whilst other trials have shown that it may help to control diabetes. Barley bran may have the effect of lowering blood cholesterol levels and preventing bowel cancer.

baroque music, therapeutic role of (Mod./New Age) Listening to baroque music, the musical style in Europe roughly corresponding to the period AD 1600–1750 and associated with composers such as Bach, Monteverdi and Purcell, is believed to increase alpha and beta BRAIN WAVES, associated with a quiet, alert state, conducive for learning, and help provide structure during activities which demand organized, multi-

level thinking, such as management planning, creative writing and planning a social event. Some studies have also demonstrated its positive impact on brain functions, such as learning, retention and retrieval of memory. See also, MOZART EFFECT, MUSIC THERAPY.

> The melting voice through mazes running; Untwisting all the chains that tie the hidden soul of harmony.
>
> —John Milton

Barrett, Professor William (New Age) A professor of physics at Dublin, and a founder of both the American and British societies for psychical research. He studied mesmeric trance and is known for his scientific research on TELEPATHY and DOWSING which he initiated in 1874. He considered the existence of telepathy proved, holding that the method of communication is probably explainable by some form of nervous induction.

barbari See BASIL.

baryta carbonica (Hom.) Also, barium carbonate, baryta. A homoeopathic remedy, used for the enhancement of memory. It has also been found useful in problems and diseases associated with old age, including lack of self-reliance, loss of memory and quick temper.

basil (Afr./Am.Ind./Eur.) *Ocimum basilicum*. Also barbari, garden basil, sweet basil, lui le, St Josephwort, tulsi. A sacred herb of India, basil is considered *royale* in France and a sign of love in Italy. It is grown in almost every household in the belief that it purifies the air with its spiritual powers. In India it is used to treat coughs and in Africa to expel intestinal worms. American colonists used basil as a snuff, sniffing it to relieve headaches, while ancient Egyptians are reported to have used it for embalming the dead. In Mexico, it was believed that carrying basil in the pocket helped accumulate money and kept a lover faithful.

Aromatic and carminative, it is used as a poultice or salve for acne, insect bites and ringworm. As a bath herb, it helps in relieving fatigue. Splashing an infusion made of basil in the eyes helps tired eyes. Pliny also knew of basil's ability to remove flatulence.

> 'Like ambrosia, tulsi is to be sought after and adored.'
>
> —The Puranas

biokinesiology (Mod.) An offshoot of AP-PLIED KINESIOLOGY, developed in the mid-1970s by John Barton, aimed at correcting stressful emotions which are considered the basis for many ailments of the body.

bashpa swedana (Ind.) Steam bath; a part of PURVAKARMA, which helps in dilating the channels of the body and, as a consequence, promotes detoxification.

basic polarity counselling (New Age) A branch of POLARITY THERAPY, focussing on the body–mind relationship by integrating concepts and practices from BIOENERGETICS and GESTALT THEORY. The counselling aims at releasing 'held feelings' and changing 'dysfunctional thought patterns' which can cause serious ailments.

basti (Ind.) Also basti karma, enema. One of the five prescribed methods under SHODHANA in which medicines in suspension are administered to the patient through ano-rectal, urethral or vaginal routes. A special apparatus, called BASTI YANTRA, facilitates the introduction of medicated material into the body.

Basti, generally recommended only during the rainy season, is of two types: NIRUHA BASTI, in which decoctions are administered, and ANUVASANA BASTI, in which oily substances are used. Abdominal swellings/pain, dysuria, oedema, headaches, gout, piles, retention of flatus, stools and/or urine, loss of vigour, fevers and splenetic diseases indicate niruha basti, whereas an increased appetite and increase of VATA are indications for anuvasana basti. This treatment is believed to helps restore the balance of the DOSHAS or humours. It is also said to prevent ageing.

basti karma (Ind.) See BASTI.

basti yantra (Ind.) An apparatus, made of the urinary bladder of an animal, used for introducing medicated materials (decoctions or oils) in BASTI.

Bates' method (Mod.) A method of re-education, aimed at restoring normal vision. Devised by William H. Bates, the method broadly consists of the following steps: splashing the eyes first with luke-warm water about twenty times, followed by cold water for the same number of times; shifting the eyeballs constantly to avoid staring; blinking every two seconds to lubricate the eyes; practising focussing repeatedly on a far and a near object, as, say, two pencils, one held in an outstretched hand at eye-level and the other held in the other hand, close to the eye; swinging the body gently while standing and letting the eyes move with the body; closing the eyes and covering them with a soft handkerchief without using the palms; and visualizing pleasant sights. Bates firmly believed that by imagining pleasant objects, the physical eyes were greatly helped.

> 'It is the effort to see that sets up the error of refraction.'
>
> —W.H. Bates

bath (Nat.) A popular prescription in holistic systems, particularly in NATUROPATHY, it is known as 'a pleasure ritual for health'. See also BALNEOTHERAPY and HYDROTHERAPY.

bath additives (Mod./Nat./New Age) The ingredients added to BATH. Adding appropriate ingredients increases the aromatic and/or therapeutic value of a bath. Traditionally, bath additives are used to moisturize the skin and improve skin tone but are now also prescribed to overcome depression. Some commonly used bath additives and their expected effects are indicated in the following table:

Common Bath additives

Bath additives	Expected effects
Epsom salts	Elimination of toxins in the body through perspiration; relaxation of muscles
Powdered nutmeg	Elimination of skin impurities
Ground ginger	Improvement of circulation

Oatmeal	Elimination of skin affections; useful in the treatment of itch, sunburn and windburn
Wheatbran	Elimination of skin affections; useful in the treatment of itch, sunburn and windburn
Common salt	Relaxation

bath herbs See HERBAL BATH.

baubologie See BIO-ARCHITECTURE.

bee glue See PROPOLIS.

bee pollen (Nat.) Also, bee pollen therapy. A compound of pollens, gathered by bees and mixed with their own salivary secretions, found in natural conditions in bee hives. Traditionally recognized for its nutritive and energy-boosting value, bee pollen can also be beneficial for seasonal allergies. It is also found to be helpful in toning up the skin and slowing the process of AGEING.

bee pollen therapy See BEE POLLEN.

bee sting therapy See APITHERAPY.

beech (Eur./Flo./Hom.) *Fagus sylvatica.* Traditionally, a strong infusion of the leaves is used to clean and heal wounds and sores. A tea made from the powdered bark and leaves makes an excellent tonic for diabetics. It is reported to be useful in ailments related to the stomach, liver, kidneys and bladder.

> 'The leaves of the beech tree are cooling and binding, and therefore good to be applied to hot swellings to discuss them... you may boil the leaves into a poultice, or make an ointment of them when the time of year serves.'
>
> —Nicholas Culpepper, seventeenth-century English herbalist

beech flower essence (Flo.) One of the thirty-nine Bach flower remedies. It is recommended as a remedy for those who are highly critical, intolerant, irritable and dwell on the negative side of life.

bee therapy See APITHERAPY.

bee venom (Nat.) Also, bee-venom therapy. The venom of bees contains anti-inflammatory substances such as adolapin and melittin, found useful in the treatment of rheumatism and osteoarthritis. The venom is administered either by actual bee stings or by injection. In the former event, the practitioner places bees, one at a time, directly on a patient's skin with a pair of long tweezers, and allows them to sting. See also, APITHERAPY.

bee venom therapy See BEE VENOM.

behaviour disorder (Mod.) Unusual behaviour, such as repetitive movements (e.g., rocking), catatonic behaviour (i.e. lack of movement) and unpredictable aggression. Various alternative remedial systems, such as BACH FLOWER REMEDIES, HOMOEOPATHY and MUSIC THERAPY are widely used to correct behaviour disorders.

behaviour modification (Mod.) The manipulation of environmental conditions so as to encourage an individual to behave in a desired manner. See BEHAVIOUR THERAPY.

behaviour rehearsal (Mod.) A form of role playing in which a patient copies the therapist's staged rehearsal of an impending situation that is expected to be problematic. The concept of behaviour rehearsal is fundamental to learning a new behaviour and is found useful in under-assertive people. It is also reported to improve athletic performance.

behaviour therapy (Mod.) An attempt to change a behaviour pattern in a person through a functional analysis of his or her behaviour. Before a therapy is chosen, an attempt is made to see what antecedents lead to the disordered behaviour and what the behaviour leads to. Where behaviour problems are a result of faulty learning or conditioning, the therapy aims to remove them by deconditioning and reconditioning methods. The methods include desensitization or counter-conditioning, flooding and modelling.

behavioural approach See BEHAVIOURISM.

behavioural psychology See BEHAVIOURISM.

behavioural kinesiology (Mod.) A version of APPLIED KINESIOLOGY as developed by psychiatrist John Diamond, in which concepts of practices of preventive medicine, psychiatry and psychosomatic medicine are included.

behaviourism (Mod.) Also, behavioural approach, behavioural psychology. A twentieth-century movement in psychology and philosophy which gave prominence to manifested behavioural aspects of thought and dismissed internal experiential and procedural aspects. As an approach to psychology, it is based on the proposition that behaviour is important and worthy of scientific research, thus overlooking the independent significance of the mind. John B. Watson, who coined the term behaviourism in the early-twentieth century, proposed abandoning attempts to make consciousness a subject of experimental investigation, to focus instead on behavioural manifestations of intelligence. The significance of this approach for psychological treatment has been profound, and is one of the pillars of pharmacological therapy. Though this approach continues to emphasize the importance of environment in determining one's behaviour, it also allows for the inclusion of cognitive processes and feelings.

The successful 'cognitive revolution' of the 1960s styled itself as a revolt against behaviourism. Though behaviourism is on the wane, recent attempts to revive it through the doctrine of Ontological Subjectivity in philosophy and bring 'consciousness research' under the aegis of Cognitive Science point to the continuing relevance of behaviourism's metaphysical and methodological challenges.

'Behavioural psychology is the science of pulling habits out of rats.'

—Douglas Busch

beheduka See VIBHITAKI.

Beliavtsev, Arcadi See BALANCE THERAPIES, FACE MODELLING.

bell stone See ARGENTUM NITRICUM.

belladonna (Hom.) *Atropa belladonna*. Also, deadly nightshade; used in HOMOEOPATHY in the treatment of delirium, nausea and parched mouth. In modern medicine, the plant is an important source of atropine, used by ophthalmologists to dilate the pupils.

belleric myrobalan See VIBHITAKI.

bellows See BHASTRIKA.

belly bean diet (Hom./Mod.) A system of DIET, aimed at weight-loss. It allows three nutritionally balanced, low-fat meals with a total calorific value of 1,000 to 2,000. The diet also recommends an additional intake of five to six glasses of water every day and an appetite control drug which contains a highly potentized homoeopathic formulation.

belocolus (Gem) A white stone with a black pupil, traditionally used in the battlefield as it was believed to impart courage and invincibility.

bemchi See BAKUCHI.

Bengal quince See BAEL.

Benner, George See HERBAL CRYSTALLIZATION ANALYSIS.

Benor, Dan (Mod.) A contemporary American doctor who reviewed the world literature on holistic healing and published over 155 controlled studies to prove that SPIRITUAL HEALING and other complementary/alternative therapies could be effective. He advocated integrative medical care to help heal psychosomatic disorders.

'When science looks at a subject, it can only do so in the way it currently knows how to. Studies in science are built upon that which came before (somewhat like a case law).'

—Dan Benor

Bensen, Herbert (Mod.) An American researcher from Harvard, who demonstrated that ritualistic techniques employed in various Christian traditions, such as the use of the ROSARY, prayer-beads, or simple prayers repeated over and over could prove useful in healing. See also, RELAXATION RESPONSE.

benzoic acid (Hom.) Also, benz. ac. A remedy for the 'confused head'.

benzoin (Chi.) *Styrax benzoin*. Also, gum benjamin, gum benzoin, Sumatra benzoin. The resin of the tree, found in Java and Sumatra, is used externally, dissolved in water, for skin irritations. Taken internally, it acts as a carminative. The compound tincture of benzoin is used as an inhalant with steam to clear the respiratory passages.

berber (Hom.) Berberis. A homeopathic remedy for fear and anxiety. See also, BARBERRY.

Bergson, Henri (Mod.) See LIFE FORCE.

Berne, Eric (Mod./West.) An American researcher who in the 1950s pioneered the concept of TRANSACTIONAL ANALYSIS, an innovative approach to modern PSYCHOTHERAPY. His popular 'parent–adult–child' theory is still the subject of debate and development. The concept has a wide range of applications in both clinical and non-clinical settings (i.e., organizational, management, personality development, relationships and behaviour). It can also help improve one's dealings with others and understand oneself better in the scheme of things.

Be-Set-Free-Fast (BSFF) (Mod./Vib.) A descriptive acronym for Behavioural and Emotional Symptom Elimination Training for Resolving Excess Emotion. A method aimed at eliminating the emotional roots of self-limiting belief-systems, such as fear, anger, sadness and trauma which hinder one's personal growth and productivity. The method aims to directly address unresolved negative emotions which linger in the depths of one's subconscious mind and have a deep-rooted influence on behaviour, experience and achievements. The training method was developed in recent years by Larry Phillip Nims, a clinical psychologist.

> 'Anger is a brief madness.'
>
> —Horace

BEST See BIO ENERGETIC SYNCHRONIZATION TECHNIQUE.

beta waves (Mod.) A category of BRAIN WAVES, with frequencies of 13–40 Hz, which characterize an alert, aroused, attentive and focussed state of MIND, concentration, cognition, visual acuity and hand–eye coordination. Beta-centred training programmes are offered by BIOFEEDBACK therapists for the treatment of attention deficit disorder, and helps in improved performance in examinations, sports, talks or presentations.

Beyond Medicine (Mod./Vib.) A multidimensional approach to alternative medicine, involving a group of non-medical modalities.

Beyond Therapy (Mod.) A system of DREAMWORK, promoted by physical therapist Ken Costello, based on the concept that everyone is a spiritual being with a 'whispering inner self'. A dreamwork is basically an enquiry into dreams, aimed at self-correction and self-healing.

Bezman, William (Mod.) An American clinical hypnotherapist and specialist in psychiatric nursing, who created the healing paradigm called Hypnosynergestic Therapy, which combines hypnosis, energywork and spirituality to enable people to make changes desired by them in their lives.

bhadrasana (Yoga) An ASANA, involving the stretching of urino-genital areas, considered helpful in stimulating the prostate gland in men. It is also beneficial for those who suffer from sciatica and sacral infections.

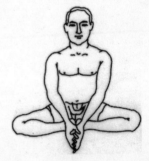

Bhadrasana

bhakti (Yoga) Devotion and dedication towards an object of worship (god), considered to be healing. As the devotee directs his total attention towards the object of worship, he develops a defence against the painful events in his life.

> 'Bhakti is an emotional—rather than intellectual—response to problems of existence.'
>
> —Krishnajoo Razdan

Bhakti Yoga (Yoga) A system of YOGA, centred on love and devotion. The system views the whole universe, with both animate and inanimate components, as being pervaded by divinity.

bhallataka (Ind.) *Semecarpus anacardium*. Also bhelwa, marking nut, oriental cashew nut. An important phytomedicine known to AYURVEDA and SIDDHA MEDICINE from ancient times. The fruit of this plant is considered an aphrodisiac and has also been in use in the treatment of piles and skin diseases. Its rind has been used to treat leprosy. Unani uses its leaves in the treatment of fever, piles and general debility. Its oil, also considered an aphrodisiac, is also a wood preservative and is also used in the treatment of leucoderma and epilepsy. A black resin, obtained from the pericarp of the fruit is used as marking ink to write on cloth.

bharadvajasana (Yoga) An ASANA that comprises the rotation of spine, thereby enhancing the flexibility of the back and hips.

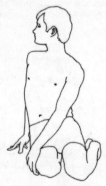

Bharadvajasana

bhasma (Ind.) A sacred ash obtained from the worship of fire, said to be charged with the intonations of MANTRAS. See VIBHUTI.

bhastrika (Yoga) Also, bellows; kundalini bhastrika. A form of PRANAYAMA, involving a very fast, non-stop inhalation and exhalation for at least five times. The method combines KAPALBHATI and UJJAYI. The practitioner's lungs are used like the bellows of a blacksmith. Traditionally, this exercise has been in use to raise KUNDALINI and hence is also known as kundalini bhastrika. It consists of a series of pumping followed by the retention of breath as in KAPALBHATI. Al-

though air is forced both in and out, the emphasis is on its expulsion.

A series of such expulsions, each following the other in quick succession, is referred to as a round. While beginners restrict a round to about five expulsions, it can be gradually increased to ten or more, depending on the desired effect.

The effects include increased ventilation, increased blood circulation, decongestion of the nasal passage, increased thinking capacity coupled with the elimination of mental inhibition or lethargy. As every expulsion is like an explosion in the body, this exercise needs to be performed under medical supervision. Over-exercising may cause severe dizziness. A series of normal breaths should be taken before undertaking a second round. This method is aimed at suffusing the internal organs of the body with abundant life-energy (PRANA).

bhavana (Ind.) Maceration of powders in fluids. Most medicinal preparations containing plant materials are taken macerated in liquid, oil, milk or GHRITA.

bhavatita dhyana See TRANSCENDENTAL MEDITATION.

bheda (Ind.) The term is used in AYURVEDA to denote the sixth stage of disease manifestation, often characterized by complications.

bhelwa See BHALLATAKA.

bharajak pitta (Ind.) The metabolic function associated with the skin.

bhishakapriya See GUDUCHI.

bhramara mudra (Yoga) A MUDRA formed by bending the index finger and touching to its base and tip of the thumb which also touches the side of the middle finger. The other fingers remain extended.

bhramari (Yoga) A form of PRANAYAMA wherein during exhalation, a smooth, continuous humming sound is created for the full duration and the vibrations that follow are closely watched till they cease to exist. Bhramari, which involves a concentrated and fixed breathing exercise, is aimed at strengthening the respiratory and circulatory mechanisms, calming the mind and increasing the power of concentration. This breathing technique is recommended particularly in advanced stages of meditation (SAMADHI).

bhringaraja (Ind.) *Eclipta alba.* A herb known in India from ancient times for its efficacy in preventing hair loss and premature graying. In the Philippines, the leaf powder is used in healing wounds and its decoction in the treatment of hepatitis. The famous oil of bhringaraja is prepared usually in combination with gooseberry (amla), soapnut powder (shikakai) and MARGOSA (NEEM), with coconut oil as its base.

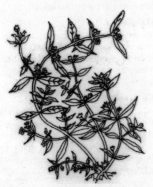

Bhringaraja

bhrumadhya (Yoga) The point at the centre of the eyebrows, identified as the seat of intuition and the THIRD EYE.

bhrumadhya drishti (Yoga) A form of TRATAKA, in which the eyes are directed towards the THIRD EYE, between the two eyebrows, or BHRUMADHYA.

bhuiamla See BHUMYAMALAKI.

bhujangasana (Yoga) Literally, serpent's posture; an ASANA considered useful in strengthening the spine and reducing abdominal fat.

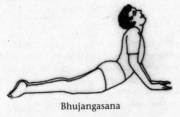

Bhujangasana

bhumyamalaki (Flo./Ind.) *Phyllanthus niruri.* Also, bhuiamla, stone-breaker. A native of South America, this plant grows wild in the central and southern parts of India and Sri Lanka. Its strong roots not only break stones, hence the name stone-breaker, but are also medicinal, along with its leaves, fruits and latex. The expressed juice of the whole plant is used in the treatment of chronic liver ailments. In Indian deserts, the roots mixed with commiphora mukul is given to camels to cure indigestion.

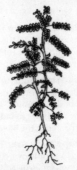

Bhumyamalaki

bhunimba (Ind.) *Swertia chirayita.* Also, chirayata, Nepalanimba. A medicinal plant common in the temperate Himalayas. This bitter plant is used as a tonic in the treatment of fevers. It is also used to treat skin diseases.

bhuta siddhi (Yoga) Control achieved over the Five Elements which are the constituents of both the body (microcosm) and the universe (macrocosm). See also, MAHABHUTA.

bhutagni (Ind.) Digestive fire. The concept of fire or agni is unique in AYURVEDA. Agni, whose origin is traced to the sun, is considered the source of all transformations in living beings. It is believed that while the maintenance of health due to metabolic processes and healing takes place due to the normal state of agni, its abnormal state contributes to pathological changes. The absence of agni is said to result in the death of the living entity. It is also believed that the life-force (PRANA) is dependent on agni.

bhutashuddhi (Yoga) A technique of KUNDALINI YOGA, aimed at purifying the mind, speech and body. Chanting MANTRA helps in purification of one's speech, and action becomes purified through the use of hand gestures, MUDRAS, and breath-control, PRANAYAMA. It is believed that thoughts get purified through MEDITATION and VISUALIZATION.

bhuta vidya (Ind.) Demonology; the science of dealing with invisible micro-organisms or evil-spirits. This ancient science is also concerned with the treatment of mental problems, using diet, herbs and yoga.

bibhitaki See VIBHITAKI.

Biblical counselling (Eur.) The use of devotional instructions in the Bible to treat psychological disorders. It also aims at facilitating healing, love and transformation.

Biblical nutrition (Eur.) An ancient viewpoint on food, nutrition, diet and health. Processed foods, chemical additives and non-organic foods are avoided as 'wrong' while those named in the Bible are preferred.

bibliotherapy (New Age) The use of literature to help people overcome problems such as alcoholism, drug addiction, smoking, anxiety and depression. Modern libraries have listings of bibliotherapy selections, categorized by various concerns such as disaster, trauma, divorce, death and dying, managing newborns and step-parenting.

Bi-Digital O-Ring Test Molecular Identification method (Mod./ New Age) A method of locating points/areas on the human tongue, representing specific internal organs with a view to enhance the efficacy of TONGUE ACUPUNCTURE and TONGUE DIAGNOSIS.

big band See BAND MUSIC.

bija (Eur./Occ./Yoga) Seed, source, sound, energy force, often associated with a particular CHAKRA. In Hindu philosophy, the term is often used to represent a mystic syllable or the condensed form of one's thought, which is an essential part of MANTRA.

bijakshara (Eur./Occ./Yoga) Literally, seed-letter. Certain alphabets, traditionally considered sacred, potent and healing. A bijakshara, woven around sound vibrations is considered to have latent power as does a MANTRA.

bija mantra (Eur/Occ./Yoga) Literally, seed mantras, known for their powerful intonations. Repeatedly chanted, they are believed to influence the healing process. According to TANTRISM, a bija mantra is an outcome of the primordial energy, containing latent power.

The following table indicates some important bija mantras of the Hindu tradition:

Bija mantra	The presiding deity in Hindu pantheon
Aim	Sarasvati, the goddess of learning
Aum	Universal Being
Dum	Durga
Gam	Ganapati
Hrim	Mahamaya
Hroum	Shiva
Hum	Bhairav
Klim	Krishna (Also, Kamadeva)
Krim	Kalika
Kshroum	Narasimha
Shrim	Lakshmi, the goddess of wealth

Bikram Choudhury (b. 1946) (Yoga) A yoga practitioner from India, he popularized his method of yoga all over the world in more than 400 franchise training centres. See also BIKRAM YOGA.

Bikram Yoga (Mod./New Age) Also, hot yoga. A system of twenty-six essential body postures, designed by BIKRAM CHOUDHURY and aimed at stretching muscles and tendons. Based on the eighty-four-posture Yoga Sutras of PATANJALI, he selected twenty-six essential body postures to be performed in ninety minutes in a hot and steamy environment. See also, BIKRAM CHOUDHURY.

Bilkis, Michael R. (Mod.) An MD in dermatology, he developed a complete skin-care programme aimed at curing skin ailments at three levels: the body, mind and spirit. See HEALING THE SKIN FROM WITHIN.

bilva See BAEL.

bimanual palpation (Mod.) The examination (of the body) with both hands, such as the clinical examination of the floor of the mouth or uterus.

bindegewebmassage (New Age) Also, connective tissue massage. A form of BODY-WORK developed in Germany in the 1930s by Elisabeth Dicke. Akin to ACUPUNCTURE, this method of healing is based on the principle that a powerful link exists between the body's connective tissues (e.g. cartilage) and specific 'paths' of nervous system and internal organs.

bindi (Cos./Spa) A type of bodywork, common in spas, which combines exfoliating treatment, using marine algae, herbs and MASSAGE.

bindu (Occ./Yoga) A CHAKRA or a psychic centre, considered the centre of infinitely concentrated energy in the body; the mark worn on the forehead by Hindus, depicting the intuitive faculty, the THIRD EYE. Bindu is also the name of a YANTRA, which represents the centre-point of the universe.

bio-architecture (New Age) The study of holistic interactions between an organism and its environment. The best examples of economical and ecological architecture are found in nature and can be of great value in preserving the health of individuals and societies; the adaptation of 'nature's intelligence' in planning and executing manmade buildings and townships is aimed at implementing biological patterns and bio-materials.

Biological Structure	Characteristics	What to learn
Spider's web	Very economical and light network construction	Economically, ecologically, structurally and functionally efficient design; organized workforce
Beehive	A honeycomb pattern consisting of hexagons and pentagons	Aesthetic and functional design and construction by a disciplined, and organized workforce
Anthill	An internally organized building with each underground compartment performing its own function	Functionally and economically efficient design and construction, using locally available materials by a disciplined and organized workforce.
Silicone body of a sponge	A complicated pattern of rods running across, providing for a strong and elegant construction	Can be useful in designing huge containers for storage of goods.
Cell-membrane	The double-layer of lipid molecules, guarding a living cell, while allowing its inter-change with the external environment	Efficiency in ensuring safety while allowing inter-change can be a lesson to present-day customs and security personnel

Examples of some biological structures are indicated in the following table:

biochemics (Hom.) An alternative healing system invented by W.H. Schuessler of Germany, and based on the understanding that the human body is mainly composed of twelve inorganic salts whose balance alone ensures health. Any disturbance in the ratio of these salts would mean an unhealthy condition or a disease. For example, the deficiency of sodium phosphate in the body is associated with acidity, and iron phosphate with inflammation. The treatment, therefore, involves correcting the contents by supplementing them. In acute conditions, salts are administered every half an hour.

bioclimatology (Mod.) A branch of climatology which deals with the effect of climate on the health and well-being of humans.

biodynamic massage (Mod./New Age) A type of MASSAGE as developed in recent times by Gerda Boyesen, a Norwegian researcher. The massage includes counselling exercises to release pent-up emotions of the patients.

bioelectricity (Mod.) The force behind the working of the body and mind. In nature, bio-electricity circuits are miniaturized beyond the dreams of any micro-chip researcher. The electric charges in a cell stand separated from its neighbouring cell by a membrane, one-millionth the width of a finger nail.

bioenergetic analysis See BIOENERGETICS.

bioenergetic healing (New Age/Vib.) A form of HEALING, based on the belief that bioenergy brought into one's hands is curative. This method was designed by Zeev Kolman, an Israeli researcher. See also, REIKI.

bioenergetic medicine See bioenergetics.

bioenergetic movement work (Eur./New Age) A method of HEALING aimed at freeing ENERGY BLOCKS in the body.

bioenergetics (New Age/Vib.) Also, bioenergetic analysis, bioenergetic medicine, bioenergetic therapy. A complementary therapy which combines work with the body and mind to help people resolve their emotional problems and realize more of their potential for joy in living. As every chronic stress or trauma produces a state of muscular tension in the body and emotional blockage in the mind, restricting their motility (the spontaneous movement of muscles and thought processes, limiting the patient's self-expression), it becomes necessary to release them. Bioenergetics acts as a way of

enhancing aliveness and emotional well-being. The technique was developed by Alexander Lowen. See also, BIOENERGY.

bioenergetic synchronization technique (Eur./New Age/Vib.) Also, BEST. A painless, relaxation technique aimed at releasing one's internal healing power. Though the technique combines CHIROPRACTIC and POLARITY THERAPY, it is devoid of a traditional chiropractic approach. The technique, developed by M.T. Morter, is based on the belief that health is regulated by one's innate intelligence.

bioenergetic therapy See BIOENERGETICS.

bioenergy (Eur./Vib./Yoga) The energy system in the body, discovered several millennia ago by the Indians and Chinese. There is evidence that this was known in many other parts of the world as well, including Africa, Arabia, Brazil and Egypt. The term bioenergy also refers to the bio-mass energy systems which produce heat/electricity and biofuels. See LIFE-FORCE, MERIDIAN, PRANA, QI.

bioenergy healing (Chi./Vib./Yoga) A healing system, developed in China around the twelfth century AD. It was based on the belief that all illness can be attributed to the blockage or depletion of vital energy (CHI or QI) in the body. As energy gets blocked because of malfunctioning in the energy centres (CHAKRAs) which do not properly transform the energy into various channels, locating problem areas and decongesting energy cobwebs through gentle hand movements is expected to result in strengthening the body's immune mechanism.

bioenergy self-treatment (New Age/Vib.) A self-exercise devised by F.P. Gallo and H. Vincenzi to overcome emotional upsets or negative feelings, caused by mild shock or trauma. This exercise can be done in privacy. The steps comprise being reminded of a mild tragedy or traumatic event in your life (Say, a 5 on a 0–10 scale) and then firmly tapping the BHRUMADHYA, the centre-point between the eyebrows, with the index fingers but without causing any pain. Continue thinking about the bad memory and keep tapping till it becomes difficult for you to be in touch with the bad feelings. At this point, if you still find a trace of discomfort or feeling, start tapping the treatment point again till you feel fairly comfortable. If the problem recurs, a few more rounds may be necessary before this problem is eliminated from the system. Other treatment points recommended for tapping are the portion below the nose, the portion below the lower lip and at the centre of your chest. It is however necessary that you take the help of a bioenergy psychotherapist before mastering this technique.)

biofeedback (Mod./New Age) Also, biofeedback monitoring, biofeedback technique. A way of monitoring and learning how the body reacts when tense or relaxed. It is a technique that measures bodily functions like breathing, heart rate, blood pressure and muscle tension. This technique permits a patient to monitor his internal organs and control some of their functions. In other words, a patient exercises more control over so-called involuntary functions by practising biofeedback.

bio-feedback training (Mod./New Age) A training in BIOFEEDBACK which teaches how one can consciously control bodily functions which are otherwise involuntary (e.g. BREATHING, heart rate and blood pressure) through information generated by electronic devices.

biofield See AURA.

biofield healing (Eur./New Age/Vib.) A method of energy healing, in which the practitioner uses his hands on the patient's body, to manipulate his BIO-FIELD.

'Self-healing, mind medicine, and biofield healing cannot be explained using conventional Western scientific paradigms.'

—B. J. Anderson

biogram (New Age) Literally, living world. A healing theory, propounded in recent years by Richard Johnson. The theory relates a person's experience and emotion to the biochemical response in his or her body. For every experience, the body creates a correlating chemical, which is the body's 'language' into which the experience has translated. As a person gets angry or melancholic, his or her whole body experiences it via a biochemical. The biogram theory has found its way into a wide range of therapeutic interventions. See BIOGRAM THERAPY.

biogram healing See BIOGRAM THERAPY.

biogram therapy (New Age) Biogram mind–body healing, biogram system. An organized and systematic method of healing, developed in recent times by Richard Johnson. Aimed at teaching how to be in control of one's emotional and physical well-being, it deals with healing through mind–body communication. It is based on the theory that emotional problems can be corrected by helping to change the biological conditions associated with them. This therapy is also oriented towards pain management and behaviour modification in children.

biokinesiology (New Age/Vib.) (From BIO meaning life, and KINES meaning movement). A non-invasive, energy-assessment method to evaluate the psycho/physiological health of an organism as a whole and its many systems. Developed in 1970s by John Barton, the method originates from the principle that stressful emotions are the root cause for many ailments. Through this method, one aims at preventing or correcting possible energy imbalances in the body.

bio-lifting (Mod./New Age) A non-surgical facial lifting treatment performed with galvanic stimulation. Cosmetic products, such as eye contour cream, contain botanical extracts of plants such as tiger grass and are currently marketed as anti-ageing formulations for ironing out wrinkles and reducing dark circles under the eyes.

biological dentistry (Mod./New Age) An integrated approach to general dentistry aimed at the overall health of an individual. It is aimed not only at the elimination of toxic conditions and materials from the mouth, but also the restoration of its structural and functional components. In other words, the oral cavity, which is a unique organization of several kinds of tissues, is addressed in its entirety. Being a holistic approach, biological dentistry takes into account aesthetics, biochemical and biomechanical mechanisms, compatibility, functional integrity, hormonal balance, meridians, pathology, proper occlusion, proprioceptive integrity and toxicology.

biological phenomena (Mod./New Age) The characteristics of biological functions and activities at the organic and molecular levels in all living matter. The phenomena in biology can be explained in two ways: mechanistically and vitalistically. The mechanists explain them in terms of the laws and principles of physics and chemistry. The vitalists, on the other hand, visualize the existence of a nonphysical entity, a causal agent which directs such life-processes.

biological transducers (Mod./New Age/Vib.) Cells and tissues in the body, which act as transducers, converting one form of energy into another. Thermal receptors in the skin, mechano-receptors in muscles, taste receptors in the tongue, olfactory nerve cells, rods and cones in the retinal of the eyes are some examples which are capable of converting input energy (or the information received through external stimuli) into an output energy (or electrical signals).

biomagnetic therapy (Grk./Vib.) An alternative system of healing, known to the ancient Greeks, finding mention in the work of Hippocrates, the father of medicine. The Greeks, in fact, discovered lodestone, the first natural magnet. Some therapists explain that in the living cell, the outside has a negative charge with respect to the inside of the cell. It is believed that this combination of opposite charges enables the cell to function normally. Whenever this equilibrium is affected, disease occurs. The use of magnets is believed to repair any such dysfunction by restoring equilibrium. Simply placing a magnet over an area of acute pain is believed to relieve pain, without any side-effects. Pregnant women and people with wounds, infections or cancer and those who use pace makers are, however, cautioned by therapists not to use magnets. Modern medicine too employs magnetic fields in diagnosis: Magnetic resonance imaging (MRI) uses magnetic fields to formulate 3-D images of the brain and an electroencephalograph (EEG) focusses on electrical activity in the brain.

biomass (Mod.) A broad term, used especially to describe biological material of recent origin. Considered a form of stored solar energy, biomass includes trees, crops, algae and other plants, as well as agricultural and forest residues. It also includes many materials considered waste, including food and drink manufacturing effluents, sludge, manures, industrial (organic) byproducts and the organic part of household waste.

bionics (Mod./West.) The application of biological principles to study and design electronic, mechanical, chemical and structural engineering systems. By improving machines and equipment, especially computers, scientists, in recent years, have made useful attempts to narrow the chasm between nature and technology.

biorhythms (New Age/Vib.) The physical, emotional and intellectual rhythms of a person, which determine the state of his physical, emotional or intellectual characteristics on a given date. The biorhythm system helps make a forecast of favourable and unfavourable dates, based on one's date of birth, from which three rhythmic cycles are worked out and made into a graph. The point where all the three lines come together is taken as the most favourable date as on that date, the body, emotions and mind fall in line with each other, indicating complete harmony. Where the chasm between the lines is wide, the dates are considered unhealthy or adverse.

Biorhythms are believed to be inborn and inherent cycles which regulate biological and psychological characteristics such as ambition, co-ordination, emotions, endurance, memory and temperament.

There are three biorhythm cycles: physical (which completes one cycle in twenty-three days), emotional (in twenty-eight days) and intellectual (thirty-three days). While the physical cycle (which determines strength, initiative and sex drive) is considered dominant in men, the emotional cycle (which determines sensitivity, temperament and sexuality) is considered dominant in women. The intellectual cycle is said to regulate alertness, memory and ambition. See BIORHYTHM CHART.

The following table indicates the cycle of the three important rhythms in human constitution and the number of days taken by their cycle to complete one round:

Rhythms	Number of days to complete a cycle
Physical	23
Emotional	28
Intellectual	33

biorhythm chart (New Age/Vib.) A chart indicating the positioning of the three cycles of BIORHYTHMS, helpful in determining the physical, emotional and intellectual conditions of an individual on a given date. By monitoring the highs and lows of these cycles, it is believed that one can devise appropriate daily action plans. For instance, one can avoid interactions with others during emotional lows as one can undertake tests or exams during intellectual highs.

biosonic repatterning (Nat./Vib.) Also, biosonics. A natural method of healing using tuning forks. Based on sonic ratios inherent in nature, this method is said to help a person align himself with intervals similar to those of the humming of tuning forks; when a tuning fork is tapped, musical intervals based on precise mathematical proportions, known as Pythagorean tunings, are produced. The method, developed by John Beaulieu, is based on the belief that listening to tuning forks coerces our nervous systems to attune itself to the pitch.

> 'Tuning into the sound of your nervous system is a meditation.'
>
> —John Beaulieu

biosonics (Nat./Vib.) See BIOSONIC REPATTERNING.

biotic (Mod.) Relating to life.

birth stones (Gem) Precious or rare stones, associated with each of the twelve signs of the zodiac and used in AMULETS and TALISMANS. In different cultures across the globe, birth stones have been assigned with luck, health and prosperity.

The following table lists some stones associated with signs of the zodiac.

Zodiac sign	Birthstone
Aries (March 21–April 19)	amethyst, bloodstone, coral, garnet, lapis lazuli, ruby, quartz
Taurus (April 20–May 20)	agate, emerald, peridot, jade, lapis lazuli, topaz, turquoise, quartz
Gemini (May 21–June 21)	agate, amethyst, aventurine, moonshine, peridot, pearl, moonstone
Cancer (June 22–July 22)	beryl, emerald, garnet, lapis lazuli, pearl, ruby, moonstone, sapphire, sodalite
Leo (July 23–August 22)	amber, carnelian, diamond, garnet, malachite, riverstone, ruby, peridot, topaz
Virgo (August 23–September 22)	agate, aventurine, aquamarine, blue topaz, fossil stone, howlite, jasper, peridot, rose quartz, sapphire
Libra (September 23–October 23)	amber, amethyst, aquamarine, blue topaz, chrysoprase, lapis lazuli, opal, rose quartz, tiger eye, tourmaline, turquoise
Scorpio (October 24–November 21)	citrine, garnet, kunzite, obsidian, opal, rose quartz, sapphire, smoky quartz, topaz, tourmaline
Sagittarius (November 22–December 21)	agate, amethyst, black onyx, lapis lazuli, malachite, sapphire, smoky quartz, sugilite, topaz, turquoise
Capricorn (December 22–January 19)	apache tear, hematite, garnet, jade, lapis lazuli, nephrite, onyx, ruby, turquoise

Aquarius (January 20–February 18)   amethyst, aquamarine, blue sapphire, clear quartz, fossils, jet, garnet, rose quartz

Pisces (February 19–March 20)   amethyst, aquamarine, bloodstone, jasper, pearl, sugilite

---

bisaja See ARAVINDA.

bismuth (Hom.) Bismuthum. A remedy for lonely and unstable minds.

bitter herb See RUTA GRAV.

bittergourd (Afr./Am. Ind./Chi./Ind.) *Momordica charantia*. Also, balsam apple, bitter melon, karela, *pomme de merveile*. A tropical vine whose unripe, bitter fruit is known for its culinary as well as medicinal use in various parts of the world, including tropical Africa, America, Asia and Australia. In traditional Chinese medicine, the fruit is used to treat gastrointestinal infections and breast cancer. In Surinam, it is used in fevers, stomach aches, diabetes and hypertension. In the Amazon, a leaf tea is used to expel intestinal gas and promote menstruation. It is also used topically for sores and skin infections. In Brazilian herbal medicine, it is used to induce abortions and as an aphrodisiac. It is made into a topical remedy for the skin to treat hemorrhoids, itchy rashes, eczema, leprosy and other skin problems. In Mexico, the root is considered aphrodisiac. In Peru, the leaf or aerial parts of the plant are used to treat measles, malaria, and various kinds of inflammation.

bitter apple See COLOCYNTHIS.

bitter cucumber See COLOCYNTHIS.

bitter melon See BITTERGOURD.

bittersweet See DULCAMARA.

black cardamom See YI ZHI REN.

black cohosh See CIMIC.

black hah feng shui (Vib.) A system of FENG SHUI, based on the premise that the front door of a building (referred to as 'mouth of chi') determines destiny. The front door, the primary entry point for CHI, plays an important role in creating a smooth, gentle and nurturing flow of energy inside the building, before it flows out through side doors or windows. Spaces in a home should be planned to maximize the flow of chi; long, straight corridors inside a building are discouraged as they slow it

down. The tinkling of hanging bells or wind chimes in doorways is believed to attract chi.

black hat Tantric Buddhism See BLACK TANTRIC BUDDHISM.

black henbane See HYOSCYAMUS.

Black Sect Tantric Buddhism (New Age) Also, Black Hat Tantric Buddhist feng shui, BTB. A system of intuitive application of FENG SHUI energy, combining the principles of traditional Chinese feng shui with the arcane practices and mysterious rituals of Tibetan Bon, the indigenous religion of Tibet before Buddhism was adopted there. The system is thus deeply mystical in its origin and practice.

black snake root See CIMIC.

black star (Gem) A stone, believed to be the potential healer of old ailments.

bliss body (Yoga) See ANANDAMAYA KOSHA.

> 'Realized souls live in bliss.'
>
> —A Sanskrit saying

blitz douche (Spa) Also, blitz-jet douche, jet douche. Pouring water on a person from a height of at least 20 feet at great pressure, said to be good for the immune system.

blitz-jet douche (Spa) See BLITZ DOUCHE.

blood-letting (Chi./Ind.) A method in traditional systems of medicine wherein infected blood and pus are cleared out of the body either with an incision or by introducing leeches to the affected area.

blood pressure The pressure exerted by blood on the walls of arteries. The average normal blood pressure is 120/80.

bloodstone See CORNELIAN.

blue aconite See ACONITE.

blue-colour therapy (New Age/Nat.) Blue is the colour associated with intuition and higher mental functions. It is also considered to have a curative influence in a number of ailments, including biliousness, bowel irregularity, burns, cataract, constipation, diarrhoea, dysentery, eye inflammation, glaucoma, goitre, gonorrhoea, headache, hysteria, insomnia, itching, jaundice, menstrual difficulties, shock, syphilis, tonsillitis, ulcers, vomiting and whooping cough. However, this colour may not be favourable for those suffering from cold, gout, hypertension and paralysis.

blue gum eucalyptus (Aus./Chi.) *Eucalyptus globulus*. Also, gum tree, Australian fever tree, Tasmanian blue gum. The leaves and oil of this tall evergreen tree, native to Australia and Tasmania, have long been used medicinally. Eucalyptus oil is obtained from the leaves and branch tops. In aboriginal medicine, topical ointments containing its oil have been used to heal wounds and treat fungal infections and its leaves in infusions to treat fevers. Russian researchers found that an alcoholic tincture containing eucalyptus leaves helps relieve chronic ear infections. The oil is commonly used to fight the common cold.

blue pearl (Ind./Yoga) A term used to refer to the brilliant blue light, the size of a tiny seed, visualized during meditation. It represents the subtle abode of one's inner self.

blue monkshood See ACONITE.

blue sapphire (Gem) A gemstone, believed to impart positive energy to the wearer. It is believed to strengthen bones, calm nerves and emotions and promote an attitude of detachment.

blue-water technique (New Age) A method of meditation as advanced by Lawrence LeShan, in which one's consciousness is used to search one's body for the source of hunger or pain. The meditator is said to locate the source and visualize three times blue water slowly filling the area and then draining from it.

bodhadruma See ASVATTHA.

bodhi tree See ASHVATTHA.

body-centred psychotherapy (Mod./New Age) An approach to healing which includes the body, while addressing the mind, emotions and behaviour. A combination of various techniques, viz., PSYCHOTHERAPY, MASSAGE, TOUCH THERAPY, MOVEMENT THERAPY and BREATHWORK, is applied to relieve distress

and tension. The technique is based on the premise that the mind and body function as one. Recent research seems to support the idea that the mind resides throughout the body and that every cell stores information and communicates with other cells.

> 'The body-unconscious is where life bubbles up in us. It is how we know that we are alive…'
>
> —D.H. Lawrence

body conditioning (New Age) An exercise programme, aimed at overall conditioning of the body. The programme usually consists of exercises for both strength and flexibility.

body harmony (New Age) A system of BODYWORK aimed at reawakening one's natural healing energies and developing access to inner wisdom.

body humors See DOSHA.

Body Mass Index (Mod.) BMI; an indicator for obesity or malnutrition, BMI is calculated by the formula, BMI=weight (in kg)/ height (in m). Normal BMI is 20–25, with values above 30 being associated with obesity and those below 18 indicating malnutrition.

body, mind and spirit diet See KEMETIC DIET.

body–mind centring (New Age) A form of meditation developed by Gay and Kathlyn Hendricks, based on the assumption that life's problems can be sorted out by contact with one's inner self. The inner self is the part of us that knows how we really feel.

body–mind counselling hypnotherapy (Mod.) A part of BODY–MIND THERAPY which includes the concepts and practices of JUNGIAN PHILOSOPHY and NLP.

body–mind dynamics (Mod./New Age) A form of BODYWORK, aimed at releasing pain, stress and negative emotions that interfere with the functioning of the glands, internal organs, nerves and MERIDIANS.

body–mind massage (Mod./New Age) A part of BODY–MIND THERAPY which includes SHIATSU, based on the belief that touch is sacred and has a healing potential.

body–mind shiatsu (Mod./ New Age) An integrative form of SHIATSU which uses direct pressure touch on specific anatomical meridian points to assist healing. The programme is aimed at releasing blocked energy and, as a consequence, pain and tension in the area.

body-oriented emotional release psychotherapy (Mod./New Age) A holistic healing method, as developed by Dee Casella, and which refers to the release of anger, fear and misery and reclamation of one's 'natural' self. See also, BODY-CENTRED PSYCHOTHERAPY.

body polish (Spa) A gentle buffing of the skin with salt and herbal extracts to exfoliate and smoothen it.

body psychotherapy (Mod.) A branch of psychotherapy which takes into account the complexity in mind–body interactions while acknowledging their functional unity. The techniques used include those involving touch, movement and breathing. Body psychotherapy recognizes the continuity and deep connections that exist in all psychocorporal processes. See also, BODY-CENTRED PSYCHOTHERAPY.

body reflexology (Mod./New Age) A system of REFLEXOLOGY or ACUPRESSURE, which incorporates pressing, pulling, massaging and clamping REFLEX POINTS on the buttocks, crotch, ears, face, feet, hands, nape, scalp, shins and tongue.

body sculpting (New Age) A fitness programme using weight-lifting, flexibility and endurance training, aimed at shaping the body, especially waist, thighs, upper arms and buttocks.

body system (Yoga) According to the system of YOGA, the human body-system is made of three bodies (causal, subtle and gross) and five sheaths (physical, vital, mental/emotional, cognitive/intuitive and super-conscious). The five sheaths in the body system are never disjointed (except at death) and are inextricably interlocked in a subtle but powerful network of NADIS and CHAKRAS. It is said that when a wave of unselfish and unconditional love surges within, we develop an instant access to the subtle sheaths, viz., intuitive/cognitive and super-conscious.

> 'The body will soon decay like the unbaked clay pots, thrown in water. Strengthen and purify it—bake it in the fire of yoga.'
>
> *—Gheranda Samhita*

body wisdom (New Age) A form of BODY-CENTRED PSYCHOTHERAPY, designed by Margo G. Steinfeld, based on the concept that as the body aligns, the life force becomes free, eliminating physical and emotional blockages.

bodytonics (Mod./New Age/Vib.) A series of movements, developed by Donald Burton Schnell, aimed at raising one's life force or 'spiritual vibrations'.

bodywork (New Age) A system of healing, aimed at bringing desired changes in the patient's muscles and skeletal structures, and through them in other parts of the body, with the help of the trained hands of the practitioner.

> 'As our bodies are loaned to us by God, they need to be treated with gentleness and care and according to His will.'
>
> — Tadamasa Fukaya

bodywork plus (Mod./New Age)A generic term, used to denote all manual or physical exercises related to healing; a form of holistic healing, which includes BREATHWORK, IMAGERY, ENERGY BALANCING and SHIATSU.

bodywork tantra (New Age) A form of holistic healing, developed by Harold Dull, combining CHAKRA meditation and ZEN SHIATSU. The other techniques used are TANTSU and WATSU.

body wrap (New Age/Spa) Also, herbal wrap. A spa treatment in which the body is cocooned in pieces of clothes soaked in herbal decoctions.

bonesano (New Age) A healing system blending SHAMANISM and Western mystical traditions, as developed by Jim Hopkins. It includes CREATIVE VISUALIZATION, CRYSTAL HEALING, MEDITATION and PRAYER.

bonsanista healing method See BONESANO.

Bon shamanic practices (Tib.) A host of traditional rituals, aimed at generating vital force for healing as practised in ancient Tibet before the spread of Buddhism.

Bonny, Helen A musician and educator, who popularized the practice of GUIDED IMAGERY.

Book of Changes See *I CHING*.

Book of Creation See SEFER YETSIRAH.

Book of Dyzan An Eastern occult text which deals with the history of cosmic evolution.

> 'In literature, as in love, we are astonished at what is chosen by others.'
>
> —Andre Maurois

Book of the Dead (Egy.) A collection of ancient Egyptian texts, concerned with the safe passage of the soul after death.

botanicals (Spa) Parts of plants whose extracts are used in hair and skin products.

botanomancy (Eur./Occ.) A method of DIVINATION in which the question to be asked is first carved on the branches of plants, such as vervain and brie, and later burnt in fire to seek answers.

botox injection (Cos./Mod.) The injection of botulinum toxin under the skin to relax muscles and soften wrinkles on the forehead, eye area and neck.

Bowen technique (Mod.) A programme of linked manual manoeuvres over muscles, devised by Tom Bowen, an Australian chemist. The method consists of a series of gentle moves on the muscle and connective tissue, using the thumb and fingers, along the whole body. Since there is no manipulation of hard tissue, the treatment is gentle and relaxing. Olympians and professional sportspersons who undergo this treatment are reported to claim that as a result of the technique, they perform at consistently higher levels. It is also reported that this technique results in an impressive injury recovery rate.

Brahma (Ind.) Literally, He who has grown expansive. The Creator of the Universe; the first principle (tattva), to emerge out of the Ultimate Reality (BRAHMAN); the presiding deity of the MULADHARA CHAKRA.

brahmacharya (Ind.) Sexual control. One of the five forms of self-restraints (YAMA) in the yoga system of PATANJALI.

> 'Brahmacharya does not mean total abstinence, but denotes a disciplined sexual life promoting contentment and moral strength from within.'
>
> —B.K.S. Iyengar

Brahma muhurta (Ind.) The period from 3 to 6 a.m., considered most conducive for practising YOGA and MEDITATION.

Brahmanda (Yoga) Literally Brahma's egg, the macrocosm.

Brahma granthi (Yoga) A psychic knot at the lower portion of the vertebral column.

Brahman (Yoga) The Godhead.

Brahman gate (Yoga) See AJNA CHAKRA.

Brahmarandhra (Yoga) A psychic aperture which is visualized to exist in the crown of one's head.

brahmi (Chi./Ind.) *Bacopa monnieri*. Also, herb of grace, pennell, water hyssop. A creeper found in wetlands in India and used in folk remedies in the treatment of anaemia, headaches, liver ailments and memory lapses.

> 'Brahmi controls leprosy and syphilis.'
>
> —Bhava Prakasa

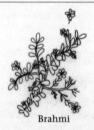

Brahmi

brain, the left and right hemispheres of (Misc.) The specificity of functional organization in the right and left hemispheres of the brain is the purview of neurologists. While the left hemisphere is concerned with more verbal, ideational and abstract thought expressions, the right atmosphere is specifically involved in the pattern perceptions such as spatial configurations, holistic images, non-verbal behaviour, and patterned auditory perceptions like music. The integrated action of the right and left hemispheres appears to be essential in adults for abstract thoughts, perceptions and creative thinking.

brain, human (Misc.) A complex organ including the brainstem or old or reptilian brain, the mid-brain or limbic system and neo-cortex, which is divided into the left, right and pre-frontal lobes. It is connected with the sense organs and energy centres, including the pineal and pituitary bodies. No other organ of the human body is as sensitive to change in energy supply as the human brain. Although it weighs hardly 2 per cent of the body-weight, it consumes over 20 per cent of the energy used by the body.

> 'In music, one must think with the heart and feel with the brain.'
>
> —George Szell

brainwaves (Misc.) Electrical impulses, responsible for activity in the brain. Brainwaves operate at different frequencies and have various rhythms and patterns. The four types of brainwaves are BETA WAVES (13–40 Hz), ALPHA WAVES (7–12 Hz), theta waves (4–7 Hz) and DELTA WAVES (up to 4 Hz). By controlling the rhythms involved in BREATHING, yogis are said to induce ALPHA rhythms in their brain which produces an altered state of consciousness, enhanced relaxation and pleasant feelings. BETA waves are dominant when the person is alert or aroused. THETA WAVES are associated with the appearance of spontaneous visual images. DELTA waves indicate either deep sleep or an ideal meditative state.

breath (Misc.) The source of life. Life starts with the first gasp of breath in the newborn as an adaptation to the outside world. With every inhalation, fresh energy is brought into the body for its sustenance. Breath is a strategic intermediary between body and mind. See also, PRANAYAMA.

> 'If the mind were the king of the senses, then the master of the mind is breath.'
>
> —*Hathayoga pradipika* (Fifteenth century AD)

breath expansion See PRANAYAMA.

breatharianism (New Age) A dietary practice, advocated by Wiley Brooks in the 1980s, based on the idea that food is poison

and that breathing is sufficient for life.

breathing (Misc.) A vital life-process wherein oxygen is absorbed as carbon dioxide gets eliminated. It is believed that proper breathing can ensure good health by easing tensions. In stress, one tends to increase the pace of breathing, using only the upper part of the chest. Long deep breaths that expand the rib cage are recommended for patients with respiratory conditions. By deliberately slowing down the cycle of breathing, as in PRANAYAMA, one becomes calm and content.

Breath energy is known variously as CHI in China, QI in Japan, PRANA in India, thymos, and later pneuma, in Greece, although each meant different things in different cultures.

The rhythm of breath is often associated with emotional and mental states. Just as the breath becomes disrupted or irregular when one is tense or agitated, by regularizing the breath and achieving proper rhythms, one can achieve peace and tranquility.

Yoga necessitates the 'conquering' of breathing before it can reach the realm of the mind. From ancient times, it was recognized that the way to relaxed breathing was by using the diaphragm, a muscle separating the abdomen from the chest. When one is anxious, however, one tends to breathe from the chest which is believed to result in fatigue.

> 'When the breath is coming rhythmically, through both nostrils, that is the time to control your mind.'
>
> —Swami Vivekananda

> 'The energy sheath consisting of breath is encased in the physical sheath and has the same form. One is filled with the other. The first has the likeness of a man and because it has the likeness of a man, the second follows it and itself takes on the likeness of a man. Through this vital sheath, the senses perform their office. From this, men and beasts derive their life. For, breath is the life of beings and so is called the life of all.'
>
> —*Taittiriya Upanishad*

breathing exercise See PRANAYAMA.

'Agitations of consciousness can be resolved by controlling the cycle of breath.'

—Sage Patanjali

breathing therapy (New Age) The conscious use of breathing to unblock, move, increase and balance energy. While doing such exercises, it is essential that one curbs thought processes and lives mindfully arises in the moment. Such exercises can be combined with VISUALIZATION, concentrating on the parts and organs of the body where the discomfort or pain arises. The aim in all these methods is to cultivate energy through appropriate breathing methods.

breathing through the left nostril (Yoga) According to the YOGA tradition, the flow of breath through the left nostrils is recommended for activities such as learning from a spiritual teacher, singing or playing music, in diseases, sorrow, dejection and fever.

breathing through the right nostril (Yoga) According to the YOGA tradition, the flow of breath through the right nostrils is recommended for more active functions such as sports, hunting, gambling, mountaineering, reading or teaching difficult subjects, in practising with swords, and in battle.

breathing through a particular nostril (Yoga) An ancient Indian manoeuvre for activating breathing through the desired nostril, i.e., either the left or right. In the system of YOGA, a particular nostril is consciously activated with a view to achieve desired results. For example, in order to achieve peak performance levels, the flow of breath is recommended through the right nostril. To achieve this, the practitioner is made to lie on his or her left side or to keep a pillow pressed tightly under his or her left arm for several minutes.

breathwork (New Age) A term coined in the 1970s by psychologist Gay Hendricks to denote the breathing process as a tool for healing, stress reduction and personal development. According to him, when a trauma occurs, the breath is first held and then becomes short and shallow. Releasing the trauma implies getting the breath gradually flowing again, as a person consciously processes the feelings that froze the breath in the first place. In moments of stress, breath can act as a remedy to build energy and endurance. Breathwork is a technique of breathing which combines movement of the body; QIGONG, HOLOTROPIC BREATHWORK, REBIRTHING and YOGA are examples of breathwork.

breema bodywork (New Age) An ancient method of health improvement, oriented towards releasing tension, promoting inner harmony, and creating ENERGY BALANCE.

brewer's yeast (Misc.) A type of fungus and a rich source of vitamins, amino acids and minerals (particularly chromium and selenium) and naturally occurring nucleic acids (DNA and RNA), believed to enhance the immune system.

bimhana (Ind.) A method to increase the body weight, as against methods to reduce the body weight by LANGHANA.

braht trayi (Ind.) Also, ASHTANGA SANGRAHA, vriddha trayi. From the Sanskrit for three great compositions. The three classics on AYURVEDA, composed, compiled, and edited by Vagabhatta II, under the title *Ashtanga Sangraha*. The compilation consists of the three volumes of CHARAKA, SUSHRUTA and *Ashtanga Hridaya* of VAGABHATTA.

British Society for Psychical Research A research body in the UK, which has for over a century performed experiments on paranormal phenomena.

broadcasting (New Age) A form of ABSENT HEALING, developed by chiropractor Ruth Drown.

bromium (Hom.) A remedy to treat depression.

bronchial mudra (Yoga) A MUDRA formed by touching the tip of the little finger to the base of the thumb, while the tip of the ring finger touches the middle joint of the thumb and the tip of the middle finger touches the tip of the thumb. This mudra is said to clear the lungs and open up the trachea. For better results, this mudra is used in conjunction with ASTHMA MUDRA.

broom (Occ.) In many parts of the world, e.g., India, Rumania and Tuscany, keeping a broom under the bed is believed to keep evil spirits at bay.

brown agate (Gem) A gem believed to drive away epilepsy, fevers and mental problems. It is said to be effective in stopping the flow of rheum in the eyes, reducing menstrual discharge and dispersing the water of dropsy.

bruhan nasya (Ind.) A treatment method in which medicated oil drops are introduced into the nostrils to nourish the brain and the senses.

brush and tone (Spa) An exfoliating technique involving dry-brushing of the skin, intended to remove dead layers of the skin and stimulate circulation. Brush and tone generally precedes mud and seaweed body masks.

bryonia (Eur./Hom.) *Bryonia alba.* Also, common bryony, wild hops, white bryony, a Eurasian vine with white flowers and black berries, long known to European herbalists. The tincture of the plant is a diuretic, prescribed for obstructions in the urinary passage and for relieving coughs and colds. In HOMOEOPATHY, Bryonia is used to treat nausea, sore throats, vomiting, diarrhoea and swelling.

BTB (New Age) See BLACK SECT TANTRIC BUDDHISM.

buddhi (Yoga) Intellect, one of the three factors constituting CHITTA or consciousness.

Buddhi Yoga (Yoga) From the Sanskrit buddhi, meaning intelligence; The yoga of contemplation. A system of YOGA, centred around the development of CONSCIOUSNESS. It is based on the idea that developing higher levels of consciousness leads one to emerge from the bondage and entanglements of the material world.

Buddhism (Misc./Tib.) A world religion which has much in common with RAJAYOGA and JNANYOGA. It emphasizes attentiveness and the witnessing of actions around. Heightening awareness on every thought, word and action, it is believed, de-automates every thought, word or action and links them with the Self.

Buddhist medicine (Tib.) A system of healing, in which MOXIBUSTION and SHIATSU massage are used. See also TIBETAN MEDICINE.

bu-hang (Chi.) A form of CUPPING.

buqi See QIGONG THERAPY.

burdock (Chi./Eur.) *Arctium lappa.* Also, great burdock. A detoxifying herb with edible roots, found in wastelands in Europe and north Asia. The juice of the plant is believed to be a cure for baldness.

It is also used in the treatment of acne, eczema, burns, bruises and ringworm. The crushed seeds are poulticed onto bruises. The leaves are poulticed onto burns, sores and ulcers. This plant is also an ingredient in the North American formula, Essiac, used to treat cancer.

business qigong (Chi./New Age) The application of QI GONG to de-stress workers so as to improve health and productivity.

Buteyko Therapy (New Age) A treatment for chronic hyperventilation syndrome (CHVS), discovered in the mid-twentieth century by Konstantin Buteyko, a Russian medical doctor. The therapy works by reversing the process by which normal episodes of acute hyperventilation become chronic. The basis of the treatment is a programme in which a patient spends about 90 minutes a day deliberately reducing his breathing by relaxing his respiratory muscles and developing and sustaining a slight hunger for air. Over a period, the patient unconsciously reduces his/her breathing.

butterfly effect (New Age) A phrase which reflects the notion of sensitive dependence on initial conditions. According to this theory, small variations of the initial condition of a dynamic system can produce long variations in the long-term behaviour of the system. The phrase reflects an idea that a butterfly's wings which create a tiny change in the atmosphere can ultimately cause (or prevent) a tornado. See also KARMA.

butterfly pea See APARAJITA.

C

Cabala See KABBALAH.

cactus (Hom.) *Cactus grandiflorus*. A homoeopathic remedy, prescribed inter alia for intense feelings of sadness and fear of death.

caduceus (Grk.) A winged staff with two snakes wrapped around it, possibly first seen in Mesopotamia as early as 2600 BC. This insignia has come to be associated with medicine and is used interchangeably with the rod of Asclepius (no wings, single snake). According to some authors, the symbol also possibly had an association with the esoteric concept of KUNDALINI which was prevalent in the pre-Vedic Indian subcontinent. The rod represents the subtle channel SUSHUMNA, while the snakes, IDA and PINGALA, symbolize the awakening of the psychic centres located in CHAKRAS, as a means of liberation from worldly bondage.

cajeput (Aus./Ind.) Native to Australia, this resinous evergreen tree with a whitish papery bark now grows widely in parts of Africa, South and Central America, Hawaii, India, the Philippines and the West Indies. Its revitalizing oil is used in Indian folk medicine to treat chronic bronchitis and laryngitis. Its softened bark is applied to boils. The Vietnamese use the oil for arthritis and rheumatism and inhale it to treat colds and rhinitis. In Myanmar, cajeput oil mixed with camphor is used to treat gout. It also acts as an anthelmintic, especially against roundworms.

caladium (Hom.) Also, calad. A remedy to treat fainting. It is also indicated in insect bites that burn intensely in small areas.

calamus (Chi./Eur./Ind.) *Acorus calamus*. Also, sweetflag, vacha. The root-paste is used in traditional medicine to treat headaches, stomach aches, coughs and fevers.

calcarea carbonica (Hom.) Also, calcium carbonate, calc carb. It is used in HOMOEOPATHY in the treatment of anxiety, depression and exhaustion.

calcarea ostrearum (Hom.) Also, calc. ostr. A remedy associated with memory and hence treats absent-mindedness.

calcium phosphate (Hom.) Also, calc. phos. A remedy, comprising the principal minerals of bones and teeth, and associated with problems in growth and development. It is considered useful for children who show slow growth and mental weakness.

caldarium (New Age) The hottest room in an ancient Roman bath where patients bathed in steaming water, a time-tested method of DETOXIFICATION.

caludronius (Gem) A colourless stone, believed to possess magical powers. It was believed that the stone countered the bad influence of evil spirits on health.

camphor (Hom.) *Camphora*. A remedy sometimes prescribed for premature greying.

cantharis (Hom.) Also, Spanish fly. A remedy to clear mental confusion and distraction which lead to low concentration. It is also used to treat abdominal cramps, convulsions, diarrhoea and vomiting.

capnomancy (Eur./Occ.) A method of DIVINATION, using smoke from sacrificial offerings. It also refers to divination by means of a trance, induced in a smoky ambience.

capoeira (New Age) A combination of aesthetic and acrobatic movements, including dance and boxing, which have an impact on stress. Performed by Brazilian slaves in ancient times, capoeira is regaining its popularity in the US.

capsicum (Hom.) *Capsicum frutes cens, c. amum.* Also, capsic. It is prescribed for peevish, irritable, easily offended and angry folks. See also, CAYENNE PEPPER.

caraway seed (Ind.) *Carum carvi.* Also, kummel, seedcake, shiajira. Native to the Mediterranean regions, caraway now grows widely in Asia, northern Europe, Russia and US. The seeds are used for culinary and medicinal purposes. The seed oil is valued as an antispasmodic and carminative. In folk use, seeds were used by women to promote breast milk and sweeten their breath.

carbo animalis (Hom.) Also, carb. an. A remedy for the confused.

carbo vegetabilis (Hom.) Also, carbo veg. A remedy prescribed in stupor and indigestion.

cardamom (Ind.) *Elettaria cardamom* Also, green cardamom. In India, cardamom is an important kitchen ingredient, eaten for its digestive properties. In traditional medicine, it is used in the treatment of gums and in preventing throat infections and congestion in lungs. It is also known to stimulate the heart and spleen.

cardiac plexus See ANAHATA CHAKRA.

carduus marianus (Hom.) Also, St. Mary's thistle, card. mar. A remedy prescribed for liver ailments.

CARE (New Age) See CHAKRA ARMOUR RELEASE OF EMOTIONS.

cornelian (Gem) A reddish-brown variety of quartz, known to the ancient Egyptians for its impact on the mind. It was believed that it made the wearer's mind free from negative thoughts.

cartomancy (Egy./Eur.) A method of DIVINATION, using a deck of cards. The practice of cartomancy, believed to have originated in ancient Egypt, developed in fourteenth-century Europe, when playing cards were first introduced. According to tradition, a deck used for cartomancy is not to be used for any other purpose. Only the owner of the deck of cards should touch them and none other. More recently, this method has given way to TAROT which uses a deck of cards which is somewhat different from the standard deck than was used for cartomancy.

castor (Egy./Ind.) *Ricinus communis.* Castor oil, extracted from the seeds of the plant is a strong purgative. The discovery of castor seeds in several pyramids dating from 4000 BC indicates its use then. Recent research indicates the analgesic and anti-viral properties of castor.

catharsis (Eur./New Age) From the Greek *katharein,* meaning to cleanse. 1. Purgation, cleaning and purification. 2. The emotional release linked to the expression of unconscious conflicts. 3. A purifying or ritualistic cleansing of emotions which restores or refreshes the spirit. 4. A technique used to relieve tension by bringing repressed feelings to consciousness. Traditionally, blood, change of garments, fire, water, wine and sacrifice were considered cleaning agents. In the Old Testament, catharsis was accomplished by means of washing and bathing. In the New Testament, purification was performed by means of baptism.

cathexis (Misc.) Concentrating one's emotional or libidinal energy on an object or an idea as in nationalism or other impassioned identification with a group or a team. When one's ego wishes to repress such desires, Freud used the term 'anti-cathexis'. Like steam is built up in a steam engine, the libido's cathexis then builds up until alternative channels are found for its release, which can lead to sublimation.

cathiodermie (Cos.) A rejuvenation treatment for the skin by applying low-voltage electric stimulation. The treatment is said to provide deep cleansing and oxygenation of outer tissue layers, besides eliminating impurities. It is also said to revitalize the skin, improving circulation.

catoptromancy See MIRROR GAZING.

cat's eye (Gem) A legendary gem, believed to endow the wearer with happiness and wealth.

causal body (Yoga) Also, karana sharira. One of the three body forms, also referred to as consciousness and expressed through one's intelligence and wisdom. The other two body forms are physical and astral. Causal body often refers to the highest or innermost subtle body which veils the soul.

caulophyllum (Hom.) Also, blue cohosh, cauloph. Prescribed for rheumatic headaches, especially in women.

cause (Yoga) Also, karana. Anything which produces an effect or result. In Indian philosophy, karana is explained in three ways: efficient cause (nimitta karana), which conceives, makes and shapes (e.g., a potter fashioning a clay pot or God creating the world); material cause (upadana karana), the material which produces the effect (e.g., clay or the primordial substratum of the material world); and instrumental cause (sahakari karana), that which serves as an instrument or mechanism (e.g., potter's wheel or universal energy).

causticum (Hom.) Also, causic. A homoeopathic remedy for strengthening one's memory.

Cayce approach to health and healing (New Age) An approach to health, developed by American psychic Edgar Cayce, which inter alia integrates BREATH WORK and ENERGY FIELD WORK.

Cayce diet (New Age) A dietary formulation, recommended for healing and the upkeep of one's health by American psychic Edgar Cayce, according to whom a healthy intake comprises at least 80 per cent ALKALINE FOOD. Certain food combinations are also to be avoided, including sugar and starchy foods, milk and citrus juice/fruit, cereals and citrus juice/fruit, coffee with milk/cream, raw apples with other foods and large quantities of starchy foods with meat/cheese. Other stipulations include steaming vegetables in their own juices, never frying foods, avoiding aluminium cookware, and eating only locally grown fruits and vegetables. Cayce was also of the view that even the most nutritious food can turn into poison if eaten in a negative frame of mind. According to him, eating should be avoided when one is angry, jealous, worried or extremely tired.

cayenne pepper (Am.Ind./Ind./Mod.) *Capsicum annum*. Also, capsicum. An annual plant cutivated in the warmer parts of Asia and Central America. Some of the many varieties include cayenne, chillies, jalapeno, hot peppers and paprika. Over the years, capsicum has been used in traditional medicine as a remedy for a host of ailments, including stomach upsets, headaches, seasickness and loss of appetite. It is also said to be an aphrodisiac. Capsaicin, an active ingredient in the plant, has been in use topically in pain-relieving creams, to treat pains caused by conditions such as arthritis. Researchers have found that capsaicin may also provide temporary relief for mouth-sore pain caused by chemotherapy and radiation. See also, CAPSICUM.

'Capsicum is the answer for vitiated conditions of KAPHA and VATA.'

—Svayamkriti

celery (Chi./Ind.) *Apium graveolens*. Celery seeds have been known in India from ancient times for their medicinal uses. They were prescribed for colds, flu, water retention, indigestion, arthritis and liver ailments, but were primarily used as a diuretic. Preliminary animal studies indicate that celery seeds help prevent the formation of cancerous tumors in mice.

celestial soul clearing (New Age/Occ.) A method of psychic HEALING which aims at the removal of earth-bound spirits, which are feared to draw energy from one's LIFE FORCE. In tribal medicine, any disease has an association with an evil spirit and the cure lies in its removal from the body, mind and spirit.

cell command therapy (New Age) A technique of HYPNOSIS, aimed at accelerating the healing process. This technique involves communication with the cells affected, suggesting that they start healing and rejuvenation. It is reported to have demonstrated effectiveness in many illnesses and conditions.

cellasene (New Age) A herbal product developed by Italian chemist Gianfranco Merizzi and promoted as a remedy for CELLULITE. The product contains evening primrose oil, dried *Fucus vesiculosi* extract, gelatin, fish oil, glycerol, soya oil, grape seed, dried sweet clover extract and dried GINGKO BILOBA extract.

celloids (Nat.) The pharmacological doses of minerals in colloidal form. Celloids were formulated in the 1930s by Maurice Blackmore.

cellulite (Mod.) A term coined in European salons and spas to describe 'fat gone wrong'; deposits of lumpy fat which causes dimpling of the skin especially on the hips, thighs and buttocks, especially in women. Not a medical term, cellulite is considered to be a special form of fat—a combination of fat, water and toxins which the body has not eliminated. The variety of treatments used to fight it include using a variety of gadgets such as electrical muscle stimulation, vibrating machines, inflatable hip-high pressurized boots, rubberized pants and heating pads, hormone and enzyme injections, body wraps and body MASSAGES.

cell-salt therapy See BIOCHEMICS.

cellular theta breath (Mod.) A method of SELF-HEALING, based on breath. The method recognizes BREATH (referred to as theta breath) as energy in transformation.

Cepa See ONION.

Celsus, Aulus Cornelius (first century AD) (Eur.) A Roman medical writer, and the author of an encyclopaedia dealing with agriculture, law, medicine, military art, philosophy and rhetoric, of which only portions on medicine have survived over time. His *De Medicina* recommended hygiene and cleanliness and urged the use of solutions such as vinegar and thyme oil for washing wounds. Celsus also wrote a detailed account on HYDROTHERAPY as was practised in his time.

Celtic magic (Chr.) Also, Celtic tribal traditions. An ancient practice involving various methods of spellwork, rituals, meditation and DIVINATION, along with the use of herbs and the elements.

Celtic shamanism (Eur./Occ.) A system of holistic healing practices inspired by Celtic tribal traditions as developed by Geo Cameron. It includes MEDITATION and CHANTING. Modern Celtic shamanism incorporates European shamanism with Celtic beliefs.

centesimal scale (Hom.) The scale used for measuring the potency of remedies in hundredths. In homoeopathy, succussions and triturations are done mainly on two scales of potencies: the decimal scale and the centesimal scale in which the remedy is diluted in the proportion of 1:100, i.e. 1 part of the drug is diluted in 99 parts of the vehicle. The centesimal potency is denoted by the letter C. Hence 1C means that the given medicine contains 1 part of the original drug substance and 99 parts of the vehicle. 2C means that the drug is 1/1000 times diluted, 6C means it is 1/1012 times diluted, and 200C means it is 1/10400 times diluted. (In practise, the letter C is dropped for centesimal scale; hence 200C is written simply as 200). See DECIMAL SCALE.

centres of energy See CHAKRAS.

cerebral cortex (Mod.) The outermost layer of the cerebral hemisphere, considered the seat of CONSCIOUSNESS, and largely responsible for human cognition. It plays an essential role in perception, memory, thought, language, mental ability, intellect and consciousness, and is responsible for all voluntary actions. The cerebral cortex in an adult human is composed of some 20 billion neurons and accounts for 40 per cent of the brain weight. Recent studies indicate that the first neurons are in place in embryos approximately thirty-one days after fertilization, much before the development of the limbs and eyes.

cereoscopy (Eur./Occ.) A method of DIVINATION, using patterns made by wax melting in boiling water.

chair massage (New Age) A form of massage, which can be given in a public place. The client sits on a chair or stool and the masseur works through the clothes, focussing on the head, neck, shoulders arms and other upper parts of the body. Sessions can last up to twenty minutes.

chaitanya (Yoga) Consciousness; spirit. In Indian philosophy consciousness is additionally endowed with quality; witness consciousness (saakshi chaitanya), devotional consciousness (bhakti chaitanya) and God consciousness (Shiva chaitanya) are some expressions commonly employed in religious literature.

chakra (Yoga) Also chakras of light, circles of energy. Literally, wheel. A subtle body-centre or a focal point of vital energy which functions in close association with the various mechanisms of the body, more particularly with the nervous and endocrine systems. There are seven major chakras, twenty-one minor and several lesser chakras located throughout the body, which when active receive and transmit precious vital energy which imparts life to an organism. They have been used in many religious, healing and mystical practices in the East. The chakras are also identified with the various levels of consciousness experienced by humans.

Some characteristics which distinguish the seven major chakras are summarized in the following table:

Chakra	Essential Characteristics
SAHASRARA or the crown chakra	Located near the pineal gland on the top of the spinal column and considered the gateway between the psychic and spiritual realms of one's existence and the point of union between the male and female principles of the body, viz., SHIVA and KUNDALINI SHAKTI.
AJNA or the eyebrow chakra	Located at the area of the pituitary glands in between the eyebrows and above the base of the nose and sconsidered to be the seat of intuition, perception and truth, facilitating decision-making on direction and the course or direction.
VISHUDDHI or the throat chakra	Located at the area of the thyroid/parathyroid glands in the throat region, and considered to be the seat of intellectual awareness, controlling overall self-expression, both verbal and non-verbal.
ANAHATA or the heart chakra	Located at the area of the thymus glands in the heart region, and considered to represent cognition and compassion.
MANIPURAKA or the solar plexus chakra	Located in the area of pancreatic glands, representing one's will-power.
SVADISHTHANA or the spleen chakra	Located in the spleen region and representing rationality and a search for sexual pleasure.
MULADHARA or the root chakra	Located at the base of the spine, near the tailbone and representing physical consciousness, memory, sex drive and survival instincts.

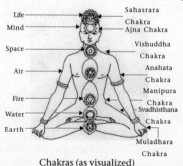

Chakras (as visualized)

'Chakra is a stage-by-stage playground of desires. Throughout life one dwells in this forest of desires, and one thinks and understands life's situations from the standpoint of the chakra in which he normally feels most comfortable.'

—Hiroshi Motoyama

chakra and cellular-memory healing (New Age) A recent approach to holistic healing, popularized by Ojela Frank, a reiki master, incorporating techniques from CON-

SCIOUS BREATHING, COUNSELLING, GUIDED IM-
AGERY and PAST-LIFE REGRESSION.

**Chakra Armour Release of Emotions
(CARE)** (New Age) A recent approach to holistic healing, recognizing the involvement
of emotions in two different energy pathways, namely chakra and armour. Armour
is a muscle spasm due to an unexpected
emotion. The approach aims at releasing
psychosomatic blocks and as a consequence, alleviates chronic pain and stubborn weight problems.

chakra bhedan (Yoga/Vib.) A system of
KRIYA involving BREATHING EXERCISES and focussing one's AWARENESS on CHAKRAs, energy
centres, and NADIs, meridians which constitute an elaborate energy network in humans. The yogic tradition considers breath a
direct means of purifying one's consciousness.

chakra breathing (New Age /Vib.) A recent selection of BREATHING EXERCISES, aimed
at cleansing CHAKRAs. The method, devised
by renowned drummer Layne Radmond, includes seated meditation to activate the
seven chakras and a standing meditation
with full yogic breath. It also includes a
walking and breathing meditation accompanied by spirited drums and music.
Tibetan singing bowls, hand-struck bells
and chimes are also played during the sessions.

chakra damage (New Age/Vib.) CHAKRA
damage is attributable to disturbances in the
gentle flow of energy. Emotional stress or
traumatic memories in one's life can result
in emotional suppression or blockages
which affect the flow of vital energy in the
body. Several healing systems work remove
such blockages and restore the chakras to
their normal functioning. According to
some masters, prolonged euphoria and too
much stimulation can also disrupt the normal energy flow.

chakra energy massage (New Age/
Vib.) A recent approach to holistic healing,
which borrows techniques from CHAKRA
HEALING and FOOT REFLEXOLOGY. In this massage, chakras are identified and addressed
for an overall positive impact on the body
system.

chakra healing (New Age/Vib.) A recent
approach to holistic healing, focussed on
CHAKRAs. The chakras and NADIs comprise a
great energy network in the body and focussing on a particular chakra is believed to
have a positive overall effect on the body
system.

chakra inner-tuning therapy (New
Age/Vib.) A recent approach to HEALING
which includes techniques such as DIET,
DREAM INTERPRETATION, MANTRAs, MEDITATION
and YOGA; a holistic approach for an overall
impact on health and healing.

chakras, lower (Occ./Vib./Yoga) Lower
consciousness states situated in the lower
portions of the body, below the FIRST CHAKRA,
MULADHARA. They are believed to harbour

Chakra below muladhara	Location in the body	Dominant emotion	Remarks
Atala; meaning without bottom, or no place	hip	fear and lust	Fear is considered a higher level of consciousness than anger or jealousy
Vitala; the region of the lost, the realm of division or confusion	thighs	rage and anger	Anger is considered a higher level of consciousness than jealousy
Sutala; great lower region, a good matter, state of spiritual darkness ruled by desire and passion	knees	jealousy	The feeling of jealousy is consid- ered a higher level of conscious ness as compared to prolonged mental confusion
Talatala; under the bottom level, 'place–nonplace' or	calves	prolonged mental	In this chakra, a person exhibits the feelings of 'me and mine'. It

		confusion	is a state of outward passion and sense indulgence.
'realm of nonbeing'			
Rasatala; literally, the state of 'sense enjoyment'	ankles	selfishness	A true home of the animal in man, as personal selfishness predominates. Persons in this consciousness level care nothing for the suffering of others.
Mahatala, the greatest lower region	feet	lack of conscience	The ego rules supreme. This is the realm of unconscionable acts, wherein perpetrators feel no remorse for the most heinous wrongdoings. Those locked in this realm have no conscience.
Patala, 'lower region of wickedness' or 'fallen state'	soles of the feet	vicious destruction, murder and malice	The realm in which one tortures others without a thought, expresses malice without a twinge of conscience, harms others in innumerable ways for sheer enjoyment and takes delight in the emotional, mental and physical suffering of fellow humans and all beings that cross their path. Hatred is the ruling force in those who live in the darkness of this area of mind.

instinctive consciousness and are the origin of negative feelings: hatred, envy, guilt and sorrow.

> 'Never in the world can hatred be stilled by hatred; it will be stilled only by non-hatred—this is the Law Eternal.'
> —Gautama Buddha

chakra meditation (New Age/Occ.) Meditating on CHAKRAS, believed to enhance one's bodily awareness and sensitivity. See CHAKRA SENSATION.

chakra puja (Occ.) An ancient, esoteric fertility practice in which an equal number of men and women gather in a circle (chakra) and engage in ritual-based sex in front of a yantra, representing the Mother Goddess. The practice centres around a highly ritualized group experience. Depending on the desired goal, such sexual activity varies widely and generally involves a great deal of purification and focussing prior to the actual sexual experience. The ritual includes invocation or prayer, utilization of MANTRA and YANTRA, purification exercises including PRANAYAMA, concentration, the use of MUDRA and BANDHA, and worship of the male (Shiva) and female (Shakti) principles.

chakrasana (Yoga) A back-bending ASANA, believed to stimulate the nerves of the spine and recommended especially for practitioners of PRANAYAMA.

chakra sensation (New Age/Occ.) Feelings derived by the practitioner, while remaining focussed on a selected CHAKRA. The sensation may vary from individual to individual, depending upon the degree of concentration. Localized warmth, localized pressure, localized throb or bubbling sensations or a combination of all could be some such sensations. See CHAKRA MEDITATION.

chakra stimulation (New Age/Occ.) A conscious attempt to infuse energy into the CHAKRAS by adopting, singly or in combination, techniques such as breathing exercises, IMAGINATION and VISUALIZATION. For example, one can imagine one's hands tearing and piercing the chakra selected by focussing awareness and flushing it with imaginary love energy for health and wellbeing. See also PSYCHIC SURGERY.

chakra therapy (New Age/Occ.) A therapeutic system based on the notion that a normal, developed, opened and healthy CHAKRA spins clockwise and a diseased CHAKRA spins anti-clockwise, with depleting energy levels. Compatible gemstones are also placed, either one after another or all at once, on chakras. Some therapists recommend clear quartz spheres or strands of frosted quartz for all chakras.

chakra yoga (Yoga) An approach to holistic healing, based on the postures of HATHA YOGA, sounding techniques and VISUALIZATION. It is aimed at maximizing one's ability to use vital energies for healing and harmony. The assumption is 'where attention goes, energy flows.'

chakralakshana See GUDUCHI.

chakrangi See GUDUCHI.

chakras of darkness See TALAs.

chakras of ignorance See TALAs.

chakras of light See CHAKRA.

chakras, Tibetan system of (Occ./Tib./Yoga) The salient feature in the Tibetan system is that the top two CHAKRAs are united as one as are the bottom two. The chakras are thus associated with five elements as indicated:

Chakras	Associated element
MULADHARA and SVADHISHTHANA the root and spleen chakras	Earth
MANIPURAKA, the solar plexus chakra	Water
ANAHATA, the heart chakra	Fire
VISHUDDHI, the throat chakra	Air
AJNA and SAHASRARA, the eyebrow and crown chakras	Ether

chakyushya (Ind.) From chaksu, meaning eyes. Chakyushya are herbs which comfort the eyes and tone the ciliary muscles. Rose, sandalwood and lemon are examples.

chamomilla (Hom.) *Matricaria recutita.* Also, chamomile. A homoeopathic remedy for a confused state of mind, restlessness and irritability.

chan mi gong (Chi./Occ.) Also, CMG. A combination of Tantric and Zen Buddhist QIGONG systems. The method is characterized by gentle, undulating wave-like motions and rhythmic rolling which help loosen the joints, hips, shoulders and spine and renders flexibility to them. The method aims at developing internal QI, regulating metabolic functions of the body and preventing sickness. The method is also aimed at the opening of the THIRD EYE by elevating one's consciousness.

chandana (Chi./Ind.) *Santalum album.* A celebrated tree, native to India. It is known for its expensive aromatic sapwood used from ancient times in perfumes and medicines. Sandalwood oil is used traditionally to treat skin diseases, acne, dysentery and gonorrhoea. In Traditional Chinese Medicine, sandalwood oil is considered an excellent sedating agent.

> The endeavours of a man who has studied science but fails to make a clear exposition are vain, like the efforts of an ass that carries a load of sandalwood without ever being able to enjoy its essence.
>
> —Charaka

chandana bala oil (Ind.) An oil, medicated with herbs such as CHANDANA and BALA, used in BAHYA SNEHANA, and aimed at pacifying aggravating PITTA.

channel See MERIDIAN.

channel purification See NADI SHUDDHI.

channeller (Occ.) Also, medium. A person who allows spiritual entities to use his or her body and mind as a link for the purpose of receiving psychic information or healing cosmic energy. The current trend is to have everyone become his or her own channeller, to have direct access to this New Age wisdom through the spirit guides. See CHANNELLING.

> Communication with creatures and spirits ... is effected in the shamanic seance; the sacred medium in trance is possessed by gods or spirits who use him or her as a means of divine transmissions.'
>
> —Joan Halifax

channelling (Occ.) A process whereby an individual (CHANNELLER) claims to have been invaded by a spirit entity which speaks through the channeller. The channeller first brings himself to a relaxed meditative state which leads him to a trance, wherein he allows himself to be occupied and controlled by a spirit. While he is in a trance, the channeller's mind and body are believed to be temporarily under the influence of the spirit. Seminars in the US teach how to channel and hear spirit guides; even phone channelling is available for a price charged to one's credit card. In the New Age publication *Spirit Speaks*, a spirit-guide explains that when a person's mind is active and thinking, it prevents spirits from 'coming through' but when the mind is emptied of thought, the 'communicating channel' is laid open for them. A passive state, like meditation, is believed to be a perfect habitation for spirits to extend their control through channellers.

> 'Humanity is learning a great lesson at this time. The lesson is, of course, to realize your godhood, your connectedness with the prime creator and all that exists. The lesson is to realize that everything is connected and that you are part of it all.'
>
> A message from Pleiadenian extraterrestials to Barbara Marciniak (*Bringers of the Dawn: Teachings from the Pleiadians*, by Mark Eastman and Chuck Missler)

chants (Occ./Yoga) Also, japa. 1. The solemn sounds of words or phrases, repeated continuously. 2. A religious prayer or song set in simple melodies. In spiritual practices around the globe, from times immemorial, chanting has been used for focussing one's mind. Apart from being a tool for MEDITATION, chanting has also been found useful for VISUALIZATION. Vibrations inherent in chanting are said to help in channellizing psychic energy and elevating CONSCIOUS-NESS. The Gregorian chants of the Benedictines, the Hindu chant of the GAYATRI MANTRA and the Tibetans' chanting routines—which are centred at lower, middle and higher frequencies of the human voice, combined with active, attentive and disciplined listening—have been found to energize the body, promoting mental and spiritual activity. Chanting, either accompanied by musical instruments or otherwise, is the time-tested method for altering the consciousness and raising the psychic power or energy.

There is an enormous body of chants in Buddhism and Hinduism, and Muslims chant the ninety-nine names of Allah, referred to as 'beautiful names'. The Sikh religion is a treasure-house of soothing religious songs, called KIRTAN. Included in Christian chants are four Western forms, the Gregorian, Gallican, Mozarabic, and Ambrosian, three Eastern forms, the Byzantine, Syrian and Armenian, and the Coptic and Ethiopian chants of northern Africa. Jewish chants are composed of Biblical texts. Chants or mantras are also greatly revered in SHAMANISM. The Navajos employ curative chants which are interwoven with myths telling how deities or supernatural beings first performed the chants. The underlying acceptance of responsibility for the suffering by the chanter besides the inherent positive vibes in chanting are supposed to result in healing effect on the chanter.

> 'Begin meditation by chanting aum aloud for ten minutes, then chant in a whisper for the next ten minutes, and then mentally chant for ten minutes. Finally, be still and meditate on the spiritual eye (the point between your eyebrows). Surrender into the vibrations of aum. Feel your awareness expanding still further into the field of pure consciousness, become one with aum.'
>
> —Steven Sturgess

chaomancy (Eur./Occ.) A form of AEROMANCY in which visions are sought from the sky, particularly in the shapes of clouds and cloud formations. The Babylonians, Hindus, and Etruscans made extensive use of this method of DIVINATION.

Charaka (Ind.) Literally, wanderer. The original commentator on AYURVEDA. He is believed to have wandered in forests, observing wild plants and animals. He put his observations together in his masterful compilation on AYURVEDA, NATUROPATHY and natural substances used for curing and preventing diseases at a time when much of mankind was unaware of their medicinal values. CHARAKA SAMHITA, the compilation named after him, is considered the bible of ayurveda. For two millenniums it remained a standard work on the subject and was translated into many foreign languages, including Arabic and Latin.

Little else is, however, known about Charaka. He is believed to have been the son of a sage who walked from place to place to cure the suffering. He was the first physician to formulate the concepts of digestion, immunity and metabolism.

> 'A physician who fails to enter into the body of a patient with the lamp of knowledge and understanding can never treat diseases. He should first study all the factors, including environment, which influence a patient's disease, and then prescribe treatment. It is more important to prevent the occurrence of disease than to seek a cure.'
>
> —Charaka

Charaka Samhita (Ind.) The original and the most authoritative commentary on AYURVEDA, dating back to 1000 BCE. This treatise contains a detailed classification and nomenclature of diseases, their definitions, etymology, etiology, prodromata, clinical history, patho-physiology, prognosis, line of treatment, drug diet and practices. Its conceptual framework is akin to that of contemporary medicine, as it includes a rational approach to the causation and cure of diseases, besides introducing objective methods of clinical diagnosis.

charm (Occ.)1. A magic spell concerned with enchanting an object to behave in a way which is not its normal way of behaviour. 2. A practice or expression believed to have magical healing powers similar to an incantation or a spell. The various types of charms include the Fidelius charm, which is said to completely hide a person or a place, the tickling charm which tickles the victim, making him or her laugh, and the memory charm which wipes out the victim's memory, damaging his or her mind permanently.

charu (Ind.) A food preparation made of steamed rice, milk, jaggery and GHEE, considered an ideal food for practitioners of PRANAYAMA.

chaturtha See TURIYA.

chebulic myrobalan See HARITAKI.

chelation therapy (Mod.) A process of removing the undesirable ionic material that causes ageing, arterosclerosis, cancer and other degenerative diseases of the circulatory system. Chelation therapy aims to remove metallic catalysts that cause the proliferation of free radicals in the body.

chelidonium (Hom.) Also, chelid. A homoeopathic remedy to treat despondent moods. It is also known to improve the function of the liver.

chelidonius (Gem) A magical stone believed to cure fevers when tied and worn around the neck in a yellow cloth.

chen pi (Chi.) *Citrus reticulata*. Also, Mandarin orange, tangerine. A small citrus tree with fruits resembling oranges. The dried tangerine peel has been traditionally used in Chinese medicine in the treatment of diarrhoea, indigestion and upset stomachs. It is also believed to enhance the circulation of fluids in the body. The peel of young green tangerines, called *qing pi*, is used as an analgesic. It is also prescribed for low blood pressure and (in combination with other herbs) in breast inflammation. Tangerine is also an important ingredient in AROMATHERAPY.

Chen style (Chi.) A type of TAI CHI, which originated more than 380 years ago during the Ching dynasty, from Chen village in the Henan province of China. It combines both gentle and vigorous movements. It is believed to represent the traditional school of TAI CHI but only recently has Chen style Tai Chi been disclosed to the public.

Cherokee herbal medicine (Am.Ind.) A traditional system of herbal healing, as practised by Cherokee Indians. The system acknowledges the medicinal use of about 400 plants. Their medicinal worth is often corelated with their strong resemblance to the body organs or the causative agents of the disease. Examples of herbs and their usage include a leaf infusion of blackberry as a general tonic, a bark infusion of black gum for relieving chest pain, a root decoction of buck brush to stimulate the kidneys, a the pollen of cattail as a source of protein, a root decoction of green briar in the treatment of arthritis, leaf infusion of mint to lower high blood pressure, inhalation of smoke from smouldering roots and leaves of mullein, a tobacco-like plant, in the treatment of asthma, a bark decoction of sumac for diarrhoea, a root decoction of wild ginger in the treatment of colic, and rose-hip tea from wild rose to stimulate the bladder and kidneys.

Cherokee medicine (Am.Ind.) Also, nvwoti. See CHEROKEE HERBAL MEDICINE. A traditional system of medicine, over 3,000 years old, as practised by the Cherokees in the mountains of North Carolina and in northern Oklahoma. The system includes various kinds of treatments including physical medicine which includes MASSAGE, called hiskoliya, MOXABUSTION, DREAMWORK and appreciation of nature. The Cherokee philosophy refers to values in life with respect to four aspects: physical, mental, spiritual and natural. The philosophy views medicine in a broad holistic manner: everything in human life can be considered as part of what is called 'medicine way'. Thus, apart from herbs and natural remedies, diet, nutrition, stress control and healthy routine are all encouraged.

chest breathing (Yoga) Rapid and shallow breathing, considered inefficient as it results in a reduced oxygen transfer to the blood and a retarded delivery of nutrients to the body tissues. YOGA therefore prescribes deep breathing (see PRANAYAMA). By placing one's right hand on the chest and the left hand on the stomach, one can gauge whether one is a chest breather. In chest breathers, the right hand rises higher than the left hand which is placed on the stomach.

chetna mudra (Yoga) A MUDRA formed by holding the right-hand thumb, with the left-hand fingers and repeating it by holding the left hand thumb with the right hand fingers. The practise of this mudra is recommended for stomach-related disorders such as constipation, indigestion and flatulence.

chi See QI.

chi energy flow Also, QI energy flow. 1. The energy flow in the living body, which is used in the traditional systems of medicine in the East for the purpose of wellbeing and healing. 2. A treatment method aimed at relieving pain and discomfort by enhancing the energy flow in the body as developed by Masato Nakagawa, the founder of SHINKIKO.

chi gong See QI GONG.

chi gung See QI GONG.

chi healing See CHI-LEL.

chi kung See QI GONG.

chi kung empowerment See QI GONG EMPOWERMENT.

chi kung meditation (Chi.) A system of holistic healing based on QI GONG and MEDITATION, as developed by Kenneth C. Cohen. It is based on the notion that in order to achieve inner peace, mental clarity and spiritual awareness, the flow of energy through one's body needs to be controlled.

chi-Lel qi gong (Chi./Mod./New Age) Also, chi-lel; zhineng qi gong . A system of holistic healing, based on QIGONG, as devised by Pang Ming, a grandmaster trained in both Western and Eastern medical systems. Chi-Lel encompasses the following: strong belief (that chi or life-energy can heal), group healing (for enhancement of the healing effects), chi healing (tapped from the exterior universe) and practise. This qigong method is practised worldwide.

chi nei tsang (Chi.) Also, CNT. An ancient method of HEALING TAO which literally means 'working the energy of the internal organs'. The self-healing method involves massaging the navel points, believed to be the reservoir of cosmic, prenatal, earthly and universal energies. The method is aimed at promoting rejuvenation, with deep, soft and gentle touches on the abdomen. The system integrates the physical, mental, emotional and spiritual aspects of our being. CNT, which uses the principles of KUNG-FU and QIGONG delves in to the very origin of health problems, including psychosomatic responses. The system draws on the energies of FIVE ELEMENTS IN CHINESE PHILOSOPHY.

Chinese herbology (Chi.) An ancient approach in TRADITIONAL CHINESE MEDICINE of using HERBS, more often to balance QI energy rather than treat individual symptoms. A mixture of herbs, rather than a single-plant remedy, is generally used.

chi-rho (Eur.) Also, Christogram. A Christian monogram and symbol for Christ, believed to exhibit healing characteristics. A christogram consists of the superimposed Greek letters *chi* (×) and *rho* (Ñ), often embroidered on altar cloths and clerical vestments.

chi self-massage (Chi.) An ancient Tao practice involving the self-application of chi energy to rejuvenate the inner organs, sense organs and teeth. The method employs energetic MASSAGE techniques which dispel negative emotions, relieve stress and strengthen the sense organs, internal organs and nervous system. While the Western concept of massage involves primarily the manipulation of muscles, chi massage emphasizes the strengthening and rejuvenating organs of the body, including the sense organs. Practising these exercises every day for a few minutes is said to strengthen the senses, especially vision, hearing and taste, and detoxifying the internal organs and glands. The routine is also reported to help control negative emotions, relieve stress and constipation, and improve one's complexion, teeth and gums, and overall stamina.

chicory (Chi./Flo.) *Cichorium intybus*. Succory, witloof chicory, radichetta, asparagus chicory. Native to Europe and western Asia, chicory is now cultivated widely. In India, the root is blended with coffee to enhance its colour. The leaf, boiled with honey for a gargle is said to cure oral cancer. The root boiled in water is said to help treat breast cancer.

chin mudra (Yoga) Formed in the same way as in JNANA MUDRA, except that in chin mudra the palms of both the hands face upwards. This mudra is believed to increase the efficacy of asanas. Mudras used in spiritual practices have been found to be of help in sensing the esoteric realities.

china See CINCHONA.

Chinese angelica See BAI ZHI.

Chinese auricular acupuncture See AURICULAR THERAPY.

Chinese auricular acu-points therapy See AURICULAR THERAPY.

Chinese auricular therapy See AURICULAR THERAPY.

Chinese date (Chi.) A component of CHINESE DIETOTHERAPY, the prevention and treatment of diseases by taking common foods tuffs. Suggested measures for weight loss include incorporating inter alia elements of YANG in otherwise YIN food.

Chinese dietotherapy (Chi.) Also, Chinese food therapy. The importance of diet in health and healing has long been recognized in TRADITIONAL CHINESE MEDICINE. Prescribing 'medicinal foods' has gone hand in hand with proscribing certain foods. The curative effect of a food or food–drug mixture, according to the system, depends on its 'energy' and 'taste'. The 'energy' of diet refers to one of four characteristics: cold, hot, warm, and cool. The 'taste' refers to one of the following: salty, sour, sweet, bitter or pungent.

The basic principle in dietotherapy involves neutralizing a given illness by prescribing diet or a food–drug combination whose 'energy' and 'taste' antagonize those found in the disease. For example, in the case of an illness of a cool nature, the energy-formula will be based on warmth. Also, sour herbs have been found to nourish the liver and gall bladder, while bitter ones are drying and detoxifying, draining QI energy downwards in the body. Bitter herbs are found to be helpful in strengthening the heart and small intestines. Sweet herbs are tonic as they are nourishing and relaxing, slowing down the QI energy. They also harmonize the spleen and stomach. Pungent herbs stimulate warmth and raise QI energy from the interior to the exterior. They also strengthen the lungs and the large intestines. Yet another theory in this system refers to the use of an organ of an animal to nourish the corresponding organ in the human body.

Chinese energetic healing See QIGONG.

Chinese food therapy See CHINESE DIETOTHRAPY.

Chinese health balls See BAODING BALLS.

Chinese herbal medicine (Chi.) Also, Chinese herbology. This system focusses on supporting the body's self-healing mechanism. Herbs are believed to nourish not only the body, but also the mind, emotions and spirit. The essence of the ingested herb is believed to reach the ACUPUNCTURE MERIDIAN and help in adjusting or correcting the vital flow of QI energy, causing healing.

The energetic classification of herbs is a science dating back to a tribal chief named Shen Nong (2700 BC). He wrote the first book on traditional Chinese herbal medicine (*The Classic of Materia Medica*, Shen Nong Ben Cao Jing), compiled around 206 BC. Each herb is listed with its properties, functions, clinical use, major combinations, dosage and pharmacological research, such as antimicrobial effect, antiviral effect, antifungal effect, effect on blood pressure, effect on smooth muscle, endocrine effect, central nervous system effect and use in gynaecology.

Chinese herbology See CHINESE HERBAL MEDICINE.

Chinese medicine (Chi.) Also, zhong yi. TRADITIONAL CHINESE MEDICINE targets the imbalance caused by the disease and not the infectious organism. It is a branch of the Taoist healing arts which includes ACUPUNCTURE, ASTROLOGY, GEOMANCY, I-CHING, MEDITATION and QIGONG. Variations of this system can be found in other parts of the globe as in KOREAN MEDICINE, TIBETAN MEDICINE and VIETNAMESE TRADITIONAL MEDICINE. See also, TRADITIONAL CHINESE MEDICINE.

Chinese peony See BAI SHAO.

Chinese physiognomy (Chi.) A diagnostic method based on the observation that specific areas of the face reflect problems affecting certain organs in the body. The art of reading personality traits from faces dates back to ancient times and is still popular among several ethnic Chinese communities. Chinese physiognomy is based on theories such as YIN-YANG, FIVE ELEMENTS IN CHINESE PHILOSOPHY and pa kua.

Chinese treatment techniques (Chi.) Historically, CHINESE MEDICINE recognizes eight popular groups: ACUPUNCTURE, Chinese Astrology, CHINESE DIETOTHERAPY, Chinese Herbal Medicine, Chinese massage therapy (TUI NA), MOXIBUSTION, TAI CHI CH'UAN, and QIGONG. In the contemporary scenario, except for ASTROLOGY and FENG SHUI, other methods are routinely used as part of medical treatment. Modern Chinese treatment methods, however, consist of herbal medicine and acupuncture as the primary methods.

> 'One disease, different treatments; different diseases, one treatment.'
> —A saying, referring to Chinese medicine

Chinese tui na therapy See TUINA.

Chinese yoga See QIGONG.

chininum sulfuricum (Hom.) Chin Sulf., sulphate of quinine. A remedy for throbbing headaches.

Chinul (1158–1210) The founder of the Korean tradition of ZEN.

chirayata See BHUNIMBA.

chiromancy (Eur.) Also, chirognomy, chirognosy, chirosophy. A diagnostic method using the individual characteristics of hands such as the shape of the hands, palms, fingers, nails and skin texture which are believed to indicate disharmony in the body. For example, flat nails indicate a predisposition to heart ailments, particularly when they are long and wide.

chiropody See PODIATRY.

chiropractic (Mod./New Age) A medical practice concerned with the diagnosis, treatment and prevention of mechanical disorders of the musculo-skeletal system and related disorders of the nervous system. The treatment includes spinal manipulation or adjustment of displaced vertebrae. Chiropractic can be considered a materialist version of ACUPUNCTURE which is aimed at unblocking the flow of QI energy. The chiropractor's 'needles' are his hands and fingers which manipulate the muscles and nerves, rather than QI. Chiropractic was introduced in the US by D.D. Palmer in 1895 and was carried forward by his son, Bartlett Joshua Palmer.

Early chiropractors believed that psychic energy, a force beyond human understanding, flowed from the brain, through the nerves, to all parts of the body and that it was interference with this force that caused disease. In 1953, the theory was revised to state that the health of body tissues is controlled by nerve impulses, and that interference in the nerve impulses causes disease.

chirosophy See CHIROMANCY.

chit (Yoga) AWARENESS, CONSCIOUSNESS, perception. See also SAT CHIT ANANDA.

chiti (Ind.) The power of universal CONSCIOUSNESS; the creative aspects of Nature.

chitra See INDRAVARUNI.

chitraka (Ind.) *Plumbago zeylanica*. A wild plant with medicinal properties, commonly found in India. Its root and root bark are used in folk medicine in the treatment of dysentery and other stomach-related problems.

chitta (Yoga) 1. The seat of the conscious, subconscious and super-conscious state. 2. Mind-stuff. 3. The three-fold mental faculty called antahkarana, comprising intellect (buddhi), mind (manas) and ego (ahamkara).

chitta shuddhi (Yoga) The purification of CHITTA. It essentially means unselfishness and egolessness. Some of the spiritual paths for purifying the mind include doing prescribed duties without hankering for their rewards, or surrendering the fruits of action or even actions to God. Purification in its true sense is an attitude of unconditional love and compassion to one and all, without discrimination.

choreotherapy See DANCE THERAPY.

chrisoletus (Gem) A magical stone, when worn as a bead strung on a donkey's hair is believed to keep the wearer from melancholy.

Christian positive thinking (Eur.) A mental attitude that admits into the mind thoughts, words and images that are conducive to growth, expansion and success. It refers to a mental attitude that expects positive and favourable results. Negative thoughts, words and attitude, on the other hand, bring up negative and unhappy moods and actions, creating conditions for failure, frustration and disappointment. In order to turn the mind towards the positive, inner work and training are addressed.

> 'I maintain Christianity is a life much more than a religion.'
>
> —R.M. Moberly

Christian science (Eur./Mod./New Age) A religion founded by Mary Baker Eddy in 1879, based on the principle that the mind is the only reality, and illness, pain and death are illusory. The religion emphasizes the importance of drawing closer to God in all healing practices. What makes Christian Science interesting is the God-centred, mind-over-matter approach that has several millions of believers around the globe.

Christian Yoga (New Age) A method of holistic healing, aimed at releasing both mental and physical limitations that hinder free access to the divine. The techniques include BREATHWORK, MEDITATION and PRAYER.

chronic pain The symptoms may appear as muscle or joint pain, fatigue, headache or other dysfunctions. The problem may actually be infectious, nutritional, structural or toxic. Using symptoms as a guide, we approach the cure. The tools to fight pain include osteopathic treatment, holistic dental treatment, orthopaedic medical techniques, such as trigger point therapy, prolotherapy (injection techniques for joint repair), oxygen therapies such as Relox™ and Hyperbaric Oxygen Therapy, and various Western and Eastern body work/massage therapies.

chu chong (Chi.) One of the four components of CHI-LEL QIGONG, it refers to verbally synchronized thinking of the group to obtain chi energy from the universe and bringing it down into a healing energy field enveloping every participant in the group, including the teacher. Other components of chi-lel are: generating a strong belief that chi energy can heal all ailments including one's own (shan shin), facilitating chi healing (fa chi) and learning easy-to-follow chi-lel movements, and practising them to achieve mastery (lan gong).

chun do sun bup energy healing (Chi.) A 6,000-year-old holistic healing practice, based on the notion that all diseases and painful experiences are caused by the disruption of energy flow in the body. By pressing into MERIDIAN points to release energy-blocks and making loud sounds with one's voice, attempts are made to shatter the blockages by a healer. The practice was originally used as a South Korean form of martial arts training that worked with the philosophy that the mind, body and spirit are interlinked. It has been identified that stress, fear and other negative emotions cause blockages along the body's MERIDIANS.

> 'We are born with a quota of energy and it's supposed to keep us going for the rest of our lives to maintain our health. But what's happening nowadays, people are losing that energy faster than they should.'
>
> —Master Park

chung moo doe (Chi.) A martial art technique, aimed at relieving pain, practised for over 1,500 years in East Asia. Originating in China, the practice was introduced to the US in the early 1970s. A combination of eight martial arts, it addresses muscles in the body, allowing them to expand. The technique is also said to allow energy to flow freely through the body, increase not only strength, flexibility, agility and stamina but also mental awareness, determination and self confidence.

churna (Ind.) A fine powder prepared by pounding dry substances, usually after passing through a filter cloth. In AYURVEDA, several herbs and their formulations are available in the form of powders.

churnasweda (Ind.) Also, podikkizhi. Massage therapy with powdered herbs to induce perspiration, often recommended for arthritic and neurological problems.

chyawanprash (Ind.) A popular herbal preparation. A RASAYANA tonic, aimed at increasing strength and youthful vigour, especially in the aged. The formulation includes the three myrobalans and several other herbs and spices, mixed with ghee and honey. Research indicates that such preparations have an antioxidant effect and a regulating effect on liver detoxification.

cicuta virosa (Hom.) Also, cicut. A remedy prescribed inter alia for dullness of the mind.

cilantro See CORIANDER.

cimex lectularius (Hom.) Also, cimex. A remedy prescribed inter alia for excessive anger.

cimicifuga racemosa (Hom.) Also, cimic. Also, black cohosh, black snake root. A remedy prescribed inter alia for anxiety and dejection.

cina (Hom.) Also, wormseed. A remedy prescribed inter alia for unruly behaviour in children.

cinchona (Ind./Hom.) *Cinchona calisaya.* Also, china, Peruvian bark, Jesuit's bark, quinine. The bark of this tree has long been known for its curative role in malarial fevers. Even before botanists identified this tree, the drug was introduced in seventeenth-century Europe by Countess Chinchon, after whom the tree was named. In Brazilian herbal medicine, quinine bark is considered a tonic, a digestive stimulant and fever reducer. It is used in anaemia, indigestion, gastrointestinal disorders, general fatigue, fevers, malaria and as an appetite stimulant. Other folk remedies in South America cite quinine bark as a natural remedy for cancer (breast, glands, liver, mesentery, spleen), amoebic infections, heart problems, colds, diarrhoea, dysentery, dyspepsia, fevers, flu, hangovers, lumbago, malaria, neuralgia, pneumonia, sciatica, typhoid, and varicose veins. In HOMOEOPATHY, China is a remedy for the low-spirited.

cinnamon (Chi./Egy./Eur./Ind.) *Cinnamomum zeylanicum.* First grown in Sri Lanka, cinnamon reached China and Egypt over 4000 years ago. Known for its medicinal properties—it is astringent, warming, stimulant, carminative, antiseptic, antifungal, anti-viral, a blood purifier and digestive aid—cinnamon was also used for embalming where body cavities were filled with spiced preservatives. Once considered more precious than gold, the Roman emperor Nero, is said to have burned a year's supply of cinnamon on his wife's funeral pyre—an extravagant gesture, signifying the depth of his loss. The demand for cinnamon launched a number of explorations which changed the course of history in a significant way. Cinnamon, along with bay leaf and cardamom form the 'three great aromatics'.

circadian rhythm From the Latin *circa*, meaning about, and *dies*, meaning day, a circadian rhythm is a rhythm which repeats itself every twenty-four hours. Under normal conditions, the sleep–wake cycle is a circadian rhythm.

circle dance An ancient form of dance, practised all over the world in tribal communities. Composed of themes based on nature, beliefs, mythology, epics and history, it brings people together in healthy social interactions.

circles of energy See CHAKRA.

circle walking See BAGUAZHANG.

circuit training (Mod.) A modern exercise plan consisting of six to ten exercises, performed one after another with a certain number of repetitions. Weight-resistance equipment is also used to increase stamina. Circuit training combines, simultaneously, aerobic and anaerobic exercises.

circular breathing See REBIRTHING.

circular movements During a massage, circular movements towards the centre or around the joints are believed to promote quick healing of the swellings.

circulation of light See SHOSHUTEN.

cistus canadensis (Hom.) Cist. can. Also, rock rose. A remedy inter alia for headaches.

citrine (Gem) Known as the success stone, this stone is believed to stabilize emotions.

clairaudience (Occ.) 'Clear hearing'. Extra-sensory hearing, associated with mystical and TRANCE experience. Clairaudience, a form of CHANNELLING, is considered a perception of messages in thought forms from an entity who exists in another realm.

clairsentience (Occ.) 'Clear sensing'. The faculty of super-physical sense-perception, which overlaps with psychic abilities such as CLAIRAUDIENCE and CLAIRVOYANCE. Clairsentience refers to the psychic perception of smell, taste, touch, emotions. While using clairsentience, psychics are said to feel other people's emotions.

clairvoyance (Occ.) 'Clear seeing'. The psychic faculty of perceiving things or events in the future or beyond normal sensory contact. Such perceptions are also said to include auditory impressions called CLAIRAUDIENCE.

clairvoyant diagnosis (Occ.) A diagnostic method performed by CLAIRVOYANCE. The ability of certain healers who conduct remote diagnosis in the absence of the patient has been ancient practice in primitive societies.

Classic Yoga See HATHA YOGA.

classical five-element acupuncture (Mod.) Also, Worsley's ACUPUNCTURE. A form of acupuncture which aims at addressing the causative factor of an illness.

classical homoeopathy (Hom.) A revolutionary healing art that involves extensive questioning of the patient by the practitioner, with a view to determine a single remedy that could be uniformly effective to all the three levels of existence: mental, emotional and physical. The system is based on the four cardinal principles (viz. similars cure similiars, the single remedy, the minimal dose, and the potentized remedy). See also HOMOEOPATHY.

classical Indian medicine (Ind.) In ancient India, two branches of knowledge were concerned with human suffering: religious philosophy and medicine. While AYURVEDA and SIDDHA evolved through practices indigenous to the subcontinent, the UNANI school traces its roots to ancient Arabic and Persian medicine.

classical Chinese medicine See CHINESE MEDICINE.

clean-me-out programme (New Age) A programme for SELF-HEALING, aimed at achieving self-healing through a complete intestinal wash and herbal formulations used for digestive rejuvenation.

cleanse group (New Age) A training course which aims at cleansing the whole being through a process of self-exploration. Cleansing techniques employed are aimed at rejuvenating the physical, mental, emotional and spiritual levels of the clients.

clear quartz (Gem) A stone believed to increase the wearer's mental clarity. Holding the quartz at one's solar plexus, while attempting even breathing for several minutes is said to be useful in calming disturbing emotions.

cleidomancy (Eur./Occ.) A method of DIVI-NATION, using a key.

clematis erecta (Hom.) Also, clemat. A remedy inter alia aimed at fear management.

cleromancy (Eur./Occ.) Also, astragalomancy. A method of DIVINATION using dice. Dice divining is an ancient method used for foretelling future events.

client-centred therapy (Mod./New Age) A form of PSYCHOTHERAPY in which the patient is in an unrestricted situation and has the freedom to explore and express attitudes, hopes and fears; a humanistic therapy based on Carl Roger's belief that an individual has an unlimited capacity for psychological growth and continues to grow unless barriers are placed in the way. This client-centred approach comes from the 'kindergarten' (a gardener whose plants are children) approach, the idea that children are like plants which if left to grow in a nurturing environment without too much input or outside influence, will flower naturally.

climacterics (Num./Occ.) An ancient belief that specific years in the course of one's life can be milestones for change, disease or danger. Septenary years such as 7, 14, 21, 28 …, for example, are associated with change. An explanation for this belief is that such changes are associated with lunar periodicities and are also linked with the growth of one's soul.

clinical kinesiology (Mod./New Age) A form of APPLIED KINESIOLOGY, developed by American chiropractor Alan Beardall, and based on the observation that various points on the skull, associated with different areas of the body, can be of use in detecting dysfunction in the respective areas. Kinesiology is a method of detecting and correcting various bio-energetic imbalances and stresses.

clinical nutrition (Mod./New Age) A modern health profession associated with healing through nutrition. The system has a wide canvas, catering to the needs of infants, growing children, teenagers, adults, the middle-aged and seniors, all of whose requirements vary from each other, depending on their health conditions, occupations, habits and lifestyles. The multi-billion dollar health industry around the globe recognizes nutrition and dietetics as essential, though many areas in nutrition remain unexplained.

cloves (Chi./Ind./Isl.) *Eugenia caryophyllata, Syzygium aromaticum.* Also, lavang. From the Latin *clavus*, meaning nail-shaped. Native to Indonesia and the Malacca Islands, its evergreen tree has bright green leaves and nail-shaped rosepeach flower buds which turn, upon drying, into deep-brown cloves.

Cloves were used by the Greeks and Romans to ease toothaches. The Chinese are reported to have used them as a breath sweetener, while talking to their emperor. An important item in the spice trade, the oil of cloves is antiseptic and stomachic and used for relieving toothaches.

> 'The flower of the heavens.'
>
> —a reference to cloves in the *Charaka Samhita*

club spa (Cos./New Age/Spa) A set-up offering a variety of spa services for the fitness-conscious. The modern spa is client-centred, proving a wide range of massage services, wraps and facials.

CNT See CHI NEI TSANG.

cobalt (Hom.) Kobaltum. A homoepathic remedy prescribed inter alia for pain in the forehead with uneasiness in the stomach.

cocculus (Hom.) A remedy prescribed inter alia for slowness of comprehension.

coconut (Ind.) *Cocus nucifera.* Considered an ideal food due to its nutritive importance. Tender coconut water and the milk extracted from the kernel are used in the treatment of stomach ulcers. Massaging the hair with coconut oil every day is said to arrest hair loss.

> 'Coconut adds beauty and prosperity to a house.'
>
> —*Matsya Purana*

co-counselling (Mod.) A type of COUNSELLING THERAPY in which the patient and the counsellor each take turns to act as counsellor. By listening and responding to the counsellor-as-patient for half a session, the patient is said to be able to learn about his or her own emotions and mental processes. See also, REEVALUATION COUNSELLING.

co-creative healing (New Age) A system of self-healing as developed by Donna La Pre, aimed at activating the healer within. It refers to the process of working with one's soul and spiritual guidance to co-create one's life. In this journey, one is said to be able to clear all obstructions to healing. In co-creative healing, the individual, with his or her inner guidance, is the ultimate authority on his or her own process or journey. This, however, does not preclude others' inputs; others' views are weighed against the self's own judgment, to honour one's truth. This method acknowledges that thoughts create reality and that every individual has his or her own natural rate of growth, change and healing, and that the pace and process may vary over time.

coffea (Hom.) A remedy inter alia for unsteady running about, sleeplessness, trembling of hands, etc.

cognition (New Age) Knowledge reached through intuitive, super-conscious faculties rather than through intellect alone.

cognitive body (Occ.) Also, wisdom sheath, vijnanamaya kosha. One of the five sheaths or layers of the human organism. See KOSHA.

cognitive behaviour therapy (Mod.) Also, CBT. An active clinical treatment for mental healthcare. The method comprises a combination of BEHAVIOURISM (based on the theories of learning) and COGNITIVE THERAPY (based on the theory that our cognitions or thoughts control a large portion of our behaviour). The therapy is reported to be useful especially in conditions such as depression and mood swings, shyness and social anxiety, obsessions and compulsions, eating disorders and obesity. While behaviour therapy helps in weakening the link between adverse situations and reactions (fear, depression or rage), cognitive therapy helps in adopting right-thinking patterns conducive to good health. CBT is said to provide powerful tools for stopping one's symptoms and finding a more satisfying track. In many ways CBT resembles coaching or tutoring. Under expert guidance, the client shares in setting treatment goals and in choosing the technique that works best.

cognitive dissonance (Mod.) The perception of incompatibility between two contradicting cognitions. The theory of cognitive dissonance holds that contradicting cognitions serve as a driving force that compels the mind to acquire or invent new thoughts or beliefs, or to modify existing beliefs, so as to reduce the amount of dissonance (conflict) between cognitions. The theory of cognitive dissonance was first propounded in 1956 by psychologist Leon Festinger.

cognitive immunology (Mod.) The study of the IMMUNE SYSTEM as an autonomous, cognitive, self-organizing and self-regulating network. Though cognitive immunology promises exciting clinical applications to the treatment of AUTO-IMMUNE DISORDERS, the field is still in its infancy and the self-organizing properties of the immune networks in the body are still a mystery to modern science. According to Francisco Varela, a sophisticated psychosomatic (mind–body) view of health will not develop until we understand the nervous system and the immune system as two interacting cognitive systems, two 'brains' in continuous conversation.

cognitive restructuring (Mod.) A theory and technique of BEHAVIOUR THERAPY, concerned with perception and belief systems. Cognitive therapy sees the state of depression as the result of sad thinking rather than believing the converse, that the latter is the resultant. The theory holds that unrealistic beliefs generate dysfunctional emotions. By setting unachievable goals, one ends up fearing failure. Cognitive restructuring helps one change beliefs from irrational to rational ones as for example in 'I might fail, but it doesn't matter as I don't have to be successful everywhere!' The rationale aims at strengthening the client's belief that self-defeating thoughts and negative statements can cause emotional distress, interfering with one's progress or performance.

cognitive therapy (Mod.) An active clinical treatment for mental healthcare based on the theory that our cognition or thoughts control most of our behaviour traits. See COGNITIVE BEHAVIOUR THERAPY.

colchicum autumnale (Hom.) Also, colchic. A remedy inter alia for weakened memory and lost perception.

cold bath (Nat.) A simple and natural way to health and hygiene. However, very cold water is not recommended for infants and the old. See also SITZ BATH.

cold double-compress (Nat.) A common health practice to induce internal heat to produce a secondary reaction to the cold. A cold wet cloth covered with a dry cloth or a water-resistant plastic or rubber is used as a COMPRESS. Sometimes a little apple cider vinegar is added to cold water to enhance its potency. Cold double compresses are used most commonly in upper respiratory infections, such as sore throats, bronchitis, influenza, pneumonia, and swollen lymph glands in the neck. They may also be applied over the trunk or abdomen, genital area, joints, limbs or feet. See also COMPRESS, HYDROTHERAPY.

cold foot-bath (Nat.) A common health practice in the treatment of sprains and inflamed bunions. However, this treatment is not recommended during menstruation, in the early stages of infection or if inflammatory conditions prevail in the chest or pelvis. See also HYDROTHERAPY.

cold hand-bath (Nat.) A common health practice aimed at getting relief from excessive perspiration, sunstroke or nose bleed. See also HYDROTHERAPY.

cold-mitten massage (Nat.) A common health practice aimed at reducing fever. See also COMPRESS.

cold shower (Nat.) A common health practice, aimed at stimulating the body or reducing fever. See also HYDROTHERAPY.

cold toe-bath (Nat.) A healthcare practice aimed at creating an intense reaction in the pelvic areas, besides decongesting the lungs and head. The toes are dipped for 30 seconds in a shallow tub containing ice-cold water. The feet are then rubbed briskly and the toes are returned to water. This process is repeated several times till the feet become ruddy. See also HYDROTHERAPY.

cold treading-bath (Nat.) See COLD WATER TREADING.

cold water (Nat.) A primary health aid widely used from ancient times for internal and external cleansing and also for its therapeutic value. See also HYDROTHERAPY, SITZ BATH.

> 'To strengthen the body: pure water to drink, cold baths, a hair-mattress to sleep, cool air to breathe and dry food.'
>
> —A Scottish saying

cold-water spray (Nat.) A restorative application of cold water.

cold-water treading (Nat.) A common health practice, aimed at improving one's energy levels and vitality. Cold water, up to the ankles, is used for treading, generally twice daily. Cold water treading, particularly on river-beds or seashores, is believed to improve one's energy levels and vitality. See also HYDROTHERAPY.

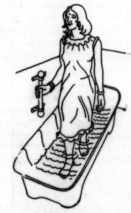

Cold-water treading

collagen (Cos./Mod.) Also, aesthetic fillers. A purified gelatinous protein found in bones and connective tissues in mammals, used in cosmetic treatments.

collagen facial (Cos./Mod.) The application of freeze-dried COLLAGEN to plump the skin and to fill in the fine lines acquired by stress and ageing. The treatment is said to last for three to four months.

collagen injection (Cos./Mod.) The injection of collagen beneath the skin with the help of a fine needle to fill out wrinkles and lines for reasons of aesthetics. Collagen is referred to as 'aesthetic fillers' as they can hide a person's age.

collar-bone breathing (Mod.) One of the two forms of CHEST BREATHING, characterized by the rising of the collar bones and shoulders during the breathing process. As only a small amount of oxygen enters into the lungs during such breathing, it is considered the wrong way of breathing. See also CHEST BREATHING.

collective unconscious (Misc.) The content of the unconscious mind that is passed down from generation to generation in humans.

colon hydrotherapy See COLONIC IRRIGATION.

colon therapy See COLONIC IRRIGATION.

colonic irrigation Also, colon cleansing, colon hydrotherapy. The flushing of intestines with water or soapy solutions administered through a rectal ENEMA, aimed at removing toxins trapped therein so that they do not get recycled into the blood stream.

colocynthis (Chi.) *Cucumis colocynthis*. A remedy inter alia for a depressed and joyless condition.

colour breathing (Mod./New Age/Occ./Yoga) Also, colour imagination. A breathing method. While inhaling, one imagines the desired colour streaming into one's body with the air, penetrating into the desired areas/CHAKRAS in the body so as to cleanse and disinfect them. Imagining oneself surrounded by a cloud of desired colour, breathing deeply and imagining that such colour is filling up the lungs and flowing through the body (or to a particular diseased spot) are the common methods adopted. This practice was popularized by *Colour Therapy,* written

by Ivah Bergh Whitten in England in 1948.

colour healing See COLOUR THERAPY.

colour imagination See COLOUR BREATHING.

colour meditation A method based on VISUALIZATION. Each of the seven CHAKRAS associated with a unique colour of the rainbow is focussed upon. Also see COLOUR THERAPY.

colour pranic healing (New Age/Occ./Yoga) Focussing colour energies on the patient to produce accelerated healing, particularly in the case of severe ailments. The treatment involves using the will and VISUALIZATION of colours.

colour projection (New Age) The use of sunlight or artificial light through a transparent coloured filter, such as a sheet or a silk. While light passing through a red filter is recommended for anaemics, those who suffer from fevers are advised to use a blue filter.

colour puncture (New Age) The application of colour light with the help of a device that resembles a pen-light, to ACUPOINTS, and aimed at healing.

colour therapy (Egy./Vib.) Also, colour healing, An ancient method of healing known to the Egyptians, Greeks and Romans, colour therapy is based on the premise that each colour has its own wavelength, its own particular energy, and can thus help in healing different conditions. The colour correspondence to CHAKRAS is shown in the following table:

Colour	Corresponding Gland	Corresponding Chakra	Ailments believed to be cured
Violet (white)	Pineal	Crown (SAHASRARA)	Mental disorders
Indigo	Pituitary	Eyebrow (AJNA)	Nervous disorders
Blue	Thyroid/ Parathyroid	Throat (VISHUDDHI)	Boils, burns, colic, cough, cuts, dysentery, inflam mation, fevers
Green (pink)	Thymus	Heart (ANAHATA)	Blood pressure, breast cancer, cold, erysipelas, influenza, syphilis, ulcers constipation, diabetes,
Yellow	Pancreas/adrenal	Solar plexus (MANIPURAKA)	Jaundice

| Orange | Spleen | Spleen (SVADISHTHANA) | Stones in kidney and gallbladder |
| Red | Sacrum/ gonads/ ovaries | Root (MULADHARA) | Arthritis, paralysis |

comarital sex therapy (New Age) A treatment aimed at addressing sexual deficiencies involving a team, consisting of a male and a female practitioner. The couple approach is aimed at bringing home the point that sexual dysfunction is not the exclusive problem of an individual, but is contextual that to the interaction between two individuals.

combination therapy (Mod./New Age) 1. An approach to healing, integrating concepts and techniques borrowed from various systems; 2. A combination of different drugs used to fight HIV.

combined spirituality and psychotherapy (New Age) An approach to healing, integrating concepts and techniques borrowed from several approaches such as CONSCIOUSNESS EXPANSION, SIMONTON METHOD, SUFI HEALING and NUTRITIONAL PSYCHOLOGY.

comfortable pranayama See SURKHA PURAKA.

common barley See BARLEY.

common bryony See BRYONIA.

Commonweal (Misc.) A non-profit health and environmental research institute in Bolinas, California, which aims at providing information from research and anecdotal experiences on the health of humans as well as their ecosystem. The institute conducts training programmes for cancer patients, physicians, medical students and other health professionals.

complementary medicine (Mod.) A system of alternative therapies, parallel to practices in modern medicine. Treatments and therapies are often used in conjunction with conventional medicine. ALTERNATIVE MEDICINE, in contrast, works as a substitute for conventional medicine.

'It's choice, not chance, that determines your destiny.'
—Jean Nidetch

compress (Nat.) A soft pad, such as of lint, soaked in a hot or cold liquid and applied to relieve inflammation. Compresses are useful for the application of cold water, hot water, liquefied medication or herbal decoctions to specific parts of the body. A cold compress consists of a cloth wrung from cold or ice water and then applied to the body. The cold single compress has a primarily vaso-constrictive effect, both locally and distally. Due to this effect, it may be used to prevent oedema following injury, inhibit inflammation, and relieve pain due to congestion. It may also be used to reduce body temperature when applied over a large area of the body. Compresses are renewed frequently (every one to five minutes) in order to maintain the primary cold effect.

Hot compresses and fomentations may create an analgesic effect, thereby decreasing pain. They are generally more effective locally for pain resulting from spasm than for pain due to congestion. Fairly hot compresses may be applied directly to the skin surface, with care taken not to burn or startle the patient. Hot applications are contraindicated on the extremities of diabetics.

compression wrap (Nat.) Wrapping a selected area of the body with an elastic bandage; a localized treatment for CELLULITE and adipose tissues, particularly on arms, thighs, legs and buttocks.

computerized radionics (Mod./New Age) An electro-diagnostic testing system which measures the body's energy system through acupuncture points on the skin. It uses BIOFEEDBACK by placing one electrode in the patient's hand while other ACUPOINTS are tested on the hand, finger, toes or teeth. This process is non-invasive and painless and helps in identifying the various causes of imbalance in the body. See AUTOMATED COMPUTERIZED TREATMENT SYSTEM.

concept therapy (New Age) A CHIROPRACTIC healing method, based on the understanding that all facets in a human being are connected and constantly interacting with one another.

condiment (Nat.) Seasoning for food, which aids in digestion and provides mineral supplements to the body.

confluent somatic therapy (New Age) Healing the whole person. CST uses the active participation of both the facilitator and the person being healed. It sees healing as an equal partnership in which the client is seen as possessing tremendous inner resources to be activated for healing. The client is made to be active and creative as opposed to passive and compliant as in most conventional medicine. This results in the client becoming empowered rather than rescued.

conium (Hom.) A remedy to treat dullness and depression.

connective-tissue massage See BINDIGEWEBMASSAGE.

conscious breathing (Tan./Yoga) A way of breathing, the chief aim of which is to reduce stress and pain. The method is based on the belief that focussing one's attention on breathing helps in achieving such benefits by diverting one's mind away from the location of the pain. See also, REBIRTHING.

conscience (Mod./New Age) A moral faculty that guides one about what is right or wrong. Sometimes called the knowing voice of the soul, the conscience can be at times distorted by the individual's training and belief patterns, and is therefore not necessarily a perfect mirror of what is right or wrong. According to SIGMUND FREUD, the conscience originates in the SUPEREGO which takes its cue from parents during childhood.

> 'In matters of conscience, the law of the majority has no place.'
>
> —Mahatma Gandhi

conscious mind (Mod./New Age) The external, everyday state of consciousness.

consciousness (Mod./New Age) Also, chitta, chaitanya, mind-stuff. 1. A state of mind, or cognition, which is characterized by self-awareness. 2. A state of AWARENESS as organized by the senses and which allows for the reception of anything that lends itself to definition and, ultimately, communication 3. Perception. 4. The condition of knowing things.

While consciousness appears to be the most obvious phenomenon, it is the most mysterious feature of the mind. The levels of consciousness vary, and includes, for example, individual consciousness (vyashti chaitanya), intellectual consciousness (buddhi chitta), and God-consciousness (Shiva chaitanya). The *Mandukya Upanishad* refers to four states of consciousness: waking, dreaming, dreamless sleep and the transcendent state or TURIYA. Myriad grades of consciousness are also known, including the simple sentience of inanimate matter, the consciousness of basic life forms, the higher consciousness of human beings to the omniscient states of super-consciousness.

> 'The waking and dream states of our life, created by our consciousness are ultimately illusory.'
>
> —*Mandukya Upanishad*

consciousness revolution (Mod./New Age) 1. A new way of viewing and experiencing one's life, based on the understanding that CONSCIOUSNESS of man, universe and God are but one and there is a perceptible (and real) INTERCONNECTEDNESS. 2. A spiritual awakening in American history which relates to a period 1964–84.

consciousness after death (Occ./New Age) The belief, prevalent in many ancient civilizations, that CONSCIOUSNESS continues even after the death of an organism indicating the point of view that consciousness is not just a mere function of the brain.

consciousness therapy (New Age) An approach to healing incorporating the concepts and practices drawn from a host of systems, viz., CHAKRA HEALING, PSYCHOSOMA, thosenes and projectiology. Attaining altered states of consciousness is described as a basic human motive and is celebrated in ancient shamanic rituals around the globe. The ancient systems like YOGA, QIGONG and TAI CHI offer refuge for the substance-dependent by offering socially acceptable and health-based methods for attaining altered states of consciousness.

contact healing (New Age) An age-old

concept and practice of transmission of vital energy from a healthy person, who can spare it, to a sick person, who is devoid of it. Usually, the contact healer places his trained hands, palms down, on the top of the patient's head or on the shoulders or waist. See also, REIKI, TOUCH THERAPY.

contact reflex analysis (New Age) A form of APPLIED KINESIOLOGY, based on the notion that the surface of the human body has about seventy-five reflex points that serve as windows to numerous conditions. It is also believed that the back of the hand is electro-negative, while the palm is positive and the fingers are neutral.

> Research has proven the human body to be like a computer, made up of the brain (electrical generator and memory bank) and thousands of miles of electrical wires called nerves. These nerves connect every organ, gland and tissue of the body. These nerves also connect with 'fuses' or 'breaker switches' called contact reflexes. By contacting these reflexes, using the body's muscular system as an indicator, we are able to monitor the function of body systems.
>
> —Dick A. Versendaal

contact yoga (New Age) A new approach to YOGA, done with a partner. The partner aids and assists in forming the correct posture and helps the other's progress.

contentment (Yoga) Satisfaction; an ideal state of mind that is believed to prevent all possible disharmony and disease in life. See also, ANANDAMAYA KOSHA.

> 'My motto is: contented with little, yet wishing for more.'
>
> —Charles Lamb

continence (Misc.) Also, sexual continence. It is believed that long-term seminal retention leads to the biological transmutation of the sperm and allows the resulting energy to be sublimated to the superior levels of the human being. It is also believed by practitioners that continence develops the ability to control instinctive desires, while imparting calmness and equanimity.

contraction points See BANDHA.

cooperative healing (New Age) A system of healing which emphasizes a cooperative relationship between the physician and the patient. According to this concept, a doctor–patient interaction has to acquire a more egalitarian status, one in which a patient's strengths and weaknesses are seriously taken note of while formulating a therapeutic intervention.

coptis rhizome See HUANG LIAN.

coral (Ind.) Hard calcareous substances, consisting of the continuous skeleton, secreted by coelenterate polyps in the seabed. Coral is regarded as a talismanic protection for children and is worn to overcome sexual inadequacies in adults. In folk medicine, coral is placed in rice-water for a few hours and the water is drunk to treat urinary problems.

core energetics (New Age) 1. A dynamic process that taps physical, mental, emotional, spiritual levels of consciousness to release blocked energies in the mind–body. 2. A form of PSYCHOTHERAPY, developed by John C. Pierrakos, aimed at therapeutic benefits by bringing together consciousness and movement.

core zero balancing See ZERO BALANCING.

coriander (Ind.) *Coriandrum sativum.* Also, cilantro, dhania. From the Latin *coriandrum*, meaning resembling a bed-bug (the reference is to the seeds of the plant). An aromatic herb with variable leaves, broadly lobed at the base of the plant, slender and feathery on the flowering stems. Fresh leaves and the dried seeds are popular in Chinese, South Asian, Middle Eastern, Mediterranean and Latin American cuisine. Coriander is used as a folk medicine for the relief of anxiety and insomnia. Researchers have recently found that coriander can assist with clearing the body of lead, aluminium and mercury.

The essential oil of this plant is known for its antibacterial action against *E. coli.*

cornelian (Gem) A flesh-coloured variety of chalcedony, a form of quartz, originally found in Arabia and Egypt, believed to be helpful in controlling bleeding and removing blotches, pimples and sores from the skin.

corpus collosum (Misc.) A bundle of nerve-fibres that link the left and right hemispheres of the CEREBRAL CORTEX. It is essential for tasks such as finger coordination, among other things.

corundrum ruby (Gem) A crystal, traditionally recommended for terminal illness.

cosmeceuticals (Cos./New Age) Also, cosmaceuticals. Combinations of cosmetics and pharmaceuticals, popular as they promote health and enhance the appearance.

cosmic Christ (New Age/Occ.) An esoteric viewpoint that Christ represents the whole cosmos. Christ is believed to be the force behind a collective Christ consciousness. According to Richard M. Burke, who coined the term in 1902, cosmic consciousness is a transpersonal mode of consciousness, an awareness of the Universal mind and one's unity with it. It refers to an awareness of the life and order in the Universe. An individual who attains the state of cosmic consciousness is described as enlightened. Burke saw this state of consciousness as the next stage in human evolution.

cosmic energy (Occ./Yoga) 1. Prana or the life-force. 2. Energy, believed to pervade the universe.

cosmic humanism (New Age) A philosophy which views man as having virtually unlimited potential, because of his inner divinity. Cosmic humanism comprises perspectives on certain disciplines, such as theology, philosophy, ethics, biology, psychology, sociology, law, politics, economics and history.

cosmic ray therapy (New Age) An approach to healing which is based on the belief that the planetary position causes a deficiency of cosmic rays, which in turn causes imbalances in one's CHAKRAS. To counter such imbalances coloured gemstones are prescribed. They are considered to be sensitive and radioactive. See also GEM THERAPY.

cosmology Knowledge of the cosmos; the area of metaphysics dealing with the origin and structure of the universe. According to Hindu cosmology, both inner and outer worlds constitute one's existence.

costus root See MU XIANG.

counselling (New Age) Also, counselling therapy; the therapeutic application of counselling. Counselling is considered an effective means to cope with situations arising from accidents or crisis, which may cause sudden, unbearable changes in a person's life.

counselling therapy See COUNSELLING.

CPT See CHRISTIAN POSITIVE THINKING.

crane-style qigong See SOARING CRANE QIGONG.

cranial chakras (New Age/Yoga) The term collectively refers to the top two chakras: the crown chakra and the eyebrow chakra. See CHAKRA.

cranial osteopathy (Mod.) Also, craniosacral therapy. Craniosacral therapy has its roots in the work of Andrew Taylor Still (1828–1917). This technique of manipulation of the bones of the skull, with an extremely light and gentle touch, was developed by William Garner Sutherland (1873–1954), an American osteopath, in consultation with Still. Looking at a disarticulated skull where the sphenoid and temporal bones joined, Sutherland noticed that it looked like the gills of a fish, designed for motion. Thus, if the bones of the skull were designed for motion, he realized that restrictions would inhibit health, which would lead eventually to pain and disease. He pursued his interest by performing experiments on himself. After many trials and errors over a period of years, he was confident enough to use these techniques on his patients, with great success.

The gentle touch, focussed on the connection between the skull and the base of the spine, along the spinal column, is said to alter the rhythms (called the breath of life by Sutherland) found in cerebrospinal fluid that surrounds the brain and the spinal cord. This technique is applied to people of various age groups, for many ailments, including headaches and migraines, learning and behavioural difficulties, trauma, hypertension and painful sinuses.

craniosacral therapy See CRANIAL OSTE-OPATHY.

creative-art therapies (New Age) The therapeutic application of creative processes and experiences, more often non-verbal. Dance, music, art, creative writing or speaking and other means of imaginative expressions are increasingly found to have a therapeutic impact in the overall development of personality and behaviour norms, useful in a social set-up. They are also found to have a role in the treatment of several ailments, such as addictions, digestive disorders, headaches, eating disorders, psychic disorders and sleep disorders. It is reported that creative activities can cause our brain cells to release neuro-chemicals (including endorphins) capable of reducing pain and improving one's ability to respond to illness. These neuro-chemicals signal the body to send blood to areas affected by the illness or injury.

> 'Without art, the crudeness of reality would make the world unbearable.'
> —George Bernard Shaw

creative imaging See VISUALIZATION.

creative visualization (New Age) A technique of visualizing positive outcomes to overcome the burden of harsh realities. Music and other creative activities in which a person is fully engaged can help train oneself towards creative visualization. According to Shakti Gawain, author of creative visualization, positive energy attracts more energy, which plays an important role in healing.

cremation (Ind.) Also, dahana, burning of the dead. Cremation, like burial, is the traditional method of disposing off bodily remains. It is believed to aid in releasing the soul quickly from any earthly or organic attachments. In recent times, cremation facilities are widely available in nearly every country, though electricity or gas-fuelled chambers are replacing the customary wood pyre.

crocus (Hom.) *Crocus sativus*. A remedy to treat alternating depression and hilarity. Also, see SAFFRON.

crow-walking (Yoga) A preparatory exercise before undertaking a long MEDITATION session, crow-walking is done by placing the palms on the knees and walking while maintaining the squatting position.

crown chakra See SAHASRARA.

cruise-ship spa (Spa) A modern spa aboard a cruise ship with professional spa services, fitness, wellness cuisine and other health and leisure facilities.

crystal (Gem) A gem, used variously in folk medicine. Placing a crystal in the room is said to improve the atmosphere, as it is believed to absorb negative energies. 'Recharging' of crystals is done by rubbing them with sea salt and washing them in flowing water before keeping them in sunlight for a few minutes.

crystal gazing See SCRYING.

crystal healing (Gem) The application of crystals for healing. The method consists of continuously wearing the stone or crystal for at least twenty-one days to initiate the process of cleansing the aura. The time factor to reap the desired benefits is reported to depend on the quality of the crystal (size, colour, energy charge), location of placement in the body, duration of wearing, and the crystal's choice appropriate to one's body constitution. Some crystals are considered better suited to healing the overall problem which underlies symptoms, than to treating just the symptoms. See also GEM THERAPY.

crystal therapeutics (Gem) An approach to healing, as designed by Ojela Frank, involving CRYSTAL HEALING, energy assessment, ENERGY BALANCING, GUIDED IMAGERY and COUNSELLING.

crystalomancy See SCRYING.

Culpeper, Nicholas (1616–54) An English botanist and author of *Complete Herbal* (1653), who was opposed to the 'closed shop' of medicine. He maintained that the use of Latin by physicians and lawyers was a conspiracy to keep power and freedom from the common man.

cumin (Chi./Eur./Ind.) *Cuminum cyminum*. Also, jeera, jiraka, Known since biblical times for its carminative action, AYURVEDA recognized the cooling effect of its fruit, and recommends it particularly for warm seasons and climates to treat constipation, indigestion and nausea.

cupping (Chi.) An ancient Chinese method, employing small glass or pottery cups. A match is lit and then quickly removed before applying the mouth of the cup to the skin. As the flame creates a vacuum, the cup sticks tightly to the skin. The vacuum produces strong suction pressure on the skin and as a consequence, increases blood supply in the region. Several cups may be applied at any one time to a particular part of the body such as back and shoulders where they remain for ten to fifteen minutes. The cup can be released by pressing the skin next to the edge of the cup so as to break the vacuum. Cupping is considered an efficient treatment for conditions such as lumbago, rheumatism, stiff neck and shoulders.

cuprum metallicum (Hom.) Also, cuprum met., copper, metallic copper. A homoeopathic remedy for mania.

curanderismo A form of Hispanic HEALING which includes the use of HERB, DIET and MAGIC.

curd therapy (New Age) The therapeutic use of curd or yoghurt. It is considered a panacea for heart and stomach problems, senility and ageing. Eaten, it checks bacterial and fungal formulations in the mucus membrane. Curd massage cures dry itching, delays wrinkles, improves complexion and moisturizes the skin.

cure (Misc.) A course of treatment.

curry leaf (Ind.) *Murraya koenigi.* Also, karipatta. A widely used aromatic in south Indian cuisine, the leaves are used in folk medicine in the treatment of constipation, indigestion, and names.

> 'Curry leaf kills germs.'
>
> —Gunapadam

cybex (Mod.) Patented exercise equipment used for isokinetic strength training.

cyclical characteristics of the phenomenal world (Mod.) The oriental systems heavily lean on the premise of non-linear or cyclical characteristics of phenomenal existence. This orientation differs from the linear and mathematical aspects employed in science. Examples of non-linear aspects that stand neglected in science are friction, turbulence, many body systems (e.g., gas molecules) and most natural processes.

There is, in recent times, an acknowledgement that what appears as chaos in nature is really not chaos and works well within a well-regulated law. It is, possibly, constraints imposed by time and space that create barriers in entirely understanding nature.

cymatic therapy (New Age) A form of SOUND THERAPY, as developed in 1960s in England by Peter Guy Manners, in which hand-held instruments are used to transmit sound waves—not through the auditory channels, but directly through the skin. The method aimed at boosting the body's regulatory and immunologic systems. It is believed that the sound could re-establish healthy resonance in unhealthy tissues and organs. The therapy is also based on the belief that life is sound and that every part of the body vibrates at a unique frequency.

> 'Every object, whether inanimate or alive, possesses a unique electro-magnetic field that exhibits antagonistic, complementary (resonant) or neutral reactions, when it interacts with other electro-magnetic fields.'
>
> —Peter Guy Manners

cymatics (Mod.) From the Greek *kyma*, meaning great wave. It is the study of the structure and dynamics of waves and vibrations, pioneered by Hans Jenny (1904–72), a Swiss medical doctor. It is believed that cymatic sound frequencies support the body's natural healing processes, particularly in arthritis, back pain, digestive problems, fractures, ligament damage, muscular problem, nerve injury and sprains.

D

dactyliomancy (Am.Ind./Occ.) A method of DIVINATION using a ring tied to a length of thread and suspended over a board or an object to divine the answer to yes-and-no questions. The idea is to let a ring swing from one's hand by a string or human hair over a circle, often the rim of a wide vase, on which letters are written. The swinging of the ring spells out the answers to questions. While Malaysians used lemons, the Cherokees used ancient arrow-heads. The ouija board is its modern version.

da huang (Chi.) *Rheum palmatum*. Also, Chinese rhubarb, Turkish rhubarb. A medicinal herb known for its laxative properties.

dadima See POMEGRANATE.

daimon (Grk.) 1. Divine power 2. Fate or God. 3. Intermediary spirits between human beings and the gods.

dalima See POMEGRANATE.

damp cold-sheet pack (Nat.) A simple method of wrapping the body in a damp, cold sheet. Wrapping in cold sheets is an ancient method to bring down the body temperature to normal levels. This method is also traditionally employed in the treatment of nervousness, skin ailments and muscular problems. It works as a tonic and sedative.

dance-movement therapy See DANCE THERAPY.

dance therapy (New Age) Based on the premise that creative arts help in healing. The bodily movements of dance and mental engagement in music are traditionally known for their therapeutic impact. A therapist well-versed in these can employ the same to help people alter their bad moods or depression. Such work-outs with individuals, families or groups can help improve self-esteem, communication skills and social interactions. Dance movement therapy is based on the belief that movement reflects an individual's pattern of thinking and feeling. It can help those with emotional problems, conflict or distress. See also MUSIC THERAPY.

dance yoga (New Age) A relaxation exercise which combines conscious dance postures and movements. It combines free dance, trance dance, GUIDED IMAGERY, music therapy, gentle humour and MEDITATION. The aim is often to enjoy an aerobic workout without the tedium that may be associated with exercise. See PANEURHYTHMIY.

> 'Dance is the mother of all arts.'
>
> —Gunther Sachs

dancercize (New Age) An aerobic workout to upbeat music with the steps and choreography derived from contemporary dance. The method is aimed at helping improve one's range of motion, endurance, aerobic capacity, flexibility, and strength. Dancing is known to foster mind–body coordination and confidence-building and is stress-reducing.

dandasana (Yoga) Recommended for people with arthritis and rheumatism of the knees and ankles, the practise of this ASANA is aimed at enhancing emotional stability and will-power.

dang gui See ANGELICA ROOT.

Daniel's diet (New Age) A diet for detoxification and weight-loss. The programme excludes all foods other than avocados, dark-green vegetable juices, herbal teas, lemons, lime, millets, nuts, oils, sea salt, soaked and sprouted seeds, tofu, tomatoes and vegetables in addition to certain specific dietary supplements (such as pycnogenol, liquid lightning oxygen, Oç). Named after a legendary Jewish prophet who refused to eat meat and wines offered by the king of Babylon, but ate vegetables and water and remained healthy and strong, Daniel's diet became popular in the late-twentieth century among the health conscious. It is based on the premise that the excessive consumption of sugar and animal proteins causes 'over acidification' which is the root-cause for a plethora of ailments.

danta dhavanam (Ind.) The use of aromatic plants and their parts in oral hygiene.

dan tien (Chi.) Also, tan tien. The energy centre, an inch and a half below the navel, visualized as a golden ball, representing will-power. A Chinese martial artiste draws his power to break concrete barriers from this centre. It is also said to be used by healers for mustering healing power; when used in healing, dan tien is said to turn red and hot and healers also feel intense heat. The heat raised by dan tien, used for drawing energy for protection as well as for charging, is traced to the molten core of the earth, as it is considered to be in harmony with the sound of the core of the earth.

According to tradition, there are other dan tiens as well, including the middle dan tien or the soul-seat, located two and a half inches below the hollow in the throat and visualized as a diffused light around a candle and said to carry the soul's longing. It is said to have a clear, spherical appearance, distinct from the heart chakra. Meditation involves feeling the laser line, which goes from the soul-seat down through the dan tien in the pelvis, into the core of the earth. As one feels this current surge, one proceeds to the steps: bringing awareness to the point above one's head, straightening the spine, imagining a fine thread running through the top of one's head, on which the head is imagined to be hanging, reaching one's mind's eye to the imaginary opening (about a quarter inch in diameter), about three feet above the head and hearing a very high-pitched sound as one sends a laser line through that hole. The whole exercise is said to integrate the self with the godhead or undifferentiated being in the universe. Feeling the laser beam (half the width of one's little finger), going from the godhead to the molten core of the earth through one's own soul-seat is said to bridge heaven and earth, giving the practitioner powerful insight.

This experience can also be synchronized with the participation of many dedicated practitioners as a group in a hall; the laser line is said to pass through the centre of the hall, to which the participants feel connected from their dan tien. This is said to be the way to get connected to the power and truth of a system, within a system which too is within a greater system, leading towards universal alignment. By subjugating oneself, the system takes care of the problems of an individual who is not to struggle nor worry about life's ups and downs.

Dao in Also, Dao yin tu. An early major text on QIGONG, dao yin is also an ancient wsord for QIGONG.

Daoist chi kung See TAOIST QI GONG.

daphnomancy (Eur.) DIVINATION, with a branch of laurel. If the branch crackles in fire, it is taken as a good omen.

dasamula (Ind.) A set of ten medicinal roots, used in ayurvedic decoctions. The roots include BAEL, Malay bushbeech, AGNIMANTHA, patala, sonapatha, Indian nightshade, the white-fruited variety of the same plant, salaparni, prashni parni and GOKSHURA.

dasamularishta (Ind.) An ayurvedic decoction made from DASAMULA, used in the treatment of digestive problems and general weakness.

day spa (New Age) An establishment that provides a tranquil atmosphere with facilities for beautifying, relaxing and pampering clients with herbs, COSMECEUTICALS and naturopathic treatments, including aerobics, diet and fasting, HYDROTHERAPY, MASSAGE and MUSIC THERAPY for an entire day.

dayan qigong (Chi.) Also, wild goose. 1. A form of QIGONG. 2. A traditional breathing exercise, named after the wild goose and developed in China during the twelfth and thirteenth centuries. Long kept a closely guarded secret, teachers of this system were traditionally at least seventy years old; possibly, this stipulation is the reason for its limited appeal.

The exercise comprises two sets of sixty-four movements, all of which look like the postures of a wild goose in flight. The goose's great energy and strength help it undertake long migrations across continents—dayan qigong incorporates many movements (e.g., slow, fluid movements coupled with strong, quick movements) that simulate a goose's stance. Some of the faster movements act to directly stimulate acupoints; a stronger surge of energy clears the area and ensures a freer pathway for it to flow.

While performing the wild goose, it is recommended that the breath is centred in the lower abdomen and remains deep and even. This exercise is believed to help slow ageing.

Dead Sea-mud treatment (New Age) The application of mineral-rich mud from the Dead Sea for the detoxification of the skin and body and to relieve pain caused by arthritis and rheumatism. The therapeutic value of the black mud of the Dead Sea is so legendary that Mark Anthony is said to have conquered the Dead Sea for the sake of Cleopatra's needs.

deadly nightshade See BELLADONNA.

death (Misc.) 1. The end of life. 2. The final cessation of vital functions in the body. 3. A mythological figure who has existed in popular culture since the earliest days of story-telling. 4. The traditional Western image of Death, as the Grim Reaper, is personified as a skeleton, wearing black robes and carrying a scythe.

Death was once defined as the ceasing of the heartbeat and of breathing—this is now often referred to as clinical death. This definition has now, however, become obsolete, as with the advent of sophisticated equipment, a person can be kept alive on life-support devices such as heart and lung machines and cardiac pacemakers. People are now considered dead when the electrical activity in the brain stops—this condition is referred to as brain death or biological death. It is presumed that a cessation of electrical activity indicates the end of consciousness. It is also likely now that the criterion for death will be the permanent and irreversible loss of cognitive function, as occurs with the death of the cerebral cortex. In this circumstance, there is no hope of recovering brain function; oxygen deprivation for about seven minutes is enough to kill the cerebral cortex.

According to Hindu belief, death refers to the detachment of the soul from the physical body and its continuing existence in subtle realms with the same desires, aspirations and occupations in the subtle body. Death is considered by Hindus as an exalted experience, full of spiritual potential.

> 'It's not Death, a man should fear; but he should fear never beginning to live!'
>
> —Marcus Aurelius

death, determination of (Misc.) Death is sometimes difficult to determine. EEGs are known to detect spurious electrical impulses when none exist, as there have also been cases in which electrical activity in a living brain was so low that EEGs cannot detect it. Because of this, hospitals often have elaborate protocols for determining death involving EEGs at widely separated intervals. There are many anecdotal references to people coming to life after being declared dead by physicians. Stories of people actually being buried alive led one inventor in the early-twentieth century to design an alarm system, with a bell and a cord that could be pulled from inside the coffin. Persons certified to be dead and lying on the funeral pyre have also been known, though rarely, to get up and walk away!

> 'His voice goes into his mind; his mind into his breath; his breath into heat; the heat into the highest divinity.'
>
> —*Chandogya Upanishad,* describing the moment of death

death chart (Misc.) A horoscope figure, constructed for arriving at the date or time of death.

death panorama (Misc.) The out-of-body experience of the newly departed soul after death; a flashback of the events of life, as seen after death.

death, physiological (Misc.) In the human body, the physiological consequences of death follow a recognized sequence, viz., the cooling of the body soon after death (*algor mortis*), becoming pallid (*pallor mortis*), the relaxation of the internal sphincter muscles leading to the release of urine, faeces and other stomach contents, and the movement of the blood towards the lowest parts (*livor mortis*), followed by its coagulation and stiffening of muscles (*rigor mortis*). Within a day, the body starts decaying both from autolytic changes and from the attacking organisms and scavengers such as microbes, insects and mammals. As the body structure collapses internally, the skin loses its integration with underlying tissues. Bacterial action generating gases causes bloating and swelling. The rate of decay is variable, depending on several factors. Thus, a body may be reduced to skeletal remains in days, though it is possible under certain conditions for it to stay largely intact for several years.

death prayer (Occ.) 1. The shadow side of prayers. 2. A special technique designed and practised by witch doctors to deprive a person of life.

> 'Between grief and nothing, I'll take grief.'
> —William Faulkner

decimal scale (Hom.) A scale that measures the potency of homoeopathic remedies in which the presence of the original drug substance is 1 in 10. In the decimal scale, the dilutions and triturations are prepared in the proportion of one part of the medicine to nine parts of the media. (i.e. water, alcohol or lactose). The decimal scale is denoted by the letters X or D. Hence 1X or ID means the given medicine contains 1 part of the original drug substance and 9 parts of the vehicle. 2X or 2D means the remedy is 1/100 times diluted, 3X or 3D means it is 1/1000 times diluted, 6X or 6D means it is 1/106 times diluted, and 12X or 12D means a dilution of 1/1012 times diluted.

deepan (Ind.) Gastrointestinal vitality, often referred to as 'digestive fire'.

deep breathing (Yoga) An ancient yogic technique to induce relaxation and healthy feelings. Each deep breath consists of a complete and full inhalation through the nose and a deep, steady exhalation also through the nose. In a recent study, Italian researchers working with cardiac patients concluded that a breath rate of six breaths per minute can be considered the optimum breath rate. As compared to the average resting breath rate (twelve–fourteen times a minute), this represents a substantial reduction in breath rate. Patients who learn to slow down their breathing through special deep-breathing exercises reported higher levels of blood oxygen and were able to perform better on exercise tests. See also PRANAYAMA.

deep emotional release bodywork (New Age) Also, DERB. A system of holistic healing, developed by musician Jim Hyman, based on the notion that damaging experiences, including anxieties, fears, phobias and traumas get 'locked' into the emotional centres of the body and that their unlocking ensures the cure. Various techniques, such as QIGONG empowerment, DEEP EMOTIONAL BREATHWORK and EMOTIONAL RELEASE are employed here for releasing such blocked energy. Releasing it from the body and the subconscious mind is believed to help in achieving freedom from worry, pain and suffering, and leading towards joy.

deepener (New Age) Any visual, auditory, or kinesthetic device used to increase a person's level of trance, including colours, numbers, letters, or silences.

deepening (New Age) 1. In hypnosis, attaining a more profound trance state. 2. A process that makes someone who is in hypnosis more suggestible. We don't really go deeper, we become more suggestible when we are in the state of hypnosis.

deep-muscle massage (New Age) Also, Pfrimmer deep-muscle therapy. A technique of massage, created by Therese Pfrimmer in the 1940s when she discovered that massaging her own leg muscles in a deep way led to the reversal of her own paralysis. Pfrimmer deep-muscle therapy is designed to encourage corrective changes to damaged muscles and to the adjacent soft tissues. It works across the muscles, manipulating deep tissues, stimulating circulation and regenerating lymphatic flow. It also facilitates the release of entrapped nerves, as it aids in dispelling toxins and congestion accumulated in damaged muscles, thus reducing oedema and inflammation and reducing pain. The therapy is said to help in the treatment of multiple sclerosis, muscular dystrophy, Parkinson's, cerebral palsy, brain injury and stroke. It has also been found effective in the treatment of injuries, arthritis, fibrositis, neck tension and chronic fatigue.

deep relaxation (Mod./New Age) An anti-stress approach, aimed at being intimately connected to deep calm and relaxation. Since the digestive process can be an impediment, the exercise is initiated two hours after a meal. The steps include choosing a quiet place and comfortable time, finding a relaxed position, closing the eyes (but not sleeping), tuning into one's muscles and relaxing them one by one–starting from the legs to the forehead through the torso, arms, shoulders, neck, mouth, cheeks, nose, temples and eyes, tuning into one's breathing, saying a word or mantra silently while exhaling, focussing on the word or mantra to keep all thoughts at bay, continuing breathing while focussing on the word or mantra and relaxing one's muscles for at least twenty minutes.

deep-tissue massage (New Age) A technique of massage which is directed towards the deeper tissues in the muscle. This kind of massage is considered useful in the treatment of neuro-musculo-skeletal problems such as facial restriction, muscle length imbalances, ischaemia, strain injuries and repetitive stress injuries.

deism (Misc.) 1. A doctrine, based on a belief in the existence of God and based on purely rational grounds. 2. A particular faith prominent in the seventeenth and eighteenth centuries and adhered to by several American Presidents, including Benjamin Franklin and Thomas Jefferson. It holds that God created the world and its natural laws but is not involved in its functioning.

delta waves (Mod.) 1. The state of mind encountered during deep sleep. 2. Total unconsciousness. 3. A type of BRAIN WAVES, with lowest frequencies of 0.1–4Hz. Delta waves are said to be involved with our ability to integrate and let go, as it reflects the unconscious mind. Most people diagnosed with Attention Deficit Disorder have increased delta activity when trying to focus, as if the brain is locked into a perpetual drowsy state.

demispan (Mod.) An alternative to height measurement, particularly in elderly people who might have lost height due to vertebral collapse. It is the distance between the sternal notch and the roots of the middle and third fingers with the arms stretched out at shoulder height to the side of the body. Demispan, so arrived at, is used for calculating the height, as per the formula given below:

Calculation of height from demispan:

Females

height in cm =

$(1.35 \times \text{demispan (cm)}) + 60.1$

Males

height in cm =

$(1.40 \times \text{demispan (cm)}) + 57.8$

demon (Eur./Occ.) A low-level spirit associated with evil. Seven sins attributed to demons are shown in the following table:

Demon	The deadly sin with which the demon is associated
Lucifer	pride
Mammon	avarice
Asmodeus	lechery
Satan	anger
Beelzebub	gluttony
Leviathan	envy
Belphegor	sloth

demonomancy (Eur./Occ.) A method of DIVINATION, using demons.

depth hypnosis (New Age) A healing modality, as developed by Isa Gucciardi, necessitating the patient's working in an altered state achieved through HYPNOSIS, MEDITATION or SHAMANIC JOURNEYING.

dermatron (Mod./New Age) An electroacupuncture device. Electro-acupuncture devices like the Dermatron, VEGA tester and MORA are widely used in Europe and Japan. Researchers in Russia and eastern Europe are further advanced in the development of diagnostic and treatment devices based on electro-acupuncture and BIOFEEDBACK, and the health of Russian cosmonauts in space is now also reported to be monitored and appropriately balanced using such devices.

descending sun (New Age) A form of VISUAL THERAPY, based on the technique of IMAGINEERING, believed to be helpful in focussing one's attention on the source of healing within the body.

desensitization (Mod./New Age) A method adopted by behaviour therapists drawn from ancient techniques such as YOGA NIDRA in which the clients are first relaxed deeply and then, over a period of time, gradually exposed to tense situations.

destination spa (New Age/Spa) Spa services and establishments which provide for lifestyle improvements, health enhancement and self-renewal in the company of the like-minded people through professionally administered cuisines, physical fitness and educational programming.

destiny 1. The final outcome. 2. The seemingly inevitable or predetermined course of events.

detoxification (Ind./New Age) Also, detox. The removal from the body of toxins which might have accumulated as a result of addictive habits or ageing. Toxins are also produced by invading microbes and other parasites and by pollutants and chemicals in the atmosphere leading to infections which impair the body's immune and autonomous nervous systems. Through safe and effective detoxification processes, toxins can be eliminated from the body.

development counselling A COUNSELLING technique, focussing on an individual rather than an issue. It is a time-consuming measure as it aims at drastic behavioural changes in the client's attitude, not only towards his or her own self but also towards others.

devil's dung See ASAFOETIDA.

devil's stone See ARGENTUM NITRICUM.

Dhanavantari (Ind.) The legendary Hindu physician of the gods, believed to have carried ambrosia from the primeval ocean. He is also considered mankind's teacher of medicine.

dhanurasana (Yoga) This ASANA is believed to impart greater flexibility to the limbs and back and reduce obesity.

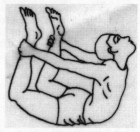

Dhanurasana

dhanyaka See CORIANDER.

dhara (Ind.) A technique of pouring down, in a steady stream, liquids such as medicated oil, milk, buttermilk and ghee, over the forehead of the patient, aimed at relieving mental tension.

dharana (Ind.) 1. Concentration 2. Inward concentration, the sixth of the eight 'limbs' prescribed by PATANJALI. Some yogic exercises, conducive for the enhancement of inner concentration are indicated in the following table:

Exercise	Meaning
nau-mukhi	shutting down of the 'nine gates'
sakti-chalini	conducting the 'thought force'

sambhavi	'lotus of Parvati'
amritpan	quaffing of 'nectar'
chakra-bhedan	piercing the chakras
sushumna-darshan	visualizing the chakras
prana-ahuti	infusing the 'vital breath'
utthan	raising the kundalini
swaroopa-darshan	visualizing the Self
linga-sanchalana	astral conduction

'An intellectual is someone whose mind watches itself.'

—Albert Camus

dharma (Yoga) 1. The duty of an individual 2. The law of being 3. Virtue 4. The righteous way of living 5. One of the four PURUSHARTHAS.

'A man's defects are the faults of his time, but virtues are his own.'

—Johann W. von Goethe

dhatri See AMLAKI.

dhatu (Ind.) The basic structural and nutritional body factor which supports and nourishes the seven body tissues, as indicated in the following table:

The seven dhatus are normally nourished by the daily intake of food. But with improper nourishment, the need for rejuvenation therapies and remedies has arisen. AYURVEDA stresses on the daily need of nutrients and a healthy lifestyle to remain healthy and achieve overall balance.

Dhatu	Equivalent term in English
rasa	plasma
rakta	blood
mamsa	muscles
meda	fat and adipose
asthi	bones
majja	nerves
sukla	reproductive cells and tissues

dhatvagni (Ind.) The digestive juices or enzymes that convert food nutrients into bodily tissues (DHATUs).

dhauti (Yoga) Also, dhouti. A mode of cleaning the alimentary canal, using a long muslin cloth, about four fingers wide and fifteen feet long.

dhenu mudra (Yoga) Formed by putting together fingers in such a way as to imitate the udder of a cow, this MUDRA is one of the five mudras made while presenting an offering to an image in Hindu rituals.

dhi (Yoga) 1. Intellect 2. The aspect of SATTVA that imparts the ability to conceive and imagine.

dhouti See DHAUTI.

dhroni (Ind.) A smooth, narrow wooden plank often used as a bed for body massage. The plank is designed to match, more or less, the body contours of the clients.

dhumra-paana (Ind.) Tapers or pastilles of medicinal leaves and substances, lit for inhaling their smoke.

dhupana (Ind.) An ancient Indian method of fumigation, aimed at sterilizing the atmosphere by burning pastilles of medicinal herbs.

dhyana (Yoga) 1. Ideating 2. A state of meditation, the seventh 'limb' of the eight-limbed yoga of PATANJALI.

'Dhyana is the uninterrupted flow of concentration of the mind on an object.'

—Sage Patanjali

Dhyana Yoga (Yoga) From the Sanskrit, for perfect contemplation. A system of yoga, considered the abstract, profound and unitive discipline of MEDITATION, DHYANA forms the 'seventh limb' of ASHTANGA YOGA of Patanjali.

diagnostic methods in alternative medicine (Mod./New Age) Several diagnostic methods such as interrogation, observations, TONGUE DIAGNOSIS, PULSE-DIAGNOSIS, ABDOMINAL TOUCH, URINE ANALYSIS, DOWSING, RADIONICS, AURA-ANALYSIS, KIRLIAN PHOTOGRAPHY, muscle-testing (APPLIED KINESIOLOGY), IRIDOLOGY, REFLEXOLOGY, hair analysis and the use of VEGA or MORA devices are employed in alternative medicine for detecting ailments.

diamond (Gem) A precious stone, remarkable for extreme hardness. It is believed that diamond fortifies the mind and body and cures many ailments.

> 'It is better to have an old second-hand diamond than none at all.'
>
> —Mark Twain

dianetic therapy See DIANETICS.

dianetics (Mod.) Also, dianetic therapy. A therapeutic method through which psychological trauma is lessened by repeated recall of the traumatic incident.

diaphragmatic breathing (Yoga) The natural rhythmic breathing which allows full expansion of the lungs. Recent research seems to show that there is a relationship between upper chest breathing and heart attacks. According to Donna Farhi, patients who have had heart attacks were subsequently taught how to integrate diaphragmatic breathing into their daily lives, significantly reducing their chances of having second heart attacks. Another study showed that all 153 patients of a coronary unit breathed predominantly through their chests. Learning deep, diaphragmatic breathing is protective of the heart to a great extent. See also, DEEP BREATHING.

dian xue an mo (Jap.) A system of body massage focussed on acupuncture cavities in the body.

didgeridoo vibrational healing (Aus.) An Australian aboriginal method of using the sound of a didgeridoo for healing people. A didgeridoo is a horn-like wind instrument, over three feet long, made of a hollowed, petrified bark of eucalyptus. Its sound is visualized so as to expand one's AURA.

diet 1. Habitual food 2. Prescribed course of food 3. Way of feeding. Eastern medical systems acknowledge the role of diet in restoring health for the diseased.

> 'Animals that have hoofs but not cloven and that are ruminant... those four-footed animals which walk on the fiat of their paws... any creature which swarms on the ground... do not defile yourself with them.'
>
> —Leviticus, 11:3–43.

> 'Eat, drink and be merry, for tomorrow ye diet.'
>
> —Lewis C. Henry

dietary fibre (Mod./New Age) The bulk and roughage in the diet, considered an essential part of a healthy diet.

dietary therapy (Mod./New Age) The therapeutic application of diet, which has been an essential component in all ancient medical interventions of the East.

> 'Another good reducing exercise consists in placing both hands against the table edge and pushing back.'
>
> —Robert Quillen

dietetics (Mod./New Age) The study and regulation of diets to achieve optimum health.

digitalis purpurea (Hom.) Also, digit. A homoeopathic remedy to overcome anxiety.

diksha (Yoga) 1. Initiation 2. The act and condition of solemn induction into a new realm of awareness and practices by a teacher through the bestowing of blessings and transmission of PRANA. 3. A deepened connection with the teacher and his lineage, usually accompanied by a solemn ceremony.

dimensional clearing (New Age/Vib.) A method aimed at clearing off the 'external elements' (also called thought forms, lost souls, and fragments) from the human energy field. Elements are considered the real cause of all ailments, and eliminating them through dimensional clearing is believed to make one healthy or cured.

Dimond, Prof. E. Gray An American heart specialist who popularized ACUPUNCTURE ANALGESIA in the West.

dinacharya (Ind.) Daily routine prescribed in AYURVEDA for maintaining good health.

The routine includes an appropriate diet (with reference to its quantity, quality and frequency), besides appropriate physical exercises and hygiene.

dipaniya (Ind.) Natural substances that kindle the gastric fire and augment the appetite.

direct command (New Age) A method of self-healing, wherein one repeatedly orders one's own subconscious, one's body and its parts as, for example, in 'get well soon'. It is based on the notion that an active mind makes one's intent understandable to bodily parts.

directed esoteric toning (New Age/Yoga) A form of TONING in which vowel sounds are combined with PRANA-carrying breath which is believed to result in the opening up of specific zones in body consciousness. Different vowel sounds, attributed with different effects, are indicated in the following table:

Vowel sounds	Pronounced as in	Probable impact
uu	woo	depth, relaxation
oh	go	self-confidence
ah	raw	expansion, pleasant disposal
ey	ray	communication, self-expression
ee	tree	awakening, energy
Mm	(nasal)	power, harmony

> 'The vocal nourishment that a mother provides to her child is just as important to the child's development as her milk.'
>
> —Alfred Tomatis

direct image substitution (New Age) A self-healing technique that amounts to visualizing oneself or a particular part of oneself as normal, healthy and functional. In other words, it refers to picturing, for example, an injured thumb as already healed and healthy.

direct moxibustion (Chi.) A technique of MOXIBUSTION in which small cones of MOXA, a dried herb, are placed on specific ACUPOINTS and burnt almost to the skin. This may have some undesirable side-effects, including burn marks, blisters and scars. The main effect of direct moxibustion is considered to result from actual damage to the skin, by which the release of immunological mediators is said to be stimulated. The effectiveness of direct moxibustion, particularly on immune function, has been endorsed by Shimetaro Hara (1927) of the Kyushu University, Japan.

In an attempt to prevent skin damage, slices of ginger or topical paste are also sometimes used between the skin and burning moxa. According to some experts, however, this deviation, categorized as INDIRECT MOXIBUSTION, has not been found to be as effective as the scarring direct moxibustion. See also, MOXIBUSTION.

direct suggestion (New Age) Suggestions given as commands have been considered therapeutic from ancient times. Hypnotic suggestion, for instance, is given directly, rather than in a covert way, to enhance its efficacy. Direct suggestions are found useful in several areas, including habit change, pain management, sports performance, in improving one's image, behaviour and confidence.

direct therapy (New Age) The administering by a therapist of positive suggestions and thoughts, conducive to healing. The idea is that such positive words and suggestions find acceptance in a patient's mind. This method is common, particularly in the treatment of addiction, nervous problems and pain.

directionology (Eur./Occ.) A method of DIVINATION, using direction.

directive hypnotherapy (New Age) A technique of HYPNOTHERAPY, characterized by direct and post-hypnotic suggestions to the patients. The therapist essentially orders the client to get into a trance state. See also, DIRECT SUGGESTION.

disease (Misc.) Also, vyadhi. Illness or ill-health. Fundamentally, disease represents imbalance, the consequences of the breakdown of homoeostatic control mechanisms of an organism.

According to PATANJALI, disease is the first of nine obstacles that comes in the way of any YOGA practise.

discernment (Misc.) Self-evaluation of information as opposed to 'blind-faith'. Using discernment is said to involve connecting to one's inner knowledge, before accepting any information or suggestion given by others (including healers). In other words, discernment can also mean following one's instincts.

distant diagnosis See TELEDIAGNOSIS.

distant healing (Vib.) Also, absent treatment. The transmission, from a distance, of PRANA energy from the healer to a receiver. As long as the receiver is willing to receive such energy from the healer, distance involved is considered immaterial. In distant-healing sessions, often a mutually-agreed-upon time and date is fixed well in advance. The healer develops a mental image that his prana is leaving him as he exhales and travels across the long distance which separates him from the receiver. He also visualizes the completion of such transmission. At the end of the session, the healer often recharges his prana, by practising KUMBHAKA. See TELE-THERAPY.

distant pranic healing (Vib.) A technique of PRANIC HEALING dealt with by Chok Kok Sui (1990) in his book *Pranic Healing*. See also DISTANT HEALING.

distant reiki (Vib.) A technique of REIKI in which the healer operates from a place at a distance from his patient. Reiki healers believe that the distance between the healer and the receiver in no way affects the efficacy of the system and that the remote energy healing technique is as effective as hands-on treatment.

divination (Eur./Occ.) An age-old practice of predicting the future, using supernatural sources. The practice has a formal, ritualistic character, and was used by witches, wizards, sorcerers, shamans and medicine men. Called diviners, practitioners of divination often belonged to a class of priests trained in the practise and interpretation of their divinatory skills.

Divination is based on natural phenomena, such as unexpected stormy weather, sudden cloud formations, birth aberrations, the howling of animals and nightmares, or the observation and interpretations of manmade predictive systems such as NECRO-MANCY, using TAROT cards and pouring oil into a trough of water to observe the formation of shapes

divine healing See FAITH HEALING.

divine healing from Japan (Jap./Vib.) A technique of hands-on healing as practised by Tadamasa Fukaya.

divine-will healing (New Age) An approach to healing, based on the teachings of Paramahansa Yogananda (1893–1952), whose main postulate was that people can transmit or project the divine healing light by aligning their will with the divine will. The method was popularized by Ram Smith, of the Ananda Church of Self Realization.

> 'There are two ways to live your life. One is as though nothing is a miracle. The other is as though everything is a miracle!'
>
> —Albert Einstein

divining See DOWSING.

divya See GUGGULU.

doctrine of signature (Flo.) The medieval concept that nature provides clues about the diseases which specific plants cure. According to this concept, plant parts that resemble specific body organs contain remedies that can act on ailments related to such organs. For instance, roots which resemble the male sexual organ (e.g., ashwagandha, ginger, and ginseng) were traditionally believed to work as aphrodisiacs. The heart-shaped leaves of some medicinal plant and liver-shaped liverworts were found to possess curative properties for diseases of the heart and liver respectively.

do-in 1. A combination of MERIDIAN stretching exercises, breathing exercises, CHI exercises and self-massage. 2. A traditional exercise for physical and spiritual development. 3. A do-it-yourself ACUPRESSURE massage for self-stimulation. Practising do-in is believed to increase the awareness of one's own energy, for self-treatment and to groom one to become a good SHIATSU therapist.

A shiatsu therapist is required to use his body without becoming tense himself. He has to feel the energy of the patient without feeling his own tension. Do-in and meditation are said to inculcate such qualities.

dolphin-assisted therapy A method of using dolphins to promote healthy feelings. The Human Dolphin Therapy Centre in Florida was founded on the premise that dolphins can trigger a great deal of positive and healing energy as they touch humans.

dong gong (Chi.) One of two types of QIGONG (CHI KUNG). Dong gong concerns dynamic body movements, and is distinguished from the other category, jing gong, which focusses on the meditative aspect of qigong.

Dong Hai Chuang See BAGUAZHANG.

dong quai See ANGELICA ROOT.

dosha (Ind.) 1. The body-type categorized on the basis of metabolic characteristics 2. Bodily humour, a governing principle for life, interpreted as a deficiency that contaminates the cosmic rhythm. 3. Individual constitution 4. Functional intelligence within the body responsible for all physiological and psychological processes and changes within an organism. Ayurveda distinguishes three types of doshas (TRIDOSHA): VATA, PITTA and KAPHA.

The nature and functions of the three doshas are summarized in the following table:

Dosha	Vata	Pitta	Kapha
Nature (general characteristics)	dry, cold, light, irregular, mobile, rarefied, rough	fluid, hot, light, clear, soft, subtle, sharp, malodorous	oily, cold, heavy, stable, dense, smooth
Seat (location in human body)	intestinal area, colon, bones, ears, hips, large intestines, pelvic cavity, skin and thighs	stomach area, brain, eyes, heart, liver, skin and stomach	lung area, mucus and in body structures (e.g., bones, cartilages, fats, joints, muscles)
Manifestation	movements (e.g., circulation of air, blood, food, nerve impulses, waste elimination, thought processes). Vata is related to the sensation of touch.	dynamism (e.g., control of, regulation of metabolic processes, transformation of electro-chemical sensory inputs into information and thoughts in the brain)	architecture (e.g., cells, tissues, organs regulation and other bodily fluids)
Regulation and control	breathing, movements in the muscles and tissues, movements of nerve impulses, all kinds of expansion and contraction, natural urges, sensory functions, nerve impulses, secretions, excretions, fear, anxiety, thoughts. It governs such feelings and emotions as	body temperature, hunger, thirst, anger, hate, jealousy, intelligence, perception and understanding	stability, lubrication, energy, greed, attachment, possessiveness, accumulation, forgiveness

	anxiety, fear, freshness, nervousness, pain, spasms and tremor		
When in excess	gas, high blood pressure, nerve irritation, confusion	anaemia, blindness, cataract, digestive disturbances, hormonal disturbances, jaundice, mental disorders (e.g., anger), skin ailments (e.g., acne) and ulcers	mucus build-up in sinus, nasal passage, lungs and colon; rigidity and inflexibility, fixation of thought
When in shortage	constipation, thoughtlessness	indigestion, sluggish metabolism, inability to understand	dryness in respiratory tract, burning stomach, inability to concentrate
Ideal climate	dry climates or cold autumn	hot climates	wet climates or damp weather
Seasons affecting dosha	fall and winter	summer	autumn and winter
Age-group	old age, which shows a tendency to shrink and wither.	teenage, when hormonal changes lead to growth and development	early parts of life when the body grows
Concentration in plant parts	parts that reach to the 'air' and 'space' (e.g., leaves, flowers)	sap, essential oils, gums, resins, aromatics	parts that reach to the 'earth' and 'water' (e.g., roots, root-stocks)
Energy-type	metabolic nerve energy	catabolic, fire energy	anabolic, nutritive energy
Corresponding quality (guna)	quiescence (sattva)	activity (rajas)	inertia (tamas)

douches (Eur./Nat.) Hot and cold water sprays on specific areas/parts of the body, usually for cleansing. They are rarely used for treating ailments. Several kinds of douches were popularized in Europe by Vincent Preissnitz, a naturopath, in the nineteenth century.

dowser (Occ.) A person specialized in DOWSING.

dowsing (Occ./Vib.) Also, divining, radiesthesia, rhabdomancy, water divining, water witching. 1. The practice of locating underground water with a forked stick. 2. The traditional use of a forked piece of hazel, rowan, willow wood or metal rod or of a pendulum suspended by a nylon or silk thread for detecting hidden substances (minerals, treasures, archaeological remnants or dead bodies) 3. A method for gaining insight into unmanifested physical and emotional health problems. Dowsing is also used to determine answers to questions such as the sex of an unborn child, the location of pipes, or for foretelling the future.

Numerous instruments are used by dowsers, including scissors, pliers, crowbars, and even German sausages. Perhaps, the three most common instruments used are the forked stick (Y-rod), pendulum, and the L-shaped stick (L-rod).

Some dowsers, however, do not employ any of these. They experience bodily sensations such as heat in their palms or a sharp pain in the back to address the problem. There are also reports that indicate that animals also show certain abilities to find hidden objects.

Several explanations have been offered to explain how dowsers get results. Debunkers claim that dowsers are little more than good practical geologists. Some suggest that a dowser may occasionally exercise the maximum powers of human observation (e.g., he may note the colour of soil and vegetation, slight differences in growth of plants, such as direction of root structure), and that he processes all this information and moves the dowsing instrument accordingly at an unconscious level. While this is a 'normal inference' explanation, a second explanation is that dowsers react to known radiations (e.g. electro-magnetic) in a little-understood way—this is often called the physical theory. A third, psychical explanation is that the dowser uses some form of ESP.

In contrast to the biophysical investigations just discussed, there is considerable agreement among studies of the physiology of dowsing. Various anecdotal reports indicate that some good dowsers become dizzy or sick while standing over underground water.

Dr Lynch's holistic self-health programme (New Age) An approach to healing, designed by James P.B. Lynch, a chiropractor, based on the notion that everyone possesses 'innate powers', usable for self-healing. The cornerstone of the programme and lifestyle, referred to by Lynch as the holistic triangle, consists of: a) a mental/spiritual base of education, moti-vation, and self-love; b) a physical side, which focusses on exercise and physical treatment; and c) a chemical side, which involves 'detoxification' through diet.

dragon qi gong See EIGHTEEN LOHAN TI-GER.

drakshasava (Ind.) An AYURVEDIC formulation containing red grapes and several other medicinal ingredients, including cinnamon, cardamom, black pepper and tail pepper, used traditionally to improve diges-tion. It is also said to be an effective cough remedy.

drava swedana (Ind.) 1. The use of hot liquids and compresses to promote perspiration 2. A detoxification method.

drawing (Mod.) A technique to draw out poisonous substances, such as pus, from ab-scesses and boils.

dream analysis (New Age) The analysis of dreams to interpret a meaning or forecast an event. See also DREAM INTERPRETATION.

dream interpretation (Mod./New Age) The process of assigning meaning to a dream experience. Some traditional inter-preters assign specific meaning by making future predictions (ONEIROMANCY). Dream in-terpretation also formed a part of psycho-analysis in the late-nineteenth century. Sigmund Freud's seminal work on the sub-ject drew worldwide interest on dream inter-pretation.

dreamcatcher (Am./Ind.) A willow hoop, woven by native Americans in the form of spider webs, believed to catch night-mares so as to protect the dreamer.

dreamwork (New Age) An enquiry into dreams aimed at self-healing. See DREAM IN-TERPRETATION.

dreamworkers (New Age) Practitioners of DREAMWORK.

drop (New Age) Also, drop into, dropping. A commonly used herb by hypnotists to de-note going into hypnotic trance.

drumming (Misc.) Rhythms and beats used in community congregations to pro-mote fellow-feelings and emotional and spiritual release. Dances accompanying such rhythms are said to enhance the effect.

dry brush (Spa) A brush made of natural

bristles, used to remove dead skin and impurities. It also helps in stimulating circulation. Dry brush is one of many exfoliating techniques often used before applying mud or seaweed body masks in spas.

dugdha neti (Ind.) Nasal irrigation, in which milk is used for cleansing the nasal passage. See also NETI.

dukha (Yoga) Suffering, a fundamental fact of life, caused, according to AYURVEDA, by ignorance (AVIDYA).

dulcamara (Hom.) *Solanum dulcamara.* Also, dulcam., bittersweet. A remedy for a confused state of mind and for the inclination to scold without being angry.

dulse scrub (Nat.) The external application of dulse seaweed powder, mixed with oil or water. While removing impurities and dead skin, the scrub is also said to remineralize the skin.

duo massage (New Age) A massage undertaken by two therapists.

durga See GUGGULU.

durva (Ind.) *Cynodon dactylon.* The juice of this grass is poured into the nose of a patient about ten drops in each nostril, and deeply inhaled to treat epistaxis.

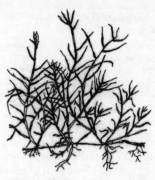

Durva

dusya (Ind.) The seat of disease manifestation in the body.

dwandaj (Ind.) A condition in which two DOSHAs have an equally dominant influence on a patient's profile.

dynamic imaging See VISUALIZATION.

eagle medicine (Am.Ind.) A part of CHEROKEE HERBAL MEDICINE which sees a divine connection in healing. It also acknowledges an ability to hover in the realm of the spirit, while remaining firmly rooted to the earth. The eagle represents the Great Spirit, and is symbolic of the joy and freedom in reaching for the sun, notwithstanding singed feathers. Cherokee medicine also includes, apart from eagle medicine, CRYSTAL HEALING, MENTAL MEDICINE, the NATURAL MEDICINE PATH and the SPIRITUAL MEDICINE PATH.

ear acupuncture See AURICULAR THERAPY.

ear bath (Mod.) Also, ear irrigation. Cleaning the ear, using tepid water and a children's syringe.

ear-candling (Egy./Tib.) Also, ear-coning. An ancient practice among Egyptians, Mayans and Tibetans, in which a hollow candle, tapering at one end, is inserted in the ear while the other end is set to flame. The vacuum so created cleans the ear.

ear-piercing (Ind.) The ancient practice of piercing the ears. It is believed that piercing the right ear brings health and the left ear, wealth. Traditionally, infants' ears in India were pierced in the belief that it helps stimulate their NADIS.

ear reflexology See AURICULAR REFLEXOLOGY.

Eastern medicine (Chi./Ind./Sufi./ Yoga) A broad grouping of all traditional systems of healing, such as AYURVEDA, CHINESE MEDICINE, SHIATSU, SIDDHA, UNANI and YOGA, and their variants, as practised in the East.

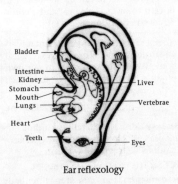

Bladder
Intestine
Kidney
Stomach
Mouth
Lungs
Heart
Teeth
Liver
Vertebrae
Eyes

Ear reflexology

Eastern mysticism (Chi./Ind./Sufi./ Yoga) A common thread between the mystic aspects of various religions and philosophies pertaining to Eastern religious and philosophical systems including Buddhism, Confucianism, Baha'i, Hinduism, KABBALAH, Taoism and ZEN. The most striking examples of eastern mysticism can be identified in concepts such as the basic oneness of the Universe and the awareness about the dynamic and expanding nature of the universe.

EAV See ELECTROACUPUNCTURE ACCORDING TO VOLL.

ecoliteracy See ECOLOGICAL LITERACY.

ecological literacy (New Age) Understanding the principles of organization of ecosystems or ecological communities and using those principles to create healthy and sustainable communities.

ecology (Mod./New Age) The study of the relationship between organisms and their environment. It is increasingly recognized that unless the relationship between humans and their environment is sustainable over time, no health system can assuage human suffering.

eco-spa (New Age/Spa) A spa set in a natural or protected area, functioning with a commitment to incorporate eco-friendly practices such as ecological architecture, water conservation, wildlife protection, organic farming, and preserving indigenous healing traditions.

eco yoga (New Age) A system of YOGA centred around the interconnectedness and interdependence of various life-forms with concern towards ecological and environmental sanctification.

> 'To not sanctify our environment is literally to deface and destroy God's physical body. We wouldn't do this to our own physical body, why would we show such little respect to His.'
>
> —Joshua David Stone

ecstasy (Misc.) 1. Literally, 'standing outside oneself'. 2. A state of being overtaken by emotions such as joy or wonder.

ECT See ELECTRO-CONVULSIVE THERAPY.

ectomorph (Mod.) One of the three body types, the ectomorph has a small and delicate frame, long fingers, toes and neck, sharp facial features, and a triangular face. See also ENDOMORPH, MESOMORPH.

EDTA (Mod.) A synthetic amino acid, used in CHELATION THERAPY.

EDxTM See ENERGY DIAGNOSTICS AND TREATMENT METHODS.

EEG See ELECTROENCEPHALOGRAM.

effleurage (New Age) A MASSAGE technique, in which quick, long strokes are used both when the massage starts and when it finishes.

EFT See EMOTIONAL FREEDOM TECHNIQUES.

ego (Misc.) 1. An essential part of one's personality that maintains a balance between the individual's impulses (id) and conscience (superego) 2. The sense of 'I' and 'mine'.

> 'Ego is a byproduct of the illusion that whatsoever you are seeing is true.'
>
> —Osho

Egyptian days (Egy.) Also, bad days, *dies Aegyptiaci*. The two days in each month considered to be 'dismal' by ancient astrologers of Egypt. Egyptian days as listed on medieval calendars are:

- January 1 and 25
- February 4 and 26
- March 1 and 28
- April 10 and 20
- May 3 and 25
- June 10 and 16
- July 13 and 22
- August 1 and 30
- September 3 and 21
- October 3 and 22
- November 5 and 28
- December 7 and 22

It was considered unlucky to begin a new enterprise on any of the days of 'misfortune' indicated on the medieval calendar.

Egyptian yoga (Egy.) A term denoting the religion and mythology of ancient Egypt. For some scholars, the postures adopted by Egyptian gods and goddesses and the teachings practised in ancient temples in the Nile valley some 10,000 years ago could be taken as the forerunner to the codified, later system of Hatha Yoga.

Ehretism (New Age) An approach to healing, as devised by Arnold Ehret and based on a mucusless diet, consisting of green vegetables and fruits. According to Ehret, mucus represents unusable food elements which cause disease and hence a mucusless diet regimen could effectively arrest the incidence of disease. For Ehret, dairy products, eggs, fats, meat and all starchy foods were mucusforming. Citing the Book of Genesis, Ehret held that fruits and starchless green leaf vegetables were the natural food of man. Ehreism also includes FASTING, ENEMA, EUGENICS, nude sunbathing and sex psychology. According to Ehret, the formula of life is:

V=P–O, where V stands for vitality, P for the power that keeps one alive and O for obstruction which includes internal impurities.

eight-limbed system of Yoga See ASHTANGA YOGA.

eight principles (Chi.) TRADITIONAL CHINESE MEDICINE recognizes eight basic ways for diagnosis and treatment protocols. The symptoms are assessed using the following eight divisions, called patterns: YIN or YANG; superficial or internal (*li-biao*); cold or hot (*han-re*); and deficient or replete (*xu-shi*).

eight types of diagnosis See ENNVAGAI THERVU.

eighteen Lohan tiger (Chi.) A series of healing exercises, aimed at developing one's internal strength. Initially practised slowly to develop relaxed power, students can practise it with focussed power (*jing*) once they learn to relax. Lohan is a term of respect for evolved Buddhist monks.

elaichi See CARDAMOM.

elakizhi (Ind./Mod.) 1. A herbal poultice intended to relieve stress by increased blood circulation in the body 2. A traditional treatment for osteoarthritis.

electricity in therapy (Mod./New Age) Electricity plays a prominent role in modern medicine. The use of charged paddles to jolt the heart back into action is common in emergency rooms. Electro-encephalograms (EEGs) record electrical brain waves and electrocardiograms (EKGs) read the rhythm of the heart. Electrical devices ranging from x-ray machines to MRI (magnetic resonance imaging) machines routinely used in diagnoses.

TRANSCUTANEOUS ELECTRICAL NERVE STIMULATION (TENS) is used for any type of localized physical pain, although it is most commonly recommended for arthritis, sciatica, neuralgia, and chronic back pain.

ELECTROACUPUNCTURE and AURICULAR ACUPUNCTURE (acupuncture limited to the ear) are advocated for the treatment of disorders throughout the body. Similarly, a device called the MORA delivers electromagnetic energy to various acupuncture points, purportedly relieving headaches, migraines, muscular aches and pains, circulation disorders, and skin disease. Another variation on this theme, ELECTROACUPUNCTURE BIOFEEDBACK, is promoted as a diagnostic tool capable of revealing the presence of toxins, food allergies, and imbalances.

ELECTRO-ACUSCOPE is known to relieve pain by running current through damaged tissues. It is generally applied to conditions such as muscle spasms, migraine, jaw pain, bursitis, arthritis, surgical incisions, sprains and strains, neuralgia, shingles, and bruises.

Microcurrent Electrical Therapy (MET) is also promoted for pain relief in the muscles and joints and to speed wound healing. A device called the Light Beam Generator is also being advocated for healing.

Some more devices have attempted to use sound and radio waves therapeutically. It is claimed that cymatic instruments are tuned to the 'frequencies' of various tissues or organs and can diagnose aberrations and restore tissues to health. Likewise, the SOUND PROBE is also employed to kill viruses, bacteria and fungi. A device called the DIAPULSE is reported to employ radio waves to reduce swelling and inflammation following surgery.

> 'Do you remember how electrical currents and "unseen waves" were laughed at? The knowledge about man is still in its infancy.'
>
> —Albert Einstein

electro-acupuncture according to Voll (Mod./New Age) Also, EAV. The diagnostic procedure in which electricity is applied to ACUPOINTS to correct energy imbalances. This procedure was developed in 1950s by German physician Reinhold Voll, who combined Chinese acupuncture theory with galvanic skin differentials to produce this system. Typically, the therapist inserts four to twenty thin disposable needles into the patient's skin, either directly into the area of pain or into traditional acupuncture points. Once the needles are in place, they are stimulated with a low-level electrical charge. The treatment generally takes fifteen to thirty minutes.

electro-acuscope See ACUSCOPE.

electro-acuscope therapy See ACUSCOPE THERAPY.

electro-acuscope myopulse therapy See ACUSCOPE MYOPULSE THERAPY.

electro-biology (Mod.) 1. A branch of biology which deals with the electrical phenomena of living organisms. 2. The study of the interaction between electro-magnetic energy and living organisms. Electro-biology involves aspects of both physical and biological science that are least understood in science.

electroconvulsive therapy (Mod.) Also, shock treatment. A brief application of electrical stimulus given as a treatment for psychiatric disorders. The treatment involves the use of electric currents to induce shock. The therapy is performed in a hospital under general anaesthesia. A very brief shock, typically lasting for a few seconds, is administered to the head to induce a short seizure. Medicine is also administered to prevent the seizure from spreading throughout the body. ECT is an effective treatment for depression. It is also used to treat bipolar disorder, catatonia and some psychic disorders.

electro-crystal therapy (New Age) A gentle and non-invasive method of balancing the human energy field. Electro-crystal therapy involves placing crystals in tubes on certain points around the body. These tubes are attached to an electro-magnetic generator which administers the balancing and normalizing energy frequencies that the human (or animal) energy system needs. The treatment, invented by Harry Oldfield in the 1970s, is considered beneficial for migraine patients. Animals and plants too are said to have benefitted by this treatment.

electro-dermal testing See ELECTRO-DI-AGNOSIS.

electro-diagnosis (New Age) Also, electro-dermal testing. A method of diagnosis employing galvanometric devices to locate energy imbalances along ACUPRESSURE MERIDIANS. The most common electro-diagnostic devices are the electrocardiogram (which addresses the heart) and the electroencephalogram (which addresses the brain).

electro-encephalogram (Mod.) A device which measures brainwaves of different frequencies within the brain. Electrodes are placed over specific areas on the scalp to detect and record electrical impulses within the brain. A diagnostic tool, EEG is also a valuable means of studying how the brain functions. For instance, the human brain uses frequencies of 13 Hz (high alpha or low beta) for 'active' intelligence. Individuals with learning disabilities have been found deficient in them in certain areas of the brain, which affects their ability to easily perform sequencing tasks and mathematical calculations. See also BRAIN WAVES.

electro-homoeopathy (Hom.) A system of herbal medicine discovered in the early nineteenth century by Italian count Caesar Mattei. As the medicine is considered to be an extract of energy, the system was so named by its founder. Each remedy is derived from the active enzymes of several plants. The system uses plant extracts in the higher energies ('vital force'), a potent invisible force, abstract in the natural form and believed to be capable of transforming diseased conditions. Some examples of electro-homoeopathic remedies are: metabolism remedies, lymph remedies, blood remedies, tissue remedies, fever and nerve remedies, intestine remedies, pectoral remedies and constitutional remedies.

electrolysis (Mod.) A technique of lasting hair-removal, proven for its safety and effectiveness for over 125 years. A hair-thin metal probe is slid into a hair follicle where electricity is delivered through the probe, causing localized damage to the areas in which hair grows.

electropathy (Mod.) A system of healing with electricity, as developed in 1865 by Italian count Caesar Mattie, based on positive and negative charges in the human body. Though the system was in practice in the late-nineteenth century, it did not make much headway.

elementals (Eur.) Nature spirits, also referred to as fairies, elves, devas, brownies, leprechauns, gnomes, sprites and pixies.

Nature spirits are broadly grouped into the following four categories, depending on the element to which they belong:

Elements	Elementals
Earth	Gnomes
Air	Sylphs
Water	Undines
Fire	Salamanders

Other elementals include elves, which live in the woods, and household spirits such as bogles, brownies and goblins.

The belief in elementals is age-old and goes back to long before the beginning of any religion. Animism, the original religion of mankind, believed that elementals inhabited all things. Most occultists and neo-pagan witches also believe that these spirits, usually invisible to people, possess supernatural powers. They are believed to inhabit forests, rivers, plants, bogs, mountains, caves and groves where they attach themselves to practically every natural thing. Indian Buddhist art has glorified such tree spirits in the form of beautiful maidens, Shalabhanjikas.

elimination diet (New Age) Also, exclusion diet. A diet regimen which prescribes the elimination or exclusion of certain foods. This procedure helps in identifying food substances that may cause food intolerances, irritable bowel syndrome, Crohn's disease, allergies, or illnesses such as migraine. Once a food causing allergies is identified, it is to be scrupulously avoided for two to three weeks and the resulting symptoms are taken note of for confirmation and avoidance thereafter.

elixir (Misc.) A pharmacological preparation containing an active ingredient (e.g., morphine) dissolved in syrup and designated to be taken orally.

emblic myrobalan See AMALAKI.

emerging (New Age) The process of returning to full alertness at the end of a HYPNOSIS session.

emchi See TIBETAN MEDICINE.

emerald (Gem) A bright green precious stone often associated with intellectual power as well as with attraction to opposite sex.

emotion 1. Feelings about an event, object, situation or person which involves changes in physiological arousal and cognition. 2. A neural impulse that moves an organism into action.

Emotion is a mental state that arises spontaneously, rather than through conscious effort. It can be differentiated from feelings by virtue of it being a psycho-physiological state that moves an organism to action. The study of emotions is part of psychology, neuroscience and, more recently, artificial intelligence.

Emotion is sometimes regarded as the antithesis of reason. Some authors differ from this view, as anger or fear can often be thought of as a systematic response to observed facts.

'Emotion has taught mankind to reason.'

—Marquis de Vauvenargues (1715–47)

emotional aura (New Age) The AURA, associated with emotional reactions. While positive feelings of a person are said to create bright rainbow colours in his or her auric fields, negative ones colour them dark. The emotional aura is also the source of passion and the total embracing, loving heart that heals and forgives.

emotional field therapy (New Age) Also, E.F.T. A pain-management version of ACUPUNCTURE, but without the use of needles. Instead, the energy meridian points are stimulated by tapping with the fingertips. The technique is based on the premise that all physical pains and ailments have direct links with unresolved negative emotions, called emotional debris.

emotional release (Mod./New Age) The release of energy blockages, considered to be the root cause of diseases.

emotional-release therapy (Mod./New Age) A technique aimed at assisting a client in expunging negative emotions and feelings that may have been encrusted in his mind for years, causing damage to his or her personal growth. Psychologists, dowsers, spiritual body workers as well as hypnotherapists are said to have adopted this technique.

'The most important thing is to be whatever you are without shame.'

—Rod Steiger

empath (New Age) A sensitive healer who takes upon himself other's pain and feelings of hurts. Natural empaths who inherit this rare ability are usually 'right-brained' as they predominantly use their creative and intuitive faculties.

empty-nest syndrome (Mod.) Psychological or emotional conditions which affect parents, more intensely the single parent, when children coming of age leave the parental home, often when the child relocates for a job or marriage. Professional counselling may be needed if parents continue to feel inconsolable with the child's departure.

encounter groups See GROUP THERAPY.

endermologie (Mod.) A treatment wherein a machine rolls, pulls, sucks and massages selected parts of the body to reduce cellulite and shape the body. When endermologie is used to treat cellulite, it may be combined with LIPOSUCTION to improve results.

endomorph One of the three basic body types, characterized by roundness, softness, fatness and heaviness, with most of the tissue mass seemingly concentrated in the abdominal area. The arms and legs of the extreme endomorph are short and tapering. See also, ECTOMORPH, MESOMORPH.

endonasal therapy (Chi.) A technique of ACUPUNCTURE, wherein the ACUPOINTS inside the nose get stimulated in the treatment of ear, nose and throat diseases. Ear conditions are also reported to respond, with varying degrees of success, to endonasal therapy technique.

endorphins (West.) A biochemical compound, belonging to a group called neurohormones. Produced by the pituitary glands, endorphins resemble opiates in their effect, as they produce analgesia and a sense of well-being, working as natural pain killers. Endorphins are released in the body during moments of great stress or pain and the modification of neural transmissions by them causes the insensitivity to pain that is experienced by people individuals under such circumstances. Certain physical activities also associated with endorphin secretion are MASSAGE therapy, ACUPUNCTURE or having a good belly laugh.

enema (Misc.) An effective treatment to counter constipation. Water is administered through the anus to cleanse the rectum and colon. Some anaesthetics may also be administered through enemas. Pregnant women were given enema to speed up delivery by inducing contractions. See also BASTI.

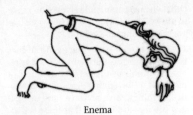
Enema

energetic medicine See VIBRATIONAL MEDICINE.

energy (Misc.) The word is used in several different contexts. In physics, energy is the capacity to work and has different forms, including thermal, chemical, electrical, radiant and nuclear energy, all of which broadly fall into two broad categories: kinetic energy or potential energy. No matter what its form, physical energy has the same unit as work.

In the context of life sciences, energy transformation is recognized as essential for the sustenance of life. Living organisms survive because of the exchange of energy within and without—though the exchange is acting in a direction to increase the entropy of the universe as a whole.

> 'It is important to realize that in physics today, we have no knowledge of what energy is.'
>
> —Richard Feynman

energy, as a healing force See ENERGY MEDICINE.

energy balancing (Yoga/New Age) An approach to healing, aimed at the removal of energy blockages and facilitating energy flow in the body. It is based on the notion that deep relaxation provides an opening for healing energy and that permeation with healing energy results in the dissolution of layers of tension.

energy blockage (New Age/Vib./Yoga) The interruption of the natural flow of subtle energy through the human (or animal) energetic system, often due to abnormal functioning in one or more of the chakras.

energy bodywork See YIN STYLE BA GUA.

energy channels See CHANNELS.

energy emission analysis (Tan./New Age/Occ.) An application of KIRLIAN PHOTOGRAPHY for holistic health.

energy intrusion (New Age/Occ./Vib.) The penetration of energy belonging to others. The luminous energy field of an individual is said to recognize it as foreign and remove it in the way the immune system functions in the body. However, at times, when an individual is exhausted, the defence system of the luminous body may fail and the intrusive energy embeds itself in the body and mind, affecting the well-being of the individual.

energy healing See PRANIC HEALING.

energy medicine See VIBRATIONAL MEDICINE.

energy psychology A method oriented towards understanding human beings in terms of their energy profile.

energy psychotherapy See VIBRATIONAL MEDICINE.

energy suckers See ANTI-NUTRIENTS.

energy tapping See BIO-ENERGY SELF-TREATMENT.

energy therapy See ENERGY MEDICINE.

energywork (Chi./New Age/Vib.) A general term for modalities, based on the notion that the human body consists of underlying energy fields that can be stimulated through various psycho–physical techniques to achieve wellness. Such modalities could be ancient and time-tested such as ACUPUNCTURE, PRANAYAMA or SHIATSU or more contemporary methods like POLARITY THERAPY and THERAPEUTIC TOUCH. In each of these modalities, attempts are made to rebalance the energy in the body through stimulation, release or distribution.

enlightenment 1. The final attainment on the spiritual path, accompanied with the merger of one's ego into the supreme Universal consciousness. 2. Becoming aware of the nature of oneself through detached observation, concentration and contemplation, by gradually reducing one's ignorance.

The systematic search for enlightenment has been a goal of knowledge from ancient times, though such attempts were not necessarily spiritual. The secular European Age of Enlightenment also has parallels in the Far Eastern religious experience (the Buddhist Bodhi, the Zen Satori, and the Hindu moksha) as well as European and Near Eastern religions (i.e., Judaism, Christianity, and Islam). Theodore Adorno and Max Horkheimer developed a wider and more pessimistic concept of enlightenment which had its dark side: while trying to abolish superstition and myths by 'foundationalist' philosophy, it ignored its own 'mythical' basis. Its striving towards totality and certainty led to an increasing instrumentalization of reason. In their view, enlightenment should be enlightened, and not pose as a 'myth-free' view of the world.

> 'Enlightenment is man's release from his self-incurred tutelage. Tutelage is the incapacity to use one's own understanding without the guidance of another. Such tutelage is self-imposed if its cause is not lack of intelligence, but rather a lack of determination and courage to use one's intelligence without being guided by another.'
>
> —Immanuel Kant

See SAMADHI, TYPE OF.

enneagram (Sufi) The nine types of human personality, as profiled in ancient Sufi typology, are summarized in the following table:

Personality Types (indicating primary role)	Characteristics	Prime Psychological Addiction (fixation or blindspot)	Personality Transformation while neutralizing Prime Psychological Addiction
Achievers and reformers	Orderly, rational and self-righteous	Anger	Path-finders
Helpers	Generous, manipulative and possessive	Pride	Partners

Succeeders, motivators and status-seekers	Ambitious, hostile and pragmatic	Deceit	Motivators
Individualists and artists	Intuitive, self-absorbed and sensitive	Envy	Builders
Observers and thinkers	Analytic, original and provocative	Greed	Explorers
Guardians and loyalists	Defensive, engaging and responsible	Fear	Stabilizers
Dreamers and generalists	Accomplished and manic	Gluttony	Illuminators
Confronters and leaders	Combative, dominant and self-confident	Lust for life and power	Philanthropists
Preservationists and peace-makers	Easy-going and receptive	Laziness	Universities

A knowledge of the enneagram types may be useful in creating a better understanding, and thereby better interaction, within a social group or team.

> 'When I first heard my enneagram type described, a whole slew of observations I had made about myself over the years suddenly fell into place. I had a short-cut conceptual system that made sense out of a lot of stuff that hadn't made much sense.'
>
> —Charles T. Tart

ennvagai thervu (Ind.) Also, Eight type of diagnosis as followed in SIDDHA MEDICINE. It refers to pulse-reading, tongue examination, observation of colour and voice changes, eye check-up, touch-factor and the examination of stools and urine.

entrainment (Misc.) 1. Synchronization and control of cardiac rhythm by an external stimulus 2. Synchronous influence of one energy system over the other. 3. The causing of synchronous activity.

entropy (Misc.) A measure of disorder or randomness of a system; a measure of how randomly distributed matter and energy are; a measure of a system's energy that is unavailable for work. A concept of classical thermodynamics, entropy is related to disorder or randomness.

enzyme (Misc.) A type of protein that acts as a chemical catalyst, regulating metabolic processes in the body.

eponymolog (Num.) A special number, derived from a person's name, believed to reflect his or her personality and path in life. This number is generally used to help judge an individual's personality traits.

Epsom salt bath (Nat.) Soaking in a tub full of hot water with a few cups of Epsom salts (commercial magnesium sulphate). By inducing perspiration, the bath draws out toxins from the body. It also has a relaxing effect on the muscles and a sedative effect on the nerves. It is also a natural emollient, exfoliator and anti-inflammatory.

To soothe aches and remove odours, the feet should be soaked in a large pan of hot water containing ½ cup Epsom salt for as long as it feels good.

Epstein, Donald M. See NETWORK SPINAL ANALYSIS; TWELVE STAGES OF HEALING.

equanimity (Misc.) 1. The yogic characteristic of remaining calm and undisturbed even amidst turbulent or testing situations in or around oneself. 2. The quality of evenness or EQUILIBRIUM of mind, come rain or shine. 3. Composure.

> 'A person in this category of mental intelligence lives in the present without being caught in the past or future, undisturbed by external circumstances.'
>
> —B.K.S. Iyengar

equilibrium (New Age/Yoga) 1. An evenly balanced state of mind. 2. A state of evenness, which harmonizes the functioning of the left hemisphere of the brain, concerned with analysis and calculation, with that of the right, assigned with creativity and emotional response. 3. A quality of ideal spiritual leadership. See also, EQUANIMITY.

> 'Having attained an equilibrium of ida and pingala, one becomes a knower of the known.'
>
> —An ancient statement, referring to yoga

equilibropathy (Chi./Yoga) Also, dulayaphap bumbud. A method of achieving dynamic balance in the body through posture control (e.g., keeping the body straight while flattening the abdomen), proper breathing (e.g., breathing slowly and deeply, without making a sound) and following four sets of prescribed physical exercises (e.g., modified QIGONG movements). The method also includes modified ACUPUNCTURE in combination with soft-tissue manipulation.

er mei qigong (Chi.) An ancient style of QI GONG, which involves either directly transmitting QI energy to heal the sick or injured or training them in selected techniques to enable them to heal themselves. Healing and ENLIGHTENMENT are the key areas focussed on in this system.

Erickson, Milton H. (1901–80) (Mod.) The American psychotherapist who did pioneering work in medical hypnosis, particularly with reference to sensory alteration and pain control. See also, ERICKSONIAN HYPNOSIS.

> 'Therapy is a way of helping patients extend their limits.'
>
> —Milton H Erickson

Ericksonian hypnosis (Mod.) An adjunct to PSYCHOTHERAPY developed by American psychotherapist Milton H. Erickson, aimed at exploring the realms of the unconscious mind and discovering new ways to resolve conflicts arising due to obstacles and problems faced. According to him, a therapist can help a client formulate specific internal processes (e.g., feelings, memories, images and internal self-talk) to help him overcome adverse situations. See also, HYPNOSIS, ERICKSON, MILTON H.

Esalen massage (Eur/New Age) Also, Swedish Esalen. A modified version of a century-old SWEDISH MASSAGE, Esalen is often practised as an exchange in which the giver also becomes the receiver. Except when done by professional therapists in public practice, the massage is done in the nude between partners. It is based on the assumption that one who is not comfortable with being seen naked will communicate the tension to the giver and both will find relaxation difficult. Esalen underscores touching, caring, energy awareness and emotional and spiritual healing, aimed at integrating the body, mind and spirit to bring in greater harmony in the lives of people. See also, SWEDISH MASSAGE.

esoteric (Occ.) 1. Difficult to understand 2. Secret 3. Private or restricted to a chosen few. A term used to denote the knowledge or understanding possessed exclusively by a few, and often guarded as secret. Knowledge relating to several systems of alternative medicine have unfortunately remained hidden or are secrets well guarded by a few individuals, families, communities or societies.

esoteric clearing (New Age/Occ./Vib.) A healing method, aimed at erasing wrong emotional and mental conditions (referred to as 'invisible foreign entities'), said to sap one's vital energy.

esotericism (New Age/Occ./Vib.) 1. Esoteric teachings or practices. 2. Knowledge meant only for a closed group of persons either for exclusivity or to protect themselves against prejudice. While esotericism tends to focus on personal enlightenment, organized exoteric religions concentrate on rituals and moral laws that govern society. Esotericism, however, also involves traditions and institutional frameworks.

ESP See EXTRA-SENSORY PERCEPTION.

ESP cards (Occ.) A pack of twenty cards with five symbols, including stars, squares, circles, crosses and waves, used for consultation. The cards are used for answering questions relating to subjects such as recovery from ailments and overcoming misfortune. They are also used by some parapsychologists who test for elusive phenomenon.

E.S.T. See ERHARD SEMINARS TRAINING.

essence (Misc.) The ultimate, real and unchanging nature of a thing or being.

ESSENCE (New Age) A technique of GUIDED

IMAGERY developed on the premise that by eliminating one's emotional barriers and blockages, healing can be achieved.

essence repatterning (Mod.) A strategic approach to create new avenues (for desired changes, including health and emotional well-being, and improving relationships) by re-educating oneself with regard to the present outcomes and results one does not want; the specifics of what one wants instead; specific steps to de-activate limiting patterns (that create undesired outcomes); and simultaneously, specific steps to re-activate one's innate success patterns.

This exercise is said to transform virtually any area of one's life. As one addresses specific areas in which one wants to make positive changes, positive results can be created in other areas as well; this dynamics is a consequence of the link between one's limiting pattern and one's early conditions.

Essence repatterning draws on the latest research in brain technology, quantum physics, psycho–neuro–immunology, and accelerated learning techniques. The approach also advocates regular documenting of changes to enable one to periodically review progress.

Essene (Misc.) A sect of pre-Christian Jewish physicians. The Hebrews called them the School of Prophets; to the Egyptians, they were the Healers. The Essenes devoted their lives to activities like healing the sick and providing food and shelter to strangers passing through their settlements. They differentiated between souls which were sleeping, drowsy and awakened. They considered that their task was to help, comfort and relieve sleeping souls, to try to awaken drowsy souls, and to welcome and guide awakened souls. As healers, they aimed at tapping the VITAL ENERGY, employing methods like AFFIRMATION, COLOUR THERAPY, SPIRITUAL HEALING and VISUALIZATION.

essential oils (Nat.) 1. Volatile oils extracted from flowers, grasses, fruits, leaves, roots or trees, which maintain the odours, tastes and thus the essence of the plant they are extracted from.

Essential oils contain complex chemicals which are capable of acting on a psycho–physical level. The molecular composition of essential oils allows for easier penetration of the skin, helping stimulate circulation and lymph flow, besides detoxification and vitalizting tissues. Commonly used in AROMATHERAPY, several essential oils have been scientifically evaluated for their antibacterial, antifungal and antiviral action.

The following table indicates common ailments, said to respond to certain essential oils as indicated:

Ailment	Suggested essential oil
Allergies	blue tansy, chamomile, helich rysum, lavender, yarrow
Asthma	amni visnaga, blue tansy
Arthritis	black pepper, cajeput, cinnamon, clove bud, eucalyptus, ginger, lavender, lemon, marjoram, nutmeg, rosemary, wintergreen
Fungal infection	lemongrass, myrrh, palma rosa, patchouli, tagetes, tea tree
Backaches	black pepper, cajeput, chamomile, eucalyptus, ginger, lavender, lemon, peppermint, marjoram, nutmeg, rosemary, thyme
Boils	bergamot, lavender, lemon, tea tree
Bronchial Congestion	inula, frankincense, black spruce, balsam, larch, pine
Bruises and wounds	black pepper, chamomile, fennel, lavender, lemon, rosemary
Burns	carrot seed, frankincense, lavender tea tree
Candida	cajeput, chamomile, eucalyptus, holy basil, lemon, tea tree
Fatigue	geranium, lemon, pink grapefruit, rosemary, sweet basil

Painful experience	frankincense, lavender, lemongrass, sweet marjoram, myrrh, peppermint, rose, roemary
Congestion in chest	eucalyptus, frankincense, inula, sweet basil, black pepper, lemon myrtle, peppermint, pine
Constipation	fennel, yarrow, black pepper, sweet marjoram, rosemary, carrot seed, peppermint, pine, sweet orange
Coughs	hyssop, cardamon seed, balsam fir, inula (for dry, unproductive cough), pine, greek sage, oregano
Cramps and muscle spasms	sweet marjoram, black pepper, roman chamomile, clary sage, cypress, geranium, lavender, marjoram, thyme
Cuts and scrapes	lavender, chamomile, tea tree, helichrysum
Dandruff	tea tree oil (added to shampoo in a 5 per cent dilution)
Diarrhoea	black pepper, cajeput, chamomile, cinnamon, eucalyptus, fennel, ginger, mandarin, neroli, peppermint
Fever	eucalyptus, lavender, and peppermint oils added to sponge bath (1 drop each)
Gas	anise, black pepper, cardamom, chamomille, fennel, oregano
Gout	juniper berry, lemon, rosemary
Headaches	basil, cajeput, chamomile, clove bud, eucalyptus, lavender, marjoram, peppermint, rosemary, thyme
Hypertension (high blood pressure)	bergamot, chamomile, lavender, marjoram, neroli, ylangylang
Hypotension (low blood pressure)	ginger, lemon, rosemary
Indigestion	anise, black pepper, cardamon, coriander, fennel, ginger, lemongrass, nutmeg
Inflammation	chamomile, coriander, fennel, nutmeg, juniper, yarrow
Insect bites	cajeput, chamomile, lavender
Insomnia	bergamot, chamomile, lavender, ledum, mandarin, sandalwood, valerian
Menstrual cramps	anise, basil, chamomille, fennel, geranium, marjoram, yarrow
Migraine	lavender, peppermint, roman chamomile, clary sage, marjoram, valerian, eucalyptus, spike lavender, neroli
Muscle aches	basil, black pepper, eucalyptus, ginger, lavender, vetiver
Muscle spasms	chamomile, fennel, frankincense, lavender, sage
Nausea	cardamom, fennel, ginger, patchouli, peppermint, spearmint
Oedema	cistus, angelica root, ravensara, rosemary, seaweed, carrot seed, sweet fennel, grapefruit, juniper, lemon, mandarin, tangerine
Peridontal problems	fennel, myrrh, peppermint, tea tree
Pressure sores (bed sores)	chamomile, helichrysum, frankincense, geranium, lavender

Rheumatism	black pepper, ginger, helichrysum, lavender, lavandin
Sciatica	black pepper, ginger, helichrysum, lavender
Sinusitis	angelica, basil, clove bud, eucalyptus, hyssop, pine, peppermint
Sore Throat	hyssop, sandalwood

ESP See EXTRA-SENSORY PERCEPTION.

estrogen (Misc.) A generic name for steroid hormones, secreted chiefly by the ovaries and placenta, which help develop secondary sex characteristics in women and has an effect on the female reproductive system.

eternity (Misc.) 1. Being eternal 2. Time without beginning or end.

> 'In the heart of this moment lies eternity.'
> —Eckhart

> 'Whatever may happen to thee; it was prepared for thee from all eternity; and the implication of causes was from eternity spinning the thread of their being... It is all part of the great web.'
> —Marcus Aurelins (second century AD)

ether (Yoga) One of the FIVE ELEMENTS that constitute the universe. It is considered the fifth and subtlest element, and is taken to be an unseen, vaporous substance.

etheric body (Vib./Yoga) An invisible field of energy which is said to maintain every atom and cell of the physical body. It is capable of sending VIBRATIONS, both positive and negative, short and long, whose appearance outside the body is referred to as AURA. The etheric body acts as the receiver, assimilator and transmitter of energy.

etheric release (New Age/Vib.) A form of ENERGY WORK, aimed at releasing suppressed or restricted emotional expressions. It is widely held that suppression and restriction of emotional expressions can prove harmful to one's health in the long run.

etheric surgery See PSYCHIC SURGERY.

etheric touch (Vib.) An approach to energy healing, aimed at projecting the healing energies for others through hands, without involving any physical contact. The approach is based on the belief that one's hands are so sensitive that they can sense energy imbalances in the body and can be made to project vibrations for boosting self-healing. See also, REIKI.

eugenics (Mod.) The study of factors, which influence hereditary qualities. Eugenics aims at eliminating deficiencies, both in mental and physical realms, and makes attempts to encourage larger families from 'superior' parents.

eupatorlun purpureum (Hom.) Eupat. purp. A homoeopathic remedy for the dull and depressed.

euthanasia (Mod.) Also, mercy killing 1. Allowing people to die by withdrawing or withholding life support systems 2. An act of killing an incurably ill person out of compassion for the person's suffering. Though it is called mercy killing, the consent of the person dying is not taken. While withholding or withdrawing life support is referred to as passive euthanasia, in active euthanasia, physicians aid in providing the means to end the life of a sufferer. In the US, active euthanasia is generally considered murder or manslaughter, whereas passive euthanasia is accepted in certain circumstances by professional medical societies and the law.

evil eye (Occ.) Spells, believed to be cast by people jealous of the fortunate. To ward off harmful effects of the evil eye, protective devices, including signs, symbols and amulets, have been used from times immemorial.

> Shyaama Gaura Sundara Dou Jori Nirakhahin Chhabi Janani Trina Tori
> —A Hindu mantra, recited to counter the evil eye

exclusion diet See ELIMINATION DIET.

exfoliating treatment (Cos.) Also, exfoliation. A skin-care procedure in which the top layer of dead skin cells is sloughed off the face and body. Dry brushing, loofah and salt scrubbing are techniques commonly used in conjunction with ingredients such as grape seed, marine sediments, sugar, clay and salt.

exfoliation See EXFOLIATING TREATMENT.

existential psychotherapy (Mod.) An approach to PSYCHOTHERAPY, which, while embracing human potential, also takes into account human limitation. Rollo May, who developed this approach, was greatly influenced by the writings of Paul Tillich, Kierkegaard, Nietzsche and Heidegger.

exorcism (Occ.) 1. Expulsion of evil spirits and demons that 'possess' a person or object. 2. An ancient ritual of binding DEMONS with oaths, words and ceremonies and casting them out, particularly in mental illness. In ancient times, exorcists used religious material, such as chants and prayers, symbols and diagrams, amulets, icons and gestures.

experiential psychology See SACRED PSYCHOLOGY.

expression therapies (New Age) 1. Therapeutic self-healing through creativity, expression and artwork. 2. A system of healing based on artistic expressions as in art, music and dance.

extispicy (Eur./Occ.) A method of DIVINATION by means of entrails. The Roman architect Vitruvius (46 BC) attempted to credit the origin of extispicy to the ancient custom of making an encampment. The entrails of animals in the area were examined to determine if the area was suitable to set up camp in.

extra-sensory perception (Occ.) The ability to perceive information without the use of senses by means of telepathy, which refers to mind-to-mind communication, clairvoyance, the awareness of remote objects, persons and events, precognition, the knowledge of events ahead, and retrocognition, the knowledge of events of the past.

eye-analysis See IRIDOLOGY.

eye of Horus (Egy.) 1. The stylized eye of Horus, a mythological falcon-headed solar and sky god, associated with health and regeneration 2. A common AMULET in ancient Egypt.

eye bright See EUPHRASIA.

eyebrow centre gazing See SAMBHAVI MUDRA.

eyebrow chakra See AJNA CHAKRA.

face modelling (Cos.) A type of FACIAL, as developed by Arcadi Beliavtsev, and promoted by the Arcadi Centre in Amsterdam. The technique is based on the theory that many internal organs are projected on the skin of the face and that intensive facial treatment provides healing impulses in such organs.

facial (Cos.) A skin-care treatment for the face. It includes deep Cleansing, EXFOLIATING TREATMENT, MASSAGE, moisturizing, STEAM THERAPY, toning of the face as well as the neck, shoulders and chest. The treatment is cosmetic as well as nourishes and hydrates the skin.

facial diagnosis (New Age) A subtle science based on the examination of the face (particularly, cheeks, ears, nostrils, eyes and mouth) to ascertain the health conditions of an individual; facial features attempt to ascertain whether an individual is 'in balance'. It helps locate stagnated internal organs so that prompt measures can be taken to avoid further damage. The method is based on the ancient AYURVEDIC premise that disorders and diseases get manifested in one's face in the form of lines and that facial features are considered to represent body types. While VATA persons have a crooked nose, a PITTA constitution is indicated by a sharp nose. A discolouration of the nose or on the cheeks may also indicate a malabsorption of iron or may be an indication of low digestive fire. Fluffy lower eyelids indicate impaired kidneys. Horizontal lines on the forehead may indicate stress. A vertical line between the eyebrows could signal suppressed emotions or trauma stored in the body. While such a line on the right side would indicate that these emotions have found their way to the liver, lines on the left side indicate that the spleen holds such emotions.

facial rejuvenation (Cos.) A method using dermal fillers like COLLAGEN in fine lines, deep creases, furrows, wrinkles, scars or other skin depressions in the face, particularly due to ageing. The fillers can give definition to the lips and remove unwanted features around the mouth, chin, cheeks, forehead and eyes.

facilitated communication (Mod.) Also, FC. A communication method developed in Australia by Rosemary Crossley in the 1970s. Aimed at helping people with defective communication caused by afflictions such as autism and cerebral palsy, the facilitator normally supports the client's hand, wrist or arm while the person uses a communicator to spell out words, phrases or sentences. The use of FC for people with autism is centred on the assumption that many of the difficulties faced are due to a movement disorder rather than social or communication deficits.

faith (Misc.) 1. Trust or belief 2. Conviction. In its broadest sense, the word means religion or DHARMA. It is not only an essential requirement for all religious practices and rituals, but also in all practices connected to healing. To have faith in others, one should first have faith in himself or herself.

> 'Believe in yourself! Have faith in your abilities! Without a humble but reasonable confidence in your own powers you cannot be successful or happy. Believe it is possible to solve your problems. Tremendous things happen to the believer. So believe the answer will come. It will.'
>
> —Norman Vincent Peale

faith healing (New Age) A concept and practice which emphasizes the dominant role of FAITH as fundamental to kick-starting the healing process. The premise is that if the patient develops faith in himself, a system, a healer, or an intervention, the chances of cure increase. The term is sometimes linked with religious beliefs as in, for example, Christian faith healing in which it is believed that God heals the suffering people through the power of Holy Spirit. Many people resort to faith healing, particularly those with terminal and incurable diseases, often as a last attempt for surviving.

> 'We have not lost faith, but we have transferred it from God to the medical profession.'
>
> —George Bernard Shaw

false daisy (Chi./Ind.) *Eclipta prostrata, Eclipta alba.* Also, *America takasaburou* in Japanese, bhringaraja in Sanskrit, *han lian cao* in Chinese, karisalanganni in Tamil; a plant, widely used in traditional Chinese herbal medicine, to prevent premature graying. In AYURVEDA, bhringaraja is considered the best tonic for the maintenance of healthy hair and is also used as a liver tonic. In Korea, the leaves are used as an antidote for scorpion stings and snakebites. The root-paste is used as an antiseptic and applied externally by veterinarians to ulcers and wounds on animals.

falun (Chi./Vib.) Also, law-wheel. The symbol of Buddhist healthcare, believed to help develop and absorb COSMIC ENERGY.

falun dafa (Chi./Vib.) Also, cultivation practice. A Buddhist healing technique, popularized by Li Hongzhi in 1992, aimed at integrating the body, mind and spirit. Called cultivation practice, the system refers to the improvement of one's heart and mind through the careful observation and realization of universal principles based on truthfulness, benevolence, and forbearance. 'Practice' also refers to doing exercises (five gentle exercises) which include a seated meditation to energize the body and mind.

falun gong See FALUN DAFA.

familiar (Occ.) The name given to spirits attendant upon witches, magicians and spiritual healers.

family therapy (Mod.) Therapeutic practices involving family members co-operating with each other to change unhealthy familial patterns or interactions. It is commonly found that the health profiles of members of a family are markedly similar, as a consequence of both genetic and environmental factors. Food habits, hygiene conditions, lifestyle and value systems are also broadly shared by family members, bringing forth traits identifiable within families. Serious mental disorders, including addiction, deficiency in nutrition, schizophrenia, interactional problems, including divorce, and metabolic disorders like diabetes and hypertension can be diagnosed with this approach.

The term is also used in the context of marriage therapy, a branch of psychotherapy that works with couples in intimate relationships. In England, family therapists are usually drawn from para-medical professionals such as psychologists, psychotherapists and counsellors.

fango (Spa) A mineralized mud from Italy, used in combination with oil or water for application over the human body. It serves as a heat pack and helps detoxify the skin by stimulating circulation. It also helps nourish the skin as it relieves arthritic and muscular pain.

fantastic energy foods See GREGORIAN CHANT.

fan yan sui See CORIANDER.

fang feng See LEDEBOURIELLA ROOT.

fascinate (Occ.) The act of casting an evil SPELL or the EVIL EYE.

fasting (Ind./Nat.) Also, vrata. 1. Abstinence from food. 2. The act of fasting. A time-tested purificatory exercise which calms the emotions. In the Indian spiritual and health tradition, fasting is undertaken on various occasions associated with astronomical changes, e.g., chandrayana vrata, krichara vrata, ekadasi vrata and pradosha vrata, all aimed at controlling and/or purifying the mind.

Fasting, according to naturopaths, overhauls the respiratory, circulatory, digestive and urinary systems. It destroys toxic accumulations in the body and eliminates uric acid deposits. As it calms the mind, fasting enhances the quality of DHYANA and MEDITATION. An occasional complete fast is recommended in many cultures across the world for developing one's will power. Some naturopaths recommend the intake of large quantities of tepid water during fasting as it helps in flushing out toxins through the kidneys or by sweating.

HATHA YOGA refers to fasting as GHATA SHUDDHI, and considers it the purification of the 'flesh-pot', i.e., the body. It is also believed that sexual excitement gets dissipated by fasting.

FC See FACILITATED COMMUNICATION.

feathering (New Age/Occ.) The application of feathers of some birds in energy-healing exercises. Selected feathers have been used in many ancient cultures, especially for clearing the 'cobwebs' of energies shrouding one's AURA. As feathers symbolically represent the wind element in nature, feathers wafting in the air, often combined with chants and aromatic smoke during rituals is believed to produce a healing state of CONSCIOUSNESS. Feathers used in folk healing practices are indicated in the following table:

Feathers	Expected effect
turkey feathers	cleansing aura and digestive tract
cardinal feathers	boosting energy levels and improving blood quality and circulation
down feathers	healing skin conditions and causing sweet dreams
peacock feathers	overall improvement in health conditions

feelings (Misc.) 1. Sensations perceived through touch. 2. An affective state of CONSCIOUSNESS, resulting from desires, emotions or sentiments. 3. Opinion formed by emotions, rather than reasons. 4. Intuitive awareness.

> 'All great discoveries are made by men whose feelings run ahead of their thinking.'
>
> —C.H. Parkhurst

feet shower (Nat.) The therapeutic application of water over specific areas of the soles, corresponding to a specific organ. See also, FOOT REFLEXOLOGY.

Feldenkrais method See FELDENKRAIS THERAPY.

Feldenkrais moshe See FELDENKRAIS THERAPY.

Feldenkrais technique See FELDENKRAIS THERAPY.

Feldenkrais therapy An education-based system devised by Russian-born engineer–physicist Moshe Feldenkrais (1904–84), especially devised for people with afflictions like arthritis, chronic pain, spasticity and spinal disorders. The method involves 'movement re-education' in which the facilitator uses gentle manipulation and movement training to encourage the impaired or burdened body align into a new and easy way of moving. Creating AWARENESS through movement and intensive verbal and TOUCH THERAPY form part of this method.

female ginseng See ANGELICA ROOT.

feng shui (Chi.) From the Chinese *feng*, meaning air, and *shui*, meaning water; containers of QI. A discrete belief system and an ancient Chinese practice in which the spaces in human dwellings were earmarked for specific human activities. The goal was to locate and orient a land or a dwelling space so as to be attuned with the flow of QI. A few general guidelines on location emanating from this ancient body of wisdom are summarized below:

• Avoid clutter and accumulated garbage in rooms.

• When one lies on a bed, the feet should not be in the direction of the entrance door.

• When one sits at a desk, the entrance door and most of the room should be directly in the line of sight.

• Staircases should not be constructed into the entrance door of a house.

• Straight passages and sharp corners should be avoided to keep away negative energy which is believed to travel in straight lines.

Objects believed to reflect or redirect the flowing qi energy, viz., crystals, mirrors, wind-chimes and small pools of flowing or standing water are desirable in houses.

A multi-disciplinary system of knowledge, feng shui is drawn from sciences including astronomy, environmental ecology, geography and physics. It serves both as a guiding philosophy and as practical information to ensure harmonious interaction between humans and their personal spaces.

Feng shui and VASTU are both thousands of years old, from China and India respectively. Both contain large bodies of knowledge and wisdom and have much in common despite significant differences in their approaches.

'Between heaven and earth stands man.'
—Siou Foon Lee

'The energy that rides the wind stops at the edge of water and is retained.'
—The Book of Burial (c. 300 BC)

fennel (Arab./Chi./Eur./Heb./Ind./Jap.) *Foeniculum vulgare*. Also, finocchio in Italian, hoehyang (in Korean), hui xiang in Chinese, madhurika (in Ayurveda), rezene in Turkish, saunf or shamaar in Arabic, shumar (Hebrew), uikyô in Japanese. Also, saunf. A tall glabrous aromatic herb, whose dried fruits are used in the treatment of coughs and sore throats, and complaints of the spleen and kidneys. Saunf constitutes an excellent stomach and intestinal remedy and hence is used in digestive liqueurs. It is also believed to stimulate lactation.

fennel flower See BLACK CUMIN.

fenugreek *Trigonella Foenum-graecum* (Arab./Eur./Chr./Heb./Ind./Jap.) Also, hilbeh in Heb., hulba in Arabic, hu lu ba in Chinese, methi in Urdu, methika (in Ayurveda), vendhayam (in Siddha medicine). A nutritive herb known for long for its smooth, supportive action in digestion and respiration. Ancient Egyptians are said to have eaten the greens of this plant as a vegetable, and used the seeds as incense to aid childbirth. The seed has traditionally been in use for lowering blood sugar and loosening the stools. It is also used as a gargle to relieve sore throats, and as an external dressing for swelling. The leaves and seeds of this plant are traditionally used in India to lower the blood lipids and sugar. The Chinese believe that they can work like an aphrodisiac for certain kinds of impotence due to *shenxu* ('kidney-deficient'). Cold, pain in the testes, hernia of the groin, stomach aches, and oedema in the legs are also treated with them in TRADITIONAL CHINESE MEDICINE.

'Methi balances vata, eliminates fevers...'
—*Bhava Prakasa*

Ferdinand and Walter Huneke See NEURAL THERAPY.

ferrum phosphoricum (Hom.) Also, ferrum phos., iron phosphate. 1. A constituent of red blood cells which helps to distribute oxygen in the body 2. A homoeopathic remedy to treat anaemia and low energy. feverishness, sore throat, cough and cold.

Ferreri, Carl A. See NEURAL ORGANIZATION TECHNIQUE.

Ferreri technique See NEURAL ORGANIZATION TECHNIQUE.

festering moxibustion See DIRECT MOXIBUSTION.

fever grass See LEMON GRASS.

fight-or-flight (Mod.) The instant response of the body and mind in a life-threatening situation, which forms the foundation of modern-day stress medicine. Also called acute stress response, this phenomenon was first explained by Walter Cannon, a Harvard physiologist, in 1929. The response is initiated in the hypothalamus in the human brain which when stimulated initiates a sequence of nerve-cell 'firing' and chemical (adrenaline, cortisol, etc.) release that prepares the body for running or fighting. This response was later recognized as the first stage of a general adaptation syndrome that regulates stress responses.

fifth chakra (Yoga) Also, throat chakra, vishuddha. One of the fourteen CHAKRAS, located in the throat region, which represents communication and creativity. It is believed that malfunctioning of this chakra may cause defects in the growth of an individual.

finoccio (Eur.) An Italian name for FENNEL.

fire See AGNI.

first aid (Misc.) Emergency treatment administered to an accident victim, as distinguishable from routine professional medical care.

first chakra (Yoga) Also, root chakra, muladhara. One of the fourteen CHAKRAS situated at the base of the spine, representing memory and survival.

first chapter (Yoga) Also, samadhi pada. The first of the four chapters in PATANJALI's Yoga Sutras. This chapter includes the concepts of yoga, CHITTA vrittis and KLESHA in fifty-one verses. It also deals with lower and higher types of SAMADHI.

first sheath (Yoga) Also, annamaya kosha, sthula sharira. The outermost part of the mind–body complex, the first of the FIVE SHEATHS which owes its origin to food and also ends up as food.

'The eater eating is himself eaten.'

—An ancient saying in Sanskrit

first moral restraint (Yoga) Also, ahimsa, non-violence. The system of yoga considers ahimsa or non-violence as the first and foremost prerequisite for any spiritual programme. See YAMA.

first observance (Yoga) Also, soucha. Cleanliness, considered the first step to be taken before venturing into any spiritual practice. It encompasses not only the cleanliness of the body and mind but of the environment of the aspirant; both are considered essential for a successful spiritual practise. See NIYAMA.

first psycho–physiological affliction (Yoga) Also avidya. Ignorance, considered the mother of all psycho–physiological af-flictions in human existence. See KLESHA.

fish cure of Hyderabad (Ind.) Also, fish medicine. A remedy for asthma-sufferers, administered in Hyderabad (India) on a sacred day falling in the first week of June every year. The medicine is reported to be a mixture of a herbal paste, swallowed with a tiny, live murrel fish.

'The (fish) cure, we believe, is due to the combined effects of fish, herbal medicine and miracle.'

—Baithni Harinath Goud

fish medicine See FISH CURE OF HYDERABAD.

fitness profile (Mod.) Also, fitness assessment. An evaluation of aerobic capacity, flexibility and strength as determined by a qualified instructor by conducting tests with regard to pulse rate, blood pressure and body composition.

fitness partner (Mod./New Age) A partner chosen while undertaking a fitness programme. Working out with a fitness partner is said to enhance one's confidence levels and motivation to achieve the target. To select a suitable partner, it is preferable to opt for a person with a similar fitness level and with similar goals.

Fitzgerald, William J. See ZONE THERAPY.

five activities (Ind.) Also, pancha kritya. The five activities with which nature is identified: creation, preservation, destruction, concealment of grace and bestowing of grace.

five avastas See FIVE STATES OF AWARENESS.

five animal frolics (Chi.) An ancient exercise programme developed by Hua Tou (110-207 AD), based on the stances of five animals, viz., bear, crane, deer, monkey and tiger. It is said that by mimicking these animals, practitioners are able to position and move their bodies to achieve balance and well-being. This set of exercises is also known as QIGONG, since its practise is aimed at strengthening the internal organs of the body by increasing one's QI energy levels. The expected benefits of the five exercises are summarized in the following table:

Exercise	Benefits expected	Therapeutic benefits
Bear	Aids in developing stability and greater strength in legs	Strengthens bones and kidneys
Crane	Aids in developing agility, balance and lightness	Relaxation
Deer	Aids in developing poise and grace and expansive movements	Relaxation
Monkey	Aids in developing agility, alertness and suppleness	Mental alertness and helps have one quick-witted reactions to situations
Tiger	Aids in developing strength	Strengthens kidneys and increases muscular strength

five blemishes (Ind.) Also, five evil traits, pancha doshas. Lust, rage, greed, abnormal fear and limitless sleep; these five traits are the five evils that affect one's personality. By keeping them under check, one is expected to advance in the spiritual path.

five constant duties (Ind.) Also, pancha nitya karma. Virtuous living, worship, observance of rituals and festivals, pilgrimage, and sacraments. These five constant duties form the religious practices in Hinduism, based on the philosophy of FIVE FAITHS.

five debts (Ind.) Also, pancha rina. The five debts to whom every human being is beholden, identified as one's mother, father, gurus, gods and the Universal Spirit.

five doshas See FIVE BLEMISHES.

five elements in Chinese philosophy (Chi.) In ancient Chinese philosophy, natural phenomena are classified into five elements: wood, fire, earth, metal and water. The philosophy makes use of these elements to explain the complex interactions and interrelationships between them in the manifest universe.

five elements in Japanese philosophy (Jap.) The Japanese concept of classifying natural phenomena into five elements traces its origin to China and India, respectively referred to as *gogyo* and godai. The godai of the Japanese traditions, used in the famous text *Gorin no sho* by Miyamoto Musashi refers to different aspects of swordsmanship by assigning each aspect with an element. In the ascending order of energetics, earth (*tsuchi* or CHI) is placed at the bottom, after which are placed respectively water (*sui* or *mizu*), fire (*ho ka* or *hi*), wind (*fū* or *kaze*) and the sky or void (*kû*). Sometimes CONSCIOUSNESS is treated as the sixth element, placed on top of all the five elements.

In the Buddhist architecture of Japan, these five elements are represented in the pagodas (*buttou*) through their five tiers, beginning with earth (*chi*) and ending with the sky (*ku*), forming a link between the earth and the heaven.

five elements in Indian philosophy (Ind.) Also, panchabhuta, panchamahabhuta, panchatattva. The basic principle of AYURVEDA, according to which the human body is composed of five elements: water, fire, air, earth and ether. The characteristic features of these elements vis-a-vis the human body are shown in the following:

Element	Nature of the underlying force	Associated sensation	Associated sensory organ
Water	Flow	Taste (rasa)	Tongue
Fire	Change and transmutation	Form (rupa)	Eyes
Air	Power and movement	Touch (sparsha)	Skin
Earth	Cohesion	Odour (gandha)	Nose
Ether (space)	Original source	Hearing (shabda)	Ears

five elixirs (Ind.) Also, panchamrita. A blend of milk, sour milk, ghee, honey and jaggery, offered to deities during Hindu worship.

five evil traits See FIVE BLEMISHES.

five faiths (Ind.) Also, pancha shraddha. The fundamental beliefs in Hinduism. For a seeker of salvation, the basic requirement is faith (shraddha). The five faiths are indicated in the following table:

Shraddhas or faith	Explanatory note
sarva Brahman	feeling God's presence in all living creatures
mandira	belief in the abode of gods and divine existence
karma	the sum of all action of the past, present and future; the entire cycle of cause and effect
samsaramoksha	liberation from the cycle of births
Vedas and satguru	scriptures and preceptors

five fingers (Occ.) The five fingers, used in forming MUDRAS, are attributed with symbolic significance, as indicated in the following table:

Finger	Symbolic characteristics
little finger	inertia (tamas)
ring finger	activity (rajas)
middle finger	peace (sattva)
index finger	self (jivatma)
thumb	the Supreme (paramatma)

five functions of the Divine Force (Occ.) Also, pancha kritya. Creation, preservation, destruction, obscuration and liberation.

five gems (Gem) Also, pancha ratna. Gold, diamond, sapphire, ruby and pearl. The *Aditya Purana*, however, replaces diamond, sapphire and ruby, with silver, coral and lapis lazuli.

five Ms (Occ.) Also, pancha makara, five forbidden substances. Though these substances are forbidden by the orthodoxy, TANTRISM not only accommodates them in its folds but also celebrates them as essential requirements in all its rituals. They are:

Makaras	Meaning
mada	wine
mamsa	flesh
matsya	fish
mudra	money
maithuna	sexual intercourse

five makaras See FIVE Ms.

five manifestations (Occ./Yoga) Also, pancha chitta vritti. According to the system of YOGA, the subconscious mind is characterized by the 'mental chatters' (chitta vrittis) indicated in the following table:

Chitta vritti	Characteristics
pramana	cognition (considered right knowledge)
viparyaya	misconception (considered false knowledge)
vikalpa	process of imagination
nidra	process of sleep
smriti	process of memory

five-minute focus (Occ.) A technique of VERBAL THERAPY which includes formulating a short resolve and repeating the same, often with total concentration and sincerity. Advocates of this exercise believe that this technique enhances self-healing and helps achieve the condition or situation one aims for.

five-minute massage (New Age) A simple, quick anti-stress massage, started in a Sydney pub and meant for city folk in a hurry. The massage focusses on improving the flow of energy.

five moral restraints (Yoga) Also, five observances, yama. According to PATANJALI, expunging all emotional disorders is a prerequisite for beginning the practise of YOGA or any spiritual journey. This can be achieved by adopting an attitude, conducive to achieving the following:

Moral restraint	Brief explanation
ahimsa	non-violence (freedom from violence in thoughts, words and action)
satya	truthfulness (freedom from falsehood)
asteya	freedom from avarice
brahmacharya	celibacy (living in harmony with creative principles)
aparigraha	freedom from desires

> 'What is moral is what you feel good after.'
>
> —Ernest Hemingway

five observances (Yoga) See FIVE MORAL RESTRAINTS. NIYAMA, the observances, stipulated as guidelines by PATANJALI for YOGA practitioners.

five pranas See PRANA.

five psycho–physiological afflictions (Yoga) Also, pancha klesha. Ignorance (about oneself), ego, attraction, reputation and clinging to life are considered the five psycho–physiological afflictions inborn in humans.

five rites rejuvenation (Tib.) Also, mind–body healing. An exercise programme, as developed by Tibetan Buddhist monks, with similar bodily movements to those prescribed in HATHA YOGA. Practising these exercises is said to clear the flow of QI energy through the psychic CHAKRAs.

five sense healing (Occ.) A system of healing, addressing the five sense organs, by prescribing appropriate healing inputs indicated in the following table:

Senses	Healing prescription
taste	elixir (herbs)
sight	colour therapy
hearing	tones and rhythms (music therapy)
smell	incense (aromatherapy)
touch	etheric touch (massage)

five sheaths (Ind.) Also, five layers, pancha kosha. The five layers of a human organism which, according to the *Taittriya Upanishad*, helps an individual discriminate between the self and non-self. Such a discrimination makes a person wise as he views these sheaths as his 'non-self' and disassociates himself with these 'outer' layers. The five sheaths and their characteristics are indicated the following table:

Kosha (sheath)	Explanatory notes
Annamaya kosha, the sheath of food	Made of the 'essence' of food retained in the body. The gross and inert physical body, a part of the manifested world.
Pranamaya kosha, the sheath of energy	Made of the universal energy (PRANA), this sheath helps in energizing the food sheath in carrying out every activity connected with life. Though not visible, its existence can be felt by sharpening one's inner awareness through various practices such as ASANA, QIGONG, PRANAYAMA and REIKI. While acknowledging the endless and infinite energy source available in the form of PRANA, it should be borne in mind that every activity connected to life and living ceases when PRANA leaves the body. Regulating the flow of prana is believed to be an effective method of healing. Though prana is considered neither 'intelligent' nor 'emotional', it can be regulated by a conscious entity (MIND) with which it is said to be connected.
Manomaya kosha, the sheath of the mind	Called antahkarana, the 'inner instrument' is considered to comprise two sheaths: the mind (manomaya kosha) and intellect (vigyanmaya kosha). The mind is regarded as a layer of thoughts, prompted by memories, conditionings of

either likes or dislikes, various shades of emotions and an overall wisdom. This sheath, like the sheath of food, is also liable to be abused and is prone to disease, which can be cured by consciously adopting a healing routine and/or repatterning.

Vigyanmaya kosha, the sheath of intellect

According to the Upanishads, the self of mind is the intellect. The sheath of intellect is believed to include 'gyana indriya' (the apparatus of perception), besides intellect (buddhi) and hence represents one's type or level of knowledge. All thoughts are, in a way, a product and reflection of our 'knowledge', which is our appreciation and understanding of the fundamentals of life. As each one of us has a self-identity, every one of us is a storehouse of his or her own 'knowledge'. Intellect or buddhi enables us to reflect and deliberate on any thought. One can objectify thoughts, sustain them, go deep into its assumptions and even quieten all such thoughts, almost effortlessly. By reflecting on the presumptions behind every thought, one can refine one's thought patterns in consonance with universal peace and brotherhood.

Anandamaya kosha, the sheath of bliss

Deep down in the intellect is the sheath of bliss, referred also as the 'realm of joy'. It is considered to be of three types: priya, the intensity of the joy experienced while dwelling on a desired object or person; moda, the intensity of the joy experienced as we are closer to such an object or person; and pramoda, the intensity of joy experienced when we are one with the object or person of love. It is the joy which is considered the motivating force and the summum bonum of one's existence. According to the Upanishads, however, this is not the ultimate station in one's life as we may remain bonded endlessly, as seekers. The final step is the realization of one's nature of bliss, which alone is believed to liberate an individual. It is this realization which is the subject matter of Vedanta.

Till you manage your mind, you can not really manage your prana.

—The Vedas

five states of awareness (Yoga) Also, five avastas. The system of yoga recognizes four states of consciousness in humans. A fifth state, which is beyond all the four states, is also recognized, as indicated in the following table:

State of consciousness	meaning
jagrat	wakeful state
svapna	dream state
shushupti	dreamless state where human beings are one with the universe
turiya	beyond deep sleep
turiyatita	beyond all the above four states

five states of mind According to ancient Indian philosophy, humans are capable of functioning in five different states of mind. Though a majority of them exhibit a tendency to limit themselves in the first two states of mind as indicated in the table, spirituality and dedication help in achieving the remaining three higher states, indicated in the table:

State of mind	Characteristics
mudha	dull, inert, mindless state
kshipta	totally distracted state
vikshipta	partially distracted state
ekagraha	one-pointed state
niruddha	controlled state of 'no mind'

five subtle elements (Yoga) Also, tanmatra. The subtle elements as perceived by the (five) senses, as explained in the following table. The system of AYURVEDA makes use of them for therapeutic purposes.

Tanmatra or subtle element	Mechanism
sound (shabda)	hearing/ auditory
form (rupa)	sight/ visual
odour (gandha)	smell/ olfactory
taste (rasana)	taste/ gustatory
touch (sparsha)	touch/ cutaneous

five-syllabled incantation (Ind.) Also panchakshara. The five-syllabled mantra 'Namah Sivaya', which means 'I bow to the Lord, who is the Inner Self.'

five tastes (Ind.) Bitter, pungent, salty, sour and sweet constitute the five tastes. According to both AYURVEDA and the CHINESE MEDICINE, balancing these tastes in food/ food preparations is essential for one's good health. Some of these tastes are linked to the direction of energy flow in the body and also to specific metabolic functions triggered by them:

Herbs	Characteristics/functions
Bitter herbs	Drying, detoxifying and antibiotic. Capable of draining QI downward in the body. Also strengthens heart and small intestines.
Pungent herbs	Stimulating and warming. Capable of raising QI from the interior to the exterior of the body. Also strengthens the lungs and large intestine.
Salty herbs	Softens hardness, lubricates intestines and drains downwards.
Sour or astringent herbs	Capable of consolidating QI and secretions in the body. Also nourishes the liver and gallbladder.
Sweet herbs	Relaxing and nourishing. Capable of slowing down QI in the body. Also strengthens the spleen and stomach.

five Tibetans See FIVE RITES REJUVENATION.

flax seed Linum usitatissimum (Arab./ Am. Ind./Chi./Eur./Ind./Jap.) Also, alsi, cheruchana vithu, linseed, uma and ya ma ren (in Chinese). The plant has been known since ancient times. Its fibre is the oldest textile fibres used by man. AYURVEDA uses linseed as a diuretic, laxative and cure for piles. It is also believed to improve one's eyesight. Pliny, the Elder (23–79 AD), the Roman naturalist, attributed thirty uses to flax seeds, more particularly as a laxative and poultice for swelling. Until World War II, linseed was commonly used in Europe and the US as a food and medicine.

Flax seeds blended with water develop a texture like that of egg-whites and is used as an egg-substitute by bakers.

> 'Wherever flax seed becomes a regular food item among the people, there will be better health.'
>
> —Mahatma Gandhi

Fleet, Thurman See CONCEPT THERAPY.

fliessgleichgewicht (Occ.) Literally, the flowing balance. A concept which relates to the co-existence of balance and flow, of structure and change, essential in all forms of life.

floatinn (Spa) A portable wooden building equipped with tanks, toilets and changing facilities. It is used in sports facilities, such as fitness centres and golf clubs where such amenities may otherwise be lacking.

flocco method (Occ.) An approach to RE-FLEXOLOGY, which integrates all the three maps of ear, foot and hand to get more effective results. The method was developed by Bill Flocco of the American Academy of Reflexology.

flotation (New Age/Spa) Also, flotation therapy. Flotation refers to floating for an hour or so inside an enclosed tank, about 8 feet long, 4 feet wide, with about 10 inches of water with a high concentration of salt, kept at body temperature. Aimed at deep relaxation and rehabilitation, the technique is claimed to be an analgesic and anti-stress. It is often prescribed in conjunction with NEURO-MUSCULAR THERAPY.

flower and tree remedies (Flo./Occ.) Ancient methods of healing, focussed around employing the ENERGY trapped in flowers and other botanical parts. Believed to be synchronized with the energy mechanism of humans, the concepts of FLOWER ESSENCE THERAPY and TREE REMEDIES are contemporary rediscoveries of an ancient wisdom prevalent over a millennia in various parts of the world.

flower essence (Flo./Hom./Occ.) The dilute, potentized extracts of flowers and plants, similar to homoeopathic remedies. It was first developed by Edward Bach (1886–1936), a famous English physician. See BACH FLOWER REMEDIES.

> 'Behind all disease lie our fears, our anxieties, our greed, our likes and dislikes.'
>
> —Edward Bach

flower essence society (Flo./Occ.) A society, founded in California in the mid-1970s for research on FLOWER ESSENCE. The society is reported to have more than 100 different flower essences collected from all over the world from various flowers. It has also played an important role in educating people on the importance of flower remedies useful for healing.

flower essence therapy (Flo./Occ./Vib.) A variation of BACH FLOWER REMEDIES, as developed in the 1970s by Richard Katz. Subtle, liquid extracts obtained from wild flowers or pristine garden blossoms, which are believed to be full of life energy, are administered for healing.

> '(Flower essences are) catalysts to mind-body wellness.'
>
> —Patricia Kaminski

flower power The rich 'life energy' concentrated in flowers and in other botanical parts. Systems like BACH FLOWER REMEDIES make an attempt to tap such sources of energy for the health and wellbeing of people.

flower psychometry See FLOWER READING.

flower remedies (Flo./Hom./Occ.) Flowers are well-known for their delicate and sensitive qualities. Traditional healers around the world have perceived their high energy, which readily synchronizes with those who come in contact with them. They have therefore been associated with almost every healing tradition around the world. Besides being soft and attractive, many are quite fragrant, thus nurturing multiple senses, viz., touch, sight and smell. Flowers of brinjal, cotton, dill, golden champa, hog weed, Indian coral tree, Indian laburnum, oleander, muskroot, night jasmine, Persian lilac, rose, sacred lotus, Spanish cherry, tanner's cassia and water lily, for example, find their medicinal use in the traditional Chinese and Indian medical systems. Systems such as BACH FLOWER REMEDIES also use the water 'potentized' with appropriate floral essences. The remedies are prepared by floating freshly plucked blossoms in bowls of clean spring water and allowing them to receive sunshine on a cloudless day. In this way the water is said to be potentized by the floral essence or the energy. The potentized water is then mixed in fixed proportions with brandy, which acts as a preservative, and stored in dark glass bottles.

Though plant-based, such flower remedies are homoeopathic, rather than herbal, in the way they are administered.

flower therapy See BACH FLOWER REMEDIES.

fluorite (Vib.) A mineral form of calcium fluoride, which is believed to be of help in unblocking the energy flow in the body. The practice of placing a purple cluster of fluorite in work stations is observed as an energy correction mechanism. Fluorite of different types find application in addressing various problems as indicated:

Type of fluorite	Prescribed for
yellow-green	digestive problems
blue-white	muscular problems
purple-clear	headache, migraine
green	asthma
purple fluorite cluster (placed on the crown of the head)	confusion in thinking

focussing (New Age) Also focussing therapy. A method aimed at one's personal growth and SELF-HEALING, focussing refers to achieving direct contact with the underlying wisdom of one's body, also referred to as prenatal bodily meaning.

folk medicine (Occ.) The medicinal heritage of a community or a region as handed down from one generation to another. It refers to simple procedures and prescriptions, usually unwritten and transmitted orally, as are WITCHCRAFT and SHAMANISM.

Various practices in HERBALISM and HOME REMEDIES form the bulk of folk medicine. In the ceaseless hunt for new pharmaceuticals, folk medicine is also attracting the attention of modern scientists.

folk remedies See FOLK MEDICINE.

folk shamanic (Occ.) Of, or related to, a tribal or village magic rituals, performed by a SHAMAN, a mystic priest whose proven abilities to tame nature and wildlife enable him to function like an intermediary between the common folk and divine forces.

fomentation (Ind.) Also, fomentation therapy. A substance or material used as a warm, moist medicinal compress, intended to relieve pain. Sweating during fomentation helps the elimination of toxins through the skin as fatty tissues get mobilized due to increase of heat. Though CHARAKA had referred to thirteen types of fomentation in his treatise, only the types indicated in the following table are currently popular in AYURVEDA:

Fomentation	Explanatory notes
upanaha sweda	fomentation by poultice
ushma sweda	steam bath
nadi sweda	vapour of steam or medicated decoctions locally employed
avagah sweda	tub bath in warm medicated water
pizhichil	pouring of oil on the body

fomentation therapy See FOMENTATION.

food energy (Mod.) The amount of energy in food that is available through digestion. In the early-twentieth century, the United States Department of Agriculture (USDA) developed a procedure for measuring food energy by burning completely the sample food in a calorimeter. The heat released through such combustion is measured to determine the gross energy value. This number is multiplied by a coefficient based on how the human body actually digests the food. The values for food energy are expressed in kilocalories (kcal) and kilojoules (kJ). According to this system, the recommended daily energy intake values for young adults are: 2500 kcal/d (10 MJ/d, 120 W) for men and 2000 kcal/d (8 MJ/d, 100 W) for women. Children, sedentary and elderly people, however, require less energy.

food therapy (Ind.) The use of selected food ingredients for health. AYURVEDA classifies the food ingredients into three broad categories, as indicated:

Type of food	Examples	Role
Saatvic food	Seeds, nuts, sprouts, leafy vegetables, fresh fruits, and other 'living' foods	Activation of higher realms of CONSCIOUSNESS, giving rise to positive feelings such as love, compassion and sacrifice
Rajasic food	'Lower' plants such as	Activation of metabolic

| Tamasic food | Old, overcooked or stale food; prepared and preserved food, devoid of PRANA | Activation of the lower levels of consciousness giving rise to negative feelings, including, anger, egoism, greed, lust and selfishness |

mushrooms and botanical parts such as tubers and flesh of animals — functions

> 'Let food be your medicine and medicine be your food.'
> —Hippocrates

> 'A meal a day makes one yogi
> Twice a day makes one bhogi
> Thrice a day makes one rogi
> And eating four times, one becomes drohi.'
>
> —A Siddha saying (note: yogi connotes a healthy person; bhogi a connoisseur; rogi, a sick person; and drohi, a traitor)

foot analysis (Mod.) A diagnostic method, based on the premise that the feet indicate how one walks and how varying pressure put on them can affect other parts, closely or remotely connected to locomotion. For instance, even a small blister on the sole of the foot can affect the pressure put on the feet and may cause one to walk differently or cause discomfort or pain in the knees or hips.

foot bath (Nat.) The application of cold, running water on the feet for relieving congestion in the head, depression, general fatigue or insomnia.

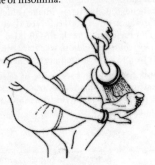

Foot bath

foot reflexology (New Age) A holistic healing method that involves pressure and

MASSAGE of the REFLEX POINTS on the feet. The reflexes on the soles of the feet act as small 'mirrors', reflecting the whole organism.

Foot reflexology focusses on unblocking VITAL ENERGY, constantly in circulation between the organs of the body. When the vital energy is blocked, the part of the body relating to such blockage becomes diseased and illness results. Such ENERGY BLOCKAGE, reflected in the feet can be addressed by using 'thumb walking' and other specific pressure techniques. The energy blocks are usually detected through the experience of discomfort, or through the presence of what is called gritty areas, or crystal deposits. Through pressure and massage, a reflexologist dissipates energy blockages and breaks down crystalline deposits. By stimulating the circulatory and lymphatic systems, foot reflexology can help the body to heal itself.

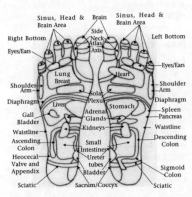

Foot reflexology

forbidden five Ms See FIVE Ms.

force (Mod.) The cause of acceleration or deceleration. See also, VITAL ENERGY.

forehead chakra See AJNA.

formless, concept of the (Occ.) Also, atattva. 1. Beyond the realm of form. Indian philosophy attempts to describe Pure Consciousness, which pervades the universe in this fashion. The 'formless' here, however, does not mean amorphous, but refers to the void emptiness beyond one's existence.

Fortean phenomena (Occ.) Paranormal events that appear to defy natural explanations, and named after a writer who had a distinct sense of humour on anomalous phenomena, Charles Hoy Fort (1874–1932).

'People with a psychological need to believe in marvels are no more prejudiced and gullible than people with a psychological need not to believe in marvels.'

—Charles Hoy Fort

Fosse, Gatter See AROMATHERAPY.

Foster, Jim See ACUTHERAPY.

four attitudes (Yoga) The attitudes conducive to controlling the mental process. in his YOGA SUTRAS, PATANJALI emphasizes the need for the conscious cultivation of the following attitudes:

Attitude	Meaning
maitri-sukha	friendliness towards happy people
karuna-dukha	compassion towards unhappy people
mudhita-punya	cheerfulness towards the virtuous
upekshanam-apunya	indifference towards the wicked

four chapters The four chapters in PATANJALI's YOGA SUTRAs which contain 196 aphorisms. The four chapters are:

samadhi pada	the chapter dealing with the theory of YOGA, as a process for mind-control
sadhana pada	the chapter containing the description of the art and technique of yoga
vibhuti pada	the chapter having guidelines on the internal disciplines of concentration, meditation and SAMADHI
kaivalya pada	the chapter dealing with the process of emancipation, overcoming the shackles of bondages in one's existence.

four ages (Yoga) According to the *Bhagavata Purana*, BRAHMA, the Creator, created the Universe, in a predetermined cycle of creation and dissolution. Each creation (kalpa) is equal to one day of Brahma and each dissolution (pralaya), one night. A creation and dissolution lasts for 4,320 million human years each. Every creation has 1,000 cycles of four ages (yuga). Each cycle of the four ages is completed in 4,320,000 human years. The four ages are:

Age	Characteristics of the age
Satya yuga	righteousness (DHARMA) reigns supreme, with 'all its four legs'.
Treta yuga	righteousness exists 'in three legs'.
Dvapara yuga	righteousness exists 'in two legs'.
Kali yuga	righteousness exists 'with only one leg', as humans turn selfish and evil, killing even their own species.

four energies (Chi.) The Chinese traditional system of HERBAL MEDICINE has identified four energies which determine the quality of herbs, as hot, cold, warm and cool. A neutral energy is also recognized. The treatment of an illness characterized as cool, will include a herb with warm characteristics. In the same way, the treatment for disorders exhibiting hot characteristics will incorporate herbs known for their cold properties.

four essentials for spiritual health (Occ.) Also, sadhana chatushtaya. The four qualities, considered essential for spiritual health have been identified in the Indian tradition as indicated in the following table:

viveka	discriminating intellect
vairagya	dispassionate dedication with detachment from worldly pursuits
shat sampat	six noble virtues (sama, dama, uparti, titiksha, shraddha and samadhana)
mumukshatva	a burning desire for self-realization

four gentlemen (Chi.) Also, four major herbs' decoction. The tonic combination of four herbs, administered in CHINESE MEDICINE for replenishing QI in the spleen and stomach. The four herbs normally prescribed are ginger, ginseng, liquorice and poria.

four great sayings (Yoga) Also, chatur mahavakyam. The four great utterances, all asserting universal oneness, as culled from the vast ancient Sanskrit treatises are given in the following table:

Original saying	Meaning	Source
tat tvam asi	Thou art That	*Chandogya Upanishad, Sama Veda*
aham brahmasmi	I am Brahman	*Brihadaranyaka Upanishad, Yajur Veda*
prajnanam brahma	Intelligence is Brahman	*Aitareya Upanishad, Rig Veda*
ayamatma brahma	This Self is Brahman	*Mandukya Upanishad, Atharva Veda*

four heads of Brahma (Yoga) The four heads of BRAHMA, Creator of the Universe, according to Hindu tradition, is symbolic of four directions. They also represent the following four distinguishable internal processes the mind is prone to:

Internal processes of the mind	Meaning
chitta	sub-conscious mind
manas	conscious mind
buddhi	intellect
ahamkara	individual principle or ego

four objectives of man (Yoga) Also, purushartha. The objectives of mankind. According to Indian philosophy, there are the following four legitimate purposes in human existence:

dharma	righteousness
artha	material wealth
kama	desire
moksha	salvation

four paths for God-realization According to the system of YOGA, there are four pathways which lead a seeker towards realizing the Truth and achieving unity with the universal principle:

karma yoga	yoga of action
raja yoga	yoga of meditation
bhakti yoga	yoga of devotion and love
jnana yoga	yoga of wisdom

four stages of the human life Also, chatur ashrama. According to the ancient Indian tradition, the four stages in a human life have been defined with corresponding appropriate activities:

Stage	Activities	Period	Remarks
Studentship (BRAHMACHARYA)	pursuit of knowledge and understanding	period of preparation for the other stages of life	5–24 years; considered conducive for

			learning and forming the right attitude
Householder (grihasta)	productive period of life; raising and maintaining home and family	period of production for family and society	24–48 years; considered the most important of all the four stages
Hermit or an elder-advisor (vanaprastha)	withdrawal from mundane responsibilities	period of service to humanity	48–72 years; a period conducive for self-discovery and learning about life's spectrum
Renouncement (SANYASA)	total detachment	period of retirement and aloofness	beyond 72 years; the mind is oriented towards the bliss in existence

Four Tantras (Tib.) Also, *Gyu-zhi*. The most important compilation on TIBETAN MEDICINE, authored by Yuthog Yonten Gonpo (1112–1203), a personal physician for a Tibetan king. *Four Tantras* contains 156 chapters, divided into four books. It classifies 1,600 types of diseases and their corresponding treatments, drawn from over 3,000 medicinal ingredients, their taste, potency and characteristics. Though indigenously Tibetan in character, the compilation is said to be greatly influenced by the medicinal knowledge of Indian and Greek traditions.

fourth chakra (Yoga) Also, ANAHATA CHAKRA, heart chakra. One of the fourteen CHAKRAS located in the area of one's heart, the fourth chakra represents cognition, compassion and love.

> 'When you begin to touch your heart or let your heart be touched, you begin to discover that it's bottomless, that it doesn't have any resolution, that this heart is huge, vast and limitless. You begin to discover how much warmth and gentleness there is, as well as how much space.'
>
> —Pema Chodron

fourth limb (Yoga) PRANAYAMA. In the 'eight-limbed' system of ASHTANGA YOGA, PRANAYAMA is considered the fourth stage. Pranayama is defined by PATANJALI as the regulation of movements in inhalation and exhalation.

fourth niyama (Yoga) Also, SVADHYAYA, self-study. One of the five forms of observances (niyama) in the yoga system of PATANJALI. It implies analytically watching one's actions and reactions to different situations and with increased awareness; reflecting on why one becomes happy, sad or angry. It refers to introspective self-analysis to preclude false knowledge.

fourth yama (Yoga) Also, BRAHMACHARYA. The continuous residence in the principle of creativity. The term also means celibacy, i.e., the control of the creative abilities and channelizing them towards scholarship.

fox glove See DIGITALIS LANATA.

fragrance for the sun signs (New Age/Occ.) The association of aromatic substances with one's sun sign. It is believed that there is a compatibility between one's sun sign and the fragrance obtained from aromatic herbs/substances as indicated in the table below:

Sun sign	Compatible aroma
Aries	Musk
Taurus	Patchouli
Gemini	lavender
Cancer	sandalwood
Leo	Rose
Virgo	coffee
Libra	orange
Scorpio	cinnamon
Sagittarius	Clove

Capricorn	myrrh
Aquarius	violet
Pisces	amber

Frank, Ojela See INITIATION HEALING; SOUL AMPLIFICATION.

free breathing See REBIRTHING.

free radicals (Mod.) Molecules having an unpaired electron, capable of snatching electrons from other molecules. Free radicals are found to be the cause for a wide range of diseases, including cancer, inflammatory and neuro-degenerative disorders and heart ailments. The process of AGEING is also attributed to be due to accumulating free radicals in the body.

free weights (Misc.) Hand-held dumbbells or barbells.

frequency (Mod.) The number of times a wave or cycle repeats itself within a second. The word wavelength describes the distance between one wave and the next. The higher the frequency, the shorter the wavelength.

Freud, Sigmund (1856–1939) (Mod.) One of the trailblazers of modern-day PSYCHOLOGY, Sigmund Freud is known as the originator of PSYCHOANALYSIS. Freud established that the human psyche is multi-faceted, and that each of us had warring factions within our subconscious.

> 'I cannot see any merit in being ashamed of sex.'
>
> —Sigmund Freud

friction (Mod./New Age) Massaging with thumbs, tips of the fingers and palms of the hand in circular movements towards the centre or around the joints. Friction limbers up joints, muscles and tendons, breaks up deposits and facilitates their clearance.

Friend, John See ANUSARA YOGA.

fringe medicine See ALTERNATIVE MEDICINE.

fritillaria (Chi.) *Fritillaria cirrhosa* Also, *Chuan bei mu* in Chinese. In TRADITIONAL CHINESE MEDICINE, the herb is used for scouring out thickened phlegm from the passages to the lungs. It is also externally applied for boils.

frontal passage (Yoga) A psychic passage, visualized to extend up the front of the trunk from the navel to the centre of the throat. The frontal passage is used extensively in the preliminary stages of training in KUNDALINI YOGA.

frozen bandage (Mod.) A healing method, recommended for athletic injuries, sciatic tensions, spasms and sprain.

fruit mono-diet (Mod./New Age) Eating only fruit as a therapeutic measure.

fruitarian diet (New Age) The administration of fruits, in place of cooked food.

Fudd, Robbert (1574–1637) British physician, author and philosopher who sought to establish parallels between man and the world, both of which he viewed as images of God. According to him, special analogies revealed by ASTROLOGY and NUMEROLOGY could be used to provide other medical insights.

Fukaya, Tadamasa See DIVINE HEALING FROM JAPAN.

fun (Arab.) An Arabic word for GARLIC.

functional foods (Mod./New Age) Food items fortified with herbs, vitamins, minerals and other supplements.

functional testing (Mod.) A form of medical assessment, functional tests help determine the way the body functions. As functional changes occur in a person's physiology much before the symptoms of diseases arise, they send early warnings so that action to prevent the disease becomes possible.

future medicine See BEYOND MEDICINE.

G

G5 (New Age) A modern-day massage machine, used in physical therapy and sports medicine industries. The electro-massage features include multiple-direction stroking, gyratory and percussive action.

Gaia (Grk.) Also, Ge. The Greek goddess who embodies planet Earth. The Gaia hypothesis proposes that the earth functions as a single living entity, maintaining conditions, conducive for its own survival.

Gaai choi (Chi) See MUSTARD.

galangal (Chi./Eur./Ind./Isl./Jap.) *Alpinia galanga*. Also, adkham in Arabic, arattai (Sid.), blue ginger, chewing John, daaih gou leuhng geung in Chinese, garanga in Japanese, kulanja (Ayur.), *lam keong*, Lengkuas, little John chew. The dried root-stock (rhizome) of this plant, a delicacy in many regional cuisines, is widely used as a household remedy in the treatment of dyspepsia, flatulence, nausea and stomach disorders. A mixture of galangal and lime juice is used as a tonic in parts of South-east Asia, and is regarded as an APHRODISIAC.

'(Galangal) is a destroyer of kapha and vata.'

—Bhava Prakasa Nighantu

Gall, Franz Joseph See PHRENOLOGY.

Galvani, Luigi See ANIMAL ELECTRICITY.

gamalel (Gem.) A natural stone or GEM, considered magical and used as a talisman. Its magical properties are attributed to astrological factors.

gan cao (Chi.) See LIQUORICE.

gandhachikitsa (Ind.) Also, ayurvedic aromatherapy. The therapeutic application of plant and floral essences in their various forms, viz., paste, powder, liquid and volatile oil for massaging the body in general and on its MARMA points in particular. They are also used for inhalation and for external applications in MASSAGE, BATH and MOXIBUSTION.

gandhapushpa See ASHOKA.

gandharva haritaki (Ind.) A medicinal formulation in AYURVEDA, which includes mercury and HARITAKI.

Gandharva Veda (Ind.) The science of therapeutic music and chanting, as was prevalent in ancient India. The practices of NADA YOGA and RAGA CHIKITSA have followed the tradition of employing music in holistic healing exercises in ancient rites, rituals and sacrifices.

gandush (Ind.) Gargling with a warm, saline solution. The liquid in the mouth cannot be swished around because the mouth is full; when it can be, the gargle is called kawal. A pinch of rock salt in a little warm sesame oil is recommended but any medicated oil (according to the DOSHA) can be used. Decoctions, fresh juices, milk, ghee also can be used for gandush.

A preparation of triphala can also be used. Triphala powder (50 gm) is added to water (400 ml) and boiled until the quantity of liquid is halved (200 ml). The strained decoction is used. Curcuma (turmeric) and salt can be added.

Ganesha mudra (Yoga) A MUDRA formed

by grappling the fingers of one hand with others and the hand kept at the level of the chest. This MUDRA is believed to help decongest the respiratory tract.

Ganzfeld stimulation (New Age) A recent experimental technique to create an environment of sensory deprivation to stimulate the receptivity of ESP.

gananga See GALANGAL.

garden basil See BASIL.

garden rue See RUE.

garden sage See COMMON SAGE.

gardeness stone See AGATE.

gargat A black stone, believed to drive away hallucination.

garlic (Chi./Heb./Ind./Isl./Jap.) *Allium sativum*. Also, da suan in Chinese, fum in Arabic, kallik in Korean, lahsuna (Ayurveda), ninniku and taisan in Japanese, sarmisak in Turkish. Known for its medicinal use for over six thousand years, it is considered an effective detoxifier, purifying the

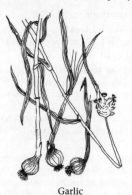

Garlic

blood and lymph. In UNANI medicine garlic is the favourite root. Hippocrates, the father of medicine, recommended the use of garlic in infectious diseases and particularly prescribed it for intestinal disorders.

> 'It is ordered that all my workers take garlic everyday to maintain their health and strength.'
>
> —Khnoom Khoufoof, who built the pyramids (4500 BC)

garnet (Gem.) A deep red transparent stone, believed to increase sexual energy, prevent skin eruptions and ensure consistency in love and friendship. When held over the ovaries or uterus, it is believed to alleviate menstrual pain.

garuda mudra (Yoga) Formed by clasping the thumbs of both the hands, this MUDRA is believed to benefit disorders of the stomach and menstrual problems in women.

gau chahng taap See BASIL.

gaussmeter (Mod.) A device consisting of a coil of wire connected to a multimeter, used for measuring magnetic fields. A voltage induced in the coil by magnetic fields is detected and measured by the meter.

Gayatri mantra (Ind.) An auspicious MANTRA, referred to as the mother of all mantras. Meditating upon the glorious splendour of the 'Great Divine Vivifier', the mantra seeks illumination of the mind, a clear recognition of the vital role the mind plays in making or marring our individual and collective existence.

The synchronization of breathing, practised while mentally reciting the four parts of this mantra is explained below:

Mantra (for mental recitation)	Breathing action to be synchronized with recitation
Om Bhur Bhuvah Svaha	Inhalation
Om Tat Savitur Virenyam Bhargo Devasya Dhimahi	Retention (antara kumbhaka)
Om Dhiyo Yo Nah Prachodayat	Exhalation
Om	Stay (bahiranga kumbhaka)

> 'Mind's in its place and in itself make a heaven of hell, a hell of heaven.'
>
> —William Shakespeare

gazing (at an object) See TRATAKA.

Geller effect (New Age) Feats of PSYCHOKINESIS, such as bending metal objects by stroking or looking at them, stopping watches or making them run faster, as performed in the 1970s by Geller Uri (6.1946), an Israeli psychic.

gelsemium (Hom.) Also, yellow jasmine. Used to treat conditions that affect vision.

gem essence (Gem.) The water derived by soaking naturally formed gems and exposing it to sunlight. In GEM THERAPY, such extracts are used in the treatment of various ailments. See also GEM THERAPY.

gem therapy (Gem.) The use of naturally formed gems believed to entrap vital energy to cure diseases. Some important gems and their traditionally acknowledged therapeutic roles are indicated in the following table:

Gem	Therapeutic role
bloodstone	arrests haemorrhage
ceraunius	sweet dreams
chelidonius	febrifugal
chrisoletus	protection against evil forces and illusions
citrine	balancing emotional upheavals
clear quartz	mental clarity
galactide	love and friendship
garatronicus	victory (in battle, etc.)
gargate	protection against hallucinations
garnet	Rejuvenation
green beryl	a remedy for eye ailments
yellow beryl	a remedy for jaundice
hamon	divine grace
hessonite garnet (gomed)	protection against anxiety, fear and illusions
hyena	a remedy for gout
jade	a remedy for heart ailments; protection during childbirth
lapis exilis	Arresting the adverse effects of ageing
moonstone	toning down passions
ruby	Chills

gemstone reiki therapy (Gem.) A practice of REIKI, with selected gemstones placed at appropriate positions on the body. Gemstones are recognized for their colour vibrations.

Gendlin, Eugene T. See FOCUSSING.

geomancy (Occ.) DIVINATION by means of figures or lines, such as natural or artificial configurations of the earth, aimed at ensuring the harmonious interaction between place and people. The term is also used to refer to the Chinese practice of FENG SHUI.

geopathic stress (Mod.) The unhealthy effects of electro-magnetic radiation emanating from the earth on its inhabitants, as discovered by German doctors in the 1920s while investigating the causes of the unusually high incidence of cancer among inhabitants living in some villages and streets. Non-uniformity in the magnetic field of the earth occurs in some areas due to geological fault lines (e.g., a deep crack in the bedrock) and allows the radiation to gush in to such areas at the surface from the deep bowels of the earth, adversely affecting the health of those who live there. Chronic illnesses, such as cancer and multiple sclerosis, headaches, stress and stress-related disorders, which are seen to afflict many who live in such areas, are attributed to the continuous disruption of the body's electrical field and its electrical control system with the earth's electro-magnetic force. Geopathic stress is suspected to be the reason for the failure of medicine which would otherwise have been effective. By changing the place of residence (or even by shifting the placement of the bed in the bedroom), the afflicted are expected to recuperate. Heavy growth of moulds, lichens and moss, previous occupants of the house/building or neighbours with serious health issues, the location of deep wells and springs in the area and repeated obvious gaps in hedges in gardens could indicate the presence of geopathic stress. The stress could be more pronounced in areas where the water table is high, such as around estuaries or in areas near oil-fields and areas of seismic or volcanic activity. Dogs, cows and horses are reported to be able to sense geopathic stress and avoid such places. According to Dr Kohfink, a German scientist and expert on geopathic stress, there has been a considerable increase in geopathic stress since the end of the Second World War, particularly after underground nuclear tests carried out in various parts of the world.

geriatric massage (New Age) MASSAGE administered to the elderly. Though the massage uses the same techniques as any general massage, it takes into account the specific age and health conditions of the individual and hence is elderly-friendly. It is characterized by shorter sessions (say, about twenty minutes), careful massaging of hands and feet, and gentle strokes.

Gerson therapy (New Age) Also, Gerson diet. A nutritional healing therapy aimed at DETOXIFICATION. It proscribes sodium salts as Gerson found a link between sodium intake and tumour growth; it was also found to interfere with body functions. It also proscribes fats and proteins, as in excess they were found to be carcinogenic. It prescribed fruit juices, potassium supplements and coffee enemas. This system of SELF-HEALING was developed by Max B. Gerson (1881–1959), referred to as a 'medical genius who walked among us' by Dr Albert Schweitzer. According to Gerson, one needs high potassium and low sodium, the same ratio which can be found in fresh live foods. As processed foods contain high levels of sodium, they are to be avoided to prevent tumour growth. Gerson therapy recognizes the importance of the liver, the filtration system, in detoxification. By the time cancer or chronic disease develops, liver function is below 35 per cent. The body isn't really restored until the liver goes back to its full activity, between 90 and 100 per cent. Consumption of alcohol, candies, ice cream, cheese, meat, and all kinds of processed foods, besides sodium chloride, fats, proteins need to be kept in check to ensure that the liver functions at its peak.

Gerson therapy is considered by many medical professionals as a basic and effective treatment not only for cancer, but also for those suffering from colitis, diabetes, heart disease, high blood pressure, multiple sclerosis, rheumatoid arthritis and several other ailments.

'We give a fresh glass of juice every hour: five glasses of apple–carrot juice, three glasses of plain carrot juice and we give liver capsules with it, four glasses of juice from leafy-type greens rich in chlorophyll, iron, nutrients, enzymes, everything the body has been lacking over the years. We also give three full vegetarian meals and a fruit plate every day. By drinking the juice, you get an enormous flooding of nutrients, minerals, enzymes, and vitamins which start to flush out the kidneys. The nutrients go into the tissues, into the cells and force out the poisons, and all those poisons are released into the blood stream. The liver filters them out. You have to help the liver get rid of them, and there is only one way—by opening the bile ducts.'

—Dr Gerson did this with the famous and much-joked-about coffee enemas.

gestalt (New Age) Also, gestalt phenomenon; a term coined by philosopher Christian von Ehrenfels in 1890 to denote experiences that require more than basic sensory capacities to comprehend. In 1912, a movement nurtured by German theorists Max Wertheimer, Wolfgang Köhler and Kurt Koffka protested against the prevailing atomistic, analytical psychological thought, a clear departure from the general intellectual climate which emphasized a scientific approach characterized by a detachment from basic human concerns. For a gestalt, reality and the science that studies it must be understood in the light of the existence of what might be called an 'implicate order' and of relationships within that order. Gestalt psychology specifically looks at contrast, organization, and dynamic processes between and within contextual reality with the goal of depicting and describing wholes and preserving meaning.

Gestalt theory (Mod.) Also, gestalt psychology; a theory of mind and brain, describing the GESTALT EFFECT. At the beginning of the twentieth century, Gestalt psychologists spoke against the limitations faced by science in handling subtler phenomena such as mind and life and warned of a science that had become void of both sense and value. According Gestalt theory, the percepts themselves are basic to experience. For example, in a set of ellipses (…), one does not see only individual dots, but a dotted line, as the dots grouped together may impart a meaning different from just a group of dots. In addition, Gestalt theorists acknowledge that memory structures information 'based on associative connections' with a 'tendency for optimal organization'. For example, a movie is just pictures in motion. The pictures themselves remain static, but when played at twenty-four frames per second, the images on the screen appear to be in motion, imparting a definitive meaning.

Kurt Koffka used Gestalt theory in applied psychology. His research with infants led to a theory that infants 'initially experience organized wholes' as opposed to discrete elements. Kohler's experiments with animal learning led him to conclude that they exhibited 'insight'. In these experiments, apes were subjected to different trials of having to obtain food that was just out of their reach. They learned how to construct a way to get the food, whether standing on a box to get it, making a long stick to reach it, through trial and error. Kohler determined that apes generated an 'interconnection based on the properties of the things themselves' and thus developed insight on how to get the food based on the available tools at a given time. Gestalt was not as concerned with what one learns as how he or she learns it. For Gestalt theorists, 'knowledge is conceived as a continuous organization and rearrangement of information according to needs, purposes and meanings'. As a challenge to conventional thinking, 'learning is not accumulation, but remodelling and insight'.

Gestalt theory is a cornerstone of learning theory. Unlike behaviouralists who insisted on observable human behaviour to determine whether learning has taken place, Gestalt theorists went after the entirety of the problem or experience. The entire structure of experience was valued, as opposed to individual sensations or perceptions.

Several theories can be built from the components of Gestalt theory. Disciplines including art, music, psychology and instructional design can be related to Gestalt theory and follow Gestalt principles in some form. In addition, Gestalt theory is continually being updated through redevelopment and reassessment.

gestalt psychology, six laws of (Mod.) Gestalt theory recognizes six laws: law of proximity, law of closure, law of symmetry, figure-ground segregation, law of good continuation and law of similarity.

gestalt psychotherapy (Mod.) A method of PSYCHOTHERAPY which focusses on the here-and-now experience and personal responsibility, based on the experiential ideals of GESTALT THEORY. Fritz Perls (1893–1970), Laura Perls (1915–90) and Paul Goodman (1911–72) paved way for this idea in the 1940s and 1950s. The objective of this humanistic psychotherapy was to make the client become more creatively alive and free him from the blocks and unresolved issues which may diminish satisfaction in one's life.

Ghatastha Yoga (Yoga) From the Sanskrit ghata, meaning pot, referring to the human body. A style of HATHA YOGA which aims at achieving the maximum yogic results with the minimal expenditure of energy. The system has selective ASANAs, which emphasize bending, twisting and stretching the spinal column, resulting in a rich supply of oxygenated blood to the areas of the brain. Ghatastha is literally 'within the pot', and refers to the great transformation that could be made by infusing energy into the human body.

Ghee kumau See ALOE.

Gheranda Samhita (Yoga) Gheranda's compendium; one of three major manuals of classical HATHA YOGA, composed in the seventeenth century.

ghrita (Ind.) Also, ghee. Clarified butter, used in AYURVEDA as an essential ingredient in some drug formulations.

ghrita neti (Ind.) Nasal irrigation with GHRITA, the regular practise of which is said to maintain a healthy secretory and drainage mechanisms of the ear, nose and throat. This is also a treatment for warding off allergic rhinitis, catarrh, cold and cough, hay fever, headache caused by eye strain, middle-ear infection, myopia and, in certain cases, deafness.

giant's funnel See ASAFOETIDA.

ginger (Chi./Heb./Ind./Isl./Jap.) *Zingiber officinale.* Also, adraka (Ayurveda); adarak (Unani), inji (Siddha), jeung in Chinese, sangvil in Hebrew, shôga in Japanese, zanjabeel in Arabic. Both fresh (sheng giang or adraka) and dried (gan jiang or sonth) rootstocks (rhizome) of this plant are used extensively in the traditional medicines of China and India. In both the countries, fresh ginger finds its application in alleviating nausea, cold and cough and phlegm, and is found useful in reducing the toxicity of other herbs (like fu zi, ban xia). The dried ginger is known for its role in fighting chronic diarrhoea, by warming up the middle portion of the body and improving circulation. It is also used to relieve pain in abdomen, chest and lower back areas.

'There's no limitation for *chukku*, that it can cure only this and not that.'

—A Tamil song, referring to ginger's use in Siddha medicine

ginkgo biloba (Chi./Jap.) In Chinese *ginkyo* refers to silver apricot. Also, bai guo in Chinese, icho in Japanese. The extract of the leaves of this plant is used in TRADITIONAL CHINESE MEDICINE in the treatment of diseases of the blood vessels, high viscosity of blood, high cholesterol, dizziness, depression, anxiety and memory impairment.

'Ginkgo has for centuries appealed to the imagination of the Oriental mind: the tree with leaves like golden ducks' feet became an object of veneration; a legacy, it might be, from a golden age and as such possessing miraculous power. We, despite our matter-of-fact Western outlook, pay homage to the sacred tree of the East because its story, written in the sands of time, gives us a vision of enduring life. The maidenhair tree appeals to the historic souls: we see it as an emblem of changelessness, a heritage from worlds of an age too remote for our human intelligence to grasp, a tree which has in its keeping the secrets of the immeasurable past.'

—Albert Seward

ginseng (Chi.) *Panax ginseng.* Also, ren shen. TRADITIONAL CHINESE MEDICINE recognizes the role of this root in the improvement of memory, cardiac functions and digestion. It is also said to regulate the circulatory and nervous systems, improve the immune system and is considered as an APHRODISIAC.

glandulars (Mod.) Concentrates of hormonal glands used in therapy. It is believed that ageing glands of patients can be rejuvenated by such concentrates.

glandular therapy (Mod.) A therapeutic method in which concentrates of hormonal glands are used. It is believed that the glands of ageing patients can be rejuvenated by such supplements, as the nourishment in glandular substances get easily absorbed.

glycolic facial (Cos.) A skin application that breaks down the glue bond that holds dry skin on the face, causing rapid exfoliation which softens lines and smoothens the skin.

goatweed See SI JOHN'S WORT.

golden apple See BENGAL QUINCE.

gokshura (Ind.) A thorny need found in wastelands. It helps eliminate toxins and

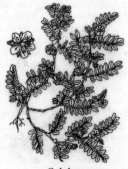

Gokshura

stones that may clog the genito-urinary tract. It is one of the TEN GREAT ROOTS that constitute the popular ayurvedic preparation DASAMULA.

golden spoons (Cos.) Two twenty-three-carat gold spoons, one warm and the other cold, used alternately, for efficient application of creams and lotions in FACIALS. This treatment is based on the principle of alternating hot and cold applications.

gommage (Cos.) Cleansing and moisturizing body treatment using creams that are applied with long massage-like strokes.

gong therapy (New Age) A system of healing based on the belief that vibrations that emanate from a gong induce healing consciousness.

gomashio (Jap./New Age) A natural flavouring used in Japanese cuisine, especially in MACROBIOTICS, as a healthy alternative to common salt. It is made of roasted sesame seeds and salt, generally in 18:1 proportion. The word *gomashio* is also used in Japanese to refer to salt-and-pepper hair.

gomed See HESSONITE GARNET.

gomutra (Ind.) Cow's urine; a time-tested ayurvedic remedy. According to AYURVEDA, eight types of animal urine have medicinal properties. They are divided into two groups: the male group and female. Included in the male group is the urine of ass, camel, elephant and horse, while the urine of the buffalo, cow, goat and sheep fall in the female group. Cow's urine is considered supreme, and has been so since pre-Vedic times; the Vedas refer to it as 'a purifying substance' among PANCHAGAVYA. Gomutra is also considered valuable in the treatment of cancer and leprosy and is traditionally used in combination with other ingredients as indicated:

Ailments	Traditional combinations
Anaemia	gomutra + TRIPHALA + cow's milk
Fever	gomutra + black pepper + yoghurt + GHRITA
Leprosy	gomutra + NEEM bark + VASAKA leaves + kuraila bark + kaner leaves
Epilepsy	gomutra + dharuharidra

In recent times, some Indian scientific research is forthcoming on urine therapy. The Centre for Scientific and Industrial Research (CSIR) has developed drugs using gomutra for the treatment of asthma. A blood-clot dissolver has been isolated from gomutra by the Institute of Microbial Technology (IMT), which can be useful in the treatment of heart ailments. A herbal formulation developed by Indian Institute of Chemical Biology (ICB) shows potential as a cure for asthma sufferers.

gong (Occ.) A metal percussion instrument, made mainly from bronze or brass, used in Eastern musical traditions and in healing rituals. They are of three varieties: flat suspended gongs, bossed gongs, played horizontally, and bowl gongs, whose rims are rubbed to enhance MEDITATION.

Gonpo, Yuthog Yonten See TIBETAN MEDICINE.

Goodheart, George J. See APPLIED KINESIOLOGY.

Gordon, Richard See AMPLIFIED ENERGY THERAPY; QUANTUM TOUCH.

grace (Occ.) The infinite power of divine love and benevolence behind the creation and maintenance of the universe. The evolved person finds himself surrounded by grace, as he or she sees all of God's actions as grace. According to the *Saiva Siddhanta*, grace paves the way for SELF-REALIZATION.

granthi (Yoga) A psychic knot of spiritual energy, which is believed to impede the flow of PRANA into SUSHUMNA. The three major granthis are: Brahma-granthi, Vishnu-granthi and Rudra-granthi.

grahachikitsa Psychiatry.

grape cure (New Age) Also, grape diet. A mono-diet of grapes or grape juice, to treat ailments including cancer, diabetes, gout, rheumatism and sex problems.

grape fast (New Age) The exclusive consumption of grapes and/or grape juices for a fixed duration, aimed at cleaning the digestive tract. It is believed to be a means of blood purification.

graphology (Occ.) The study of handwriting, especially when applied as a means of analyzing one's character. According to graphologists, details such as loops, dotted i's and crossed t's, slants, endings, letter-spacing and letter-heights reveal as much details about a person as ASTROLOGY or PALMISTRY. They are considered physical manifestations of the unconscious mind of a person.

graphotherapy (Occ.) The analysis of handwriting with a view to find out a person's attitude, feelings, emotions or situations. It is believed that some personality traits can be changed by changing one's handwriting.

great burdock See BURDOCK.

Greek medicine (Grk.) Medical practices in ancient Greece. Hippocrates' theory of the Four Humours, for example, was long the accepted basis for medical reasoning. Several Greek philosophers also contributed to our current understanding of diseases and their causes.

green beryl (Gem.) A stone worn to overcome diseases of the eyes. Yellowish beryl is often prescribed for jaundice and liver diseases.

green-colour therapy (Occ.) A system of colour therapy based on the notion that the colour green keeps bacteria, viruses and other pathogens at bay and has a therapeutic role in the treatment of a host of ailments including asthma, backache, colic, erysipelas, exhaustion, hay fever, haemorrhoids, insomnia, irritability, laryngitis, malaria, malignancy, nervous disorders, neuralgia, over-stimulation, syphilis, typhoid, ulcers and venereal disease.

green tea (Nat.) Tea leaves which are heated before oxidation (fermentation) is complete. Green tea is reported to reduce the risk of cancer and help prevent cardiovascular disease.

Gregorian chants (Occ.) A type of plainsong believed to have therapeutic value. It is associated with Pope Gregory I, and is characterized by simple melody and the emphasis on long, slow breaths.

> 'Gregorian songs are fantastic energy foods.'
>
> —Dr Alfred Tomatis

Grof, Stanislav and Christina See HOLOTROPIC BREATHWORK.

group psychotherapy (Mod.) A form of PSYCHOTHERAPY performed in groups; a modern equivalent to the ancient practice of SATSANG.

group therapy (Mod.) PSYCHOTHERAPY conducted with at least three or four non-related individuals who otherwise exhibit certain common traits, such as gender, age, mental illness, or communication problems.

Gruber work (New Age) A form of BODYWORK as promoted by Susanne Gruber, incorporating the techniques of CONNECTIVE TISSUE MASSAGE, ROLFING and YOGA.

guduchi (Ind.) The plant's various names make references to its attributes; madhurparni refers to its sweet leaves, kundali suggest that it is a creeper. Vishalya refers to the smoothness of its surface (it is without thorns, spines or other outgrowths). Although its fresh stems are more potent than the dried ones, it is easier to employ the latter. Guduchi which grows on neem trees is much sought after as it is believed to incorporate the medicinal virtues of neem as well. The stems are collected during the summer months and dried with the bark intact. The dried stems are popular as the drug tinospora or gilo.

The plant has been used in native medicine from times immemorial to treat anaemia, bleeding piles, consumption, diabetes, chronic dysentery, diarrhoea, enteric fevers, erysipelas, gonorrhoea, heart disease, helminthiasis, hypertension, itching, jaundice, leprosy, rheumatoid arthritis, skin infections, thirst, syphilis, vomiting and worm-

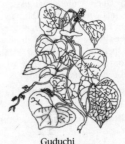

Guduchi

infection. It is also considered useful in promoting longevity, imparting vitality and youthfulness and improving the intellect. It is also used to make a bitter tonic which finds its application in the preparation of blood purifiers.

guggulu (Ind.) *Commiphora mukul* Also, guggul. A small, thorny tree found throughout the Indian subcontinent. Guggul, a commercial medicinal substance, consists of the yellowish resin produced by the stem of the plant. This resin has long been used in medicine to fight problems connected with acne vulgaris, osteo-arthritis, artherosclerosis, obesity, high levels of cholesterol and tri-glycerides .

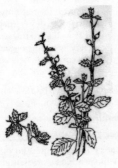

Guggulu

guided imagery (Occ.) Also, creative imagery, creative visualization, focused daydreaming, mental imagery. The technique of picturing something and actually experiencing it. Images aren't necessarily limited to visual but can be sounds, tastes, smells or a combination of sensations. Based on the assumption that the mind can affect physiological functions in the body, this technique is used in sorting out emotional problems and blockages encountered by people. According to some psychologists, picturing something and experiencing it are equivalent as far as brain activity is concerned. Recent brain scan experiments support this view. It is therefore, recommended as a relaxation method. Selected music is also played during the therapeutic sessions to enhance its effect. Guided imagery promises not only enlightenment, but also empowerment, courage and strength.

gulkand (Ind.) A delicious preparation made primarily of rose petals, mixed with other rejuvenating ingredients like honey and herbs blended in. It is used in AYURVEDA as a cooling tonic to combat fatigue, lethargy, muscular aches, biliousness, itching, and heat-related conditions. It is also rich in calcium and antioxidants. It is often recommended as a tonic for year-round use, especially for those with aggravating VATA and PITTA.

gum tree See BLUEGUM EUCALYPTUS.

guna (Ind.) Quality. Three fundamental qualities in nature (referred to as triguna) determine the inherent characteristics of all things in nature. The concept and practices relating to guna form the backbone of AYURVEDA, as all things in nature, including the human mind, are believed to be composed of one of these qualities.

The gunas are believed to pave the way for creation, maintenance and destruction of all living creatures and living systems in the universe. They are broadly grouped in to three categories:

Guna	Role	Nature
sattva (the principle of lucidity)	Binds the spirit to the body by focussing on happiness, knowledge, lofty ideals, noble desires and selfless service to humanity	Awakening and uplifting
rajas (the principle of dynamism)	Binds the spirit to the body by focussing on sensory fulfillment, craving for pride, power and position	Activity and movement
Tamas (the principle of inertia)	Binds the spirit to the body by focussing on lethargy, resistance and sleep	Obstructive and downward flowing

guna in food (Ind.) The categorization of
DIET, based on GUNA, its inherent quality, is
summarized below:

Guna	Food types	Expected Impact
Sattva (sattvic diet)	Closest to its original, natural condition: living, raw, fresh, alkaline, and uncooked foods such as fruits, greens, sprouted grains, nuts , seeds etc form this category	Promotes positive feelings such as love and compassion, accompanied by positive behaviour tendencies conducive to the preservation of family, community or society.
Rajas (rajasic diet)	Foods, rich in hot spices, condiments and salt; freshly cooked food of predominantly animal origin	Stimulating strategic alertness and committed participation in all possible activities concerning self and self aggrandisement
Tamas (tamasic diet)	Acidic, over-cooked, processed, preserved, frozen or stale food	Conducive to unhealthy lifestyle, causing harm to the self as well as to the family or society by fueling negative traits such as FIVE BLEMISHES

guptasana See VIRASANA.

Gurdjief, George Ivanovich (1866–
1949) (Occ.) A spiritual leader and founder of
a movement that subscribed to meditation
and heightened self-awareness.

guru (Yoga) A spiritual master. A title for a
teacher or guide in any subject, especially
art, dance, music and religion.

> 'The best of seers is he who guesses well.'
> —Euripides (484–06 BC)

guru bhakti (Ind.) 1. Devotion to the
teacher and dedication to his principles. 2.
The attitude of humility and commitment
to knowledge exhibited by a student in any
field of knowledge or skill.

gyan mudra See JNANA MUDRA.

gyan yoga See JNANA YOGA.

gyromancy (Occ.) A method of DIVINA-
TION in which alphabets are written on the
ground in a large circle, around the diviner,
from where the diviner will spin around on
his feet until he stumbles on a letter. From
this, he will again spin on his feet until he
stops and stumbles upon another letter,
which is recorded by the observers.

Gyu-zhi See FOUR TANTRAS.

Haelan work (Occ.) A method in pain management which helps people focus on the need to integrate their body, mind and spirit. The method includes COUNSELLING, MEDITATION, PSYCHOTHERAPY, PRAYER and THERAPEUTIC TOUCH.

habaq (Isl.) An Arabic name for BASIL.

haematite Also, black diamond. A brown stone, believed to be useful in pain management. It is worn in rings, bracelets, belts or chains, depending on the pain locus.

Hahnemann, Christian Friedrich Samuel (1755–1843) (Hom.) A German physician who was the founder of HOMOEOPATHY. The system is based on the premise 'like cures like'—which refers to the principle by which a substance which produces a set of symptoms in a healthy individual can be useful in treating a sick individual manifesting similar symptoms. The fruits of Hahnemann's labour are contained in his treatise *The Organon of the Medical Art.*

> 'The physician's highest calling, his only calling, is to make sick people healthy—to heal, as it is termed.'
>
> —Samuel Hahnemann

Hahnemannian method of attenuation (Hom.) The Hahnemannian method uses a new container at each attenuation step. It uses a measurement of 1 part of the previous homoeopathic potency and the appropriate amount of the diluent to create the next homoeopathic potency after succussion (9 parts for X or D potencies, 99 parts for C potencies). All homoeopathic drug products manufactured by this method bear the letter H in their potency designation, e.g. 6DH or 9CH, to indicate that the Hahnemannian method has been employed. See also, ATTENUATION, KORSAKOVIAN METHOD OF ATTENUATION, SUCCUSSION.

hakim (Ind.) Physician or medical professional, especially in UNANI.

Hakini (Occ.) The presiding deity of the SIXTH CHAKRA, who controls the subtle mind.

Hakini mudra (Yoga) A MUDRA formed by keeping all the fingertips of both hands juxtaposed as shown in the illustration. The mudra is believed to help strengthen the respiratory organs and overcome respiratory problems.

Hakomi method (New Age) Also, Hakomi Experiential Method of Assisted Self-Study and Mindfulness-based Psychotherapy. A method of body-centred PSYCHOTHERAPY, developed in the 1970s by Ron Kurtz. The experiential method is based on the five therapeutic principles: mindfulness, organicity, non-violence, the mind–body connection and unity. Essential to Hakomi are a loving presence, quieting the mind, and emotional nourishment. The method makes use of ENERGY WORK, MASSAGE and THERAPEUTIC TOUCH. The system recognizes the philosophy that the human body is an ever-changing, interactive and living source of information about the UNCONSCIOUS MIND.

halasana (Yoga) An ASANA which resembles a plough. This posture is believed to optimize blood flow to the neck region and benefit thyroid functioning.

hallelujah diet (Occ.) A vegetarian diet developed by Rev. George H. Malkmus (1934–), the American pastor, who claims to have eliminated his colon cancer and other serious health problems more than twenty-five years ago by 'following biblical principles for a natural diet and healthy lifestyle.' The diet prescription is rooted in the philosophy that the only nourishing substances available for the human body are in the form of sunlight, pure air, water and raw food.

hamsa (Yoga) 1.The wild goose (*Anser indicus*) associated with BRAHMA 2. PRANA 3. A MANTRA which on repetition makes the sound 'sa-ham', the sound of breath ('sa' in inhalation and 'ha' in exhalation).

hana hakka See OREGANO.

hand healing (Occ.) The use of hands in healing, common in several Eastern medical traditions. The hand healer is believed to harness cosmic, healing energy with his hands which transfer it into his client's body-areas which are thirsting for it.

hand reflexology (Occ.) A system of RE-FLEXOLOGY relating to palms. Hands, like feet, are considered to embody corresponding areas of the body which stand miniaturized in them. The use of hands and feet as re-mote- control mechanisms to various parts and organs which are not otherwise easily or directly accessible is an age-old method, re-invented by American physiotherapist Eunice Ingham (1879–1974) who developed a 'body chart' reflecting the entire body in the soles and sides of feet. See FOOT REFLEX-OLOGY.

hand sanitizer (Mod.) An alcohol gel, used as an alternative to hand-washing with soap and water. A Harvard Medical School study reported that families that used alcohol-based hand sanitizer gel had a 59 per cent less gastrointestinal illnesses as compared with families that didn't use it.

Happy Fellows of the Plant World (Flo.) A name coined by English pathologist Edward Bach (1886–1936), to refer to thirty-eight healing plants he identified; each flower remedy was associated with a particular characteristic or emotional state. See BACH FLOWER REMEDIES.

hara (Chi.) 1. The seat of QI, located slightly below the navel region. 2. The source of vital power in the body, connected to AURA.

harmonic convergence (New Age) A loosely organized assembly of practitioners of MEDITATION, gathered on 16–17 August 1987 at various sacred sites and mystical places all over the world to usher in a new era. The convergence aimed at a global awakening of love and unity with the beginning of a new age of universal peace. This highly publicized event drew light on New Age religion and popularized the ancient concepts of yoga and alternative healing.

harmonious octave (Occ.) The UNIVERSE. According to a long-existing Pythagorean belief, the Universe represents a harmonious octave, as it comprises planets, each of which has a unique individual tone.

haritaki (Ind.) Also, *Terminalia chebula*. A tree indigenous to the Indian subcontinent. It has been in medicinal use from times immemorial. Its fruit constitutes one of the three essential fruits that go into TRIPHALA, the widely used Ayurvedic compound used to treat constipation.

hatha yoga (Yoga) An important branch of the system of YOGA, according to whose philosophy, the human body is the perfect instrument for SELF-REALIZATION. The spiritual practice envisages the mechanisms of body-posture (ASANA), cleansing techniques (SHODHANA), regulation of breathing pattern (PRANAYAMA), attitudinal hand-gesture (MUDRA) and energy lock (BANDHA). The concepts and practices of this system are well documented in manuals such as *Hatha Yoga Pradipika*, a fourteenth-century text of 389 verses by Svatmarama. The text is divided into four parts. The first part contains advice on environment, conduct and postures, the second on breathing exercises and body-purification, the third on mudras, believed to confer miraculous power for the practitioner, and the fourth on the effects of yoga practice.

'Remain even-minded at all times even amidst profit or loss, pleasure or pain, sickness or health, victory or defeat, praise or criticism.'

—Bhagavad Gita

hayagriva mudra (Occ.) A MUDRA, formed by juxtaposing the tip of the middle finger of the right hand with that of the left hand, and positioning the tips of all the remaining fingers of the right hand on the palm of the left hand. The mudra is believed to increase one's concentration and mental agility.

Hay diet (New Age) A dietary regime based on food combining, developed in 1911 by William Howard Hay, an American nutritionist. Hay classified foods into three types according to their chemical requirements for efficient digestion: alkali-forming foods such as fruits and vegetables, acid-forming concentrated proteins such as meat, game,

fish, eggs or cheese and concentrated carbohydrates which include flours and grains. According to Hay's theory, although protein and starch foods are acid forming, they need different conditions for digestion and should never be combined at the same meal. Vegetables, salads and fruits (whether acid or sweet), if correctly combined, should form the bulk of the diet.

The following chart indicates the 'foods that fight'. While one can mix any food items from List A with List B, and List C with List B, according to the Hay diet items in List A should never be combined with those in List C. It is also recommended that milk is not combined with a meal but drunk separately.

List A (proteins)	List B (neutral foods)	List C (starches)
all meat	most vegetables	biscuits and crackers
All poultry	all greens and salads	bread
cheese	Seeds	cakes
eggs	nuts	rice
fish	Herbs	oats
soya beans	Cream	potatoes, pasta and noodles
yoghurt	butter and olive oil	sugar, honey and sweets

hazel-leaved psoralea (Ind./Chi.) *Psoralea corylifolia*. Also, babchi (Urdu), bakuchi (Sanskrit) bu gu zhi (Chinese), karbhogarisi (Tamil). In AYURVEDA, the one-seeded fruit of this plant finds its application in the treatment of all kinds of skin disorders including dermatitis, leucoderma, leprosy, scabies, and ulcers. In TRADITIONAL CHINESE MEDICINE, it is known for its useful role in urino-genital functioning of the body, as a cure for frequent urination, impotence, premature ejaculation and spermatorrhoea.

> '[Bakuchi], the destroyer of leprosy'
>
> —A Sanskrit phrase

head bath (Nat.) Pouring water down the head. According to a nature-cure procedure, tepid water is poured down from a great height, on the back of the head of the person, who is lying, face down, as a complementary treatment for epilepsy, hysteria and head congestion.

head belt (New Age) A belt with a magnetic device, believed to maintain proper blood circulation in the head region. It is rec-

ommended to be worn around the head, particularly in the treatment of dizziness, migraine, tension headaches and fatigue.

head reflex massage (New Age) The manipulation of REFLEX POINTS on the head—identified by the masseur—by pulling the hair and pounding the head with the fingers and fist.

healing (Mod.) 1. Restoration of health. 2. The process whereby the cells in the body regenerate and repair as the damaged necrotic area is replaced.

> 'Love is the most powerful healing force!'
>
> —James P. B. Lynch

healing meditation on twin hearts (Occ.) An advanced technique of MEDITATION, aimed at achieving UNIVERSAL CONSCIOUSNESS. The twin hearts refer to the meeting-point of the FOURTH CHAKRA, the centre of the 'emotional heart', and the SEVENTH CHAKRA, the centre of the 'divine heart'. By developing the higher subtle emotions, it is believed that one can feel divine love.

healing the skin from within (Occ.) A

complete skin-care programme, aimed at curing skin ailments at all the three levels—body, mind and spirit. The programme was developed and popularized in recent times by American dermatologist Michael R. Bilkis.

healing touch (Occ.) Long recognized for its healing effect, touch has been used as a healing mechanism in traditional systems like REIKI, as its underlying energy enables quick restoration of balance and harmony.

health (Misc.) 1. The functional, metabolic efficiency of a living organism. 2. Soundness of the condition of body, mind and spirit. 3. Health was defined in 1946 by the World Health Organization as a state of complete physical, mental and social wellbeing and not merely the absence of disease or infirmity. In recent years, this definition of health includes the ability to lead a 'socially and economically productive life'.

healtheology (New Age) A training programme which blends harmoniously the discipline of theology with health-related issues. Functioning in harmony with the universe, based on one's individual awareness and thought process, is greatly emphasized.

health harmonics (New Age) The determination of the sound frequency, considered useful for balancing and harmonizing one's body, mind and spirit. According to French physician Alfred Tomatis, who worked with understanding the function of the human ear, sounds that contain high-frequency harmonics—of frequencies around 8,000 Hz—such as those found in Gregorian chants could be extremely beneficial in stimulating the brain.

health kinesiology (New Age) An offshoot of APPLIED KINESIOLOGY, as developed by psychologist Dr Jimmy Scott, employing a variety of bio-energetic balancing methods including crystals, gems, magnets and homoeopathic remedies. This method is said to be useful in overcoming allergies, emotional traumas and learning blocks.

health patterning (New Age) A general approach to healing, aimed at facilitating unitary wellbeing through the use of techniques such as IMAGERY, MEDITATION and THERAPEUTIC TOUCH.

healthy-eating pyramid (Mod.) A weight-loss programme developed by American nutritionist Dr Walter Willett and his colleagues at the Harvard School of Public Health. It is based on scientific evidence of the link between diet and health; daily exercise and weight control are also emphasized here. The pyramid offers information to help people make better choices about what to eat.

> 'When you begin to touch your heart or let your heart be touched, you begin to discover that it's bottomless, that it doesn't have any resolution, that this heart is huge, vast and limitless. You begin to discover how much warmth and gentleness is there, as well as how much space.'
>
> —Pema Chodron

heart rate (Mod.) A term used to describe the frequency of the cardiac cycle. It is considered one of the four vital signs and is usually calculated as the number of contractions (heart beats) of the heart per minute and expressed as beats per minute (bpm). At rest, an adult human heart beats at about 70 bpm in men and 75 bpm in women, but this rate varies between people. However, the reference range is nominally between 60 bpm and 100 bpm (if it is less, the condition is called bradycardia and if greater, it is termed tachycardia). Resting heart rates can be significantly lower in athletes. The infant/neonatal rate of heartbeat is about 130–150 bpm, the toddler's about 100–130 bpm, the older child's about 90–110 bpm, and the adolescent's about 80–100 bpm. The body can increase the heart rate in response to a wide variety of conditions in order to increase the cardiac output (the amount of blood ejected by the heart per unit time). Exercise, environmental stressors or psychological stress can cause the heart rate to increase above the resting rate. The pulse is the most straightforward way of measuring the heart rate, but it can be deceptive when some heart beats do not have much cardiac output. In such cases (as for example, in some arrhythmias), the heart rate may be considerably higher than the pulse rate.

heartwood massage (New Age) A BODY-WORK programme, taught at Heartwood Institute, Garberville, California, which includes BREATHWORK, ENERGY BALANCING, HYPNOTHERAPY, GUIDED IMAGERY, POLARITY THERAPY, SWEDISH MASSAGE and ZEN SHIATSU.

Heimlich manoeuvre (Mod.) A first-aid method developed by an American physician Henry J. Heimlich (b.1920), aimed at effectively dislodging obstructions, such as food particles in the trachea which may choke the patient.

heliotherapy (Mod./Spa) A therapeutic method in which light, usually in the UVA/UVB range, is used particularly in the treatment of eczema, psoriasis and vitamin D deficiencies. Though treatment originally included sunlight, in recent years the use of tanning beds and booths are also gaining popularity. It is also reported that a small amount of endorphins, 'the body's own morphine', are released by the body while exposed to certain frequencies of light, UV in particular.

Hellerwork structural integration (New Age) An approach to maintain alignment and mobility by enabling the client to learn movement exercises designed to eliminate bad habits and teach them how to stand, walk, sit and move more efficiently. The method was developed by Joseph Heller (b.1940), a somatic educator-cum-aerospace engineer.

hemi-sync (Occ.) The trademark for a process developed by Robert A. Monroe (1915–95), a pioneer in the investigation of out-of-body experiences, who created audiopatterns containing binaural beats. The purpose of the binaural beats is to synchronize the brain waves of both hemispheres of the brain so as to help the listener achieve a meditative state. The impact is also said to be of help in lowering blood pressure, increasing stamina and controlling pain, besides weakening addictive behaviour.

Hemme approach (New Age) Hemme, an acronym for History, Evaluation, Modalities, Manipulation and Exercise, is a technique derived from aspects of osteopathy, physical medicine, chiropractic and physical therapy as developed by Dave Leflet in 1986. The technique is used in the treatment of chronic low-back pain and soft-tissue injury. Pain is relieved by restoring alignment and improving myofascial dysfunction.

henna (Ind.) *Lawsonia inermis*. A plant whose natural dye is widely used to decorate the skin and colour the hair by women, especially in the Middle East.

hemo-acupuncture (Chi.) Also, bleeding acupuncture. An ancient Chinese method employed in therapeutic veterinary acupuncture. It is based on BLOOD-LETTING as the method uses hypodermic needles on selected acupoints of animals and allows a few drops of blood to be released. This is done when there is excess heat in the animal's body.

hepar sulphuris (Hom.) Derived from the inner layers of oyster shells, hepar sulphuris is used to treat infections.

hypericum (Hom.) Also, St. John's wort. Used in the treatment of nerve damage.

herb (Nat.) A non-woody plant or plant part, usually of culinary, medicinal or aesthetic value. Culinary herbs can be distinguished from vegetables in that they are used in small quantities to provide flavour rather than bulk to food.

> 'There is no herb which is non-medicinal and no man who is useless; it is, indeed, the wise man who knows how to make use of them.'
>
> —A Sanskrit saying

herbage (Nat.) 1. A herb collection. 2. A herbaceous plant growth 3. The fleshy, edible portions of a plant.

herbal (Nat.) 1. A text or compilation of herbs, containing their descriptions and properties. 2. The aroma of herbs, as in lemon balm, lavender and thyme, and flavours which suggest the presence of herbs.

> 'A weed is a plant, whose virtues we do not yet know.'
>
> —Emerson

herbal bath (New Age/Spa) The use of herbs and their extracts in baths. Some bath herbs and their extracts traditionally used are shown in the following table:

Herb/extract	Used for
aloe vera	softening the skin
besan	in the treatment of skin ailments
chamomile	in the treatment of skin ailments and insomnia
fennel and nettle	effective cleansing
ginger	adding lustre to the skin and to give relief to sore muscles
hay flower	in the treatment of skin infections
neem	in the treatment of skin allergies, skin infections and haemorrhoids
nutmeg	inducing perspiration and in radiation detoxification
oatmeal	in the treatment of itchiness, sunburn and skin ailments
rosemary	increasing blood circulation
sage	inducing perspiration
sandal	healing and tranquilizing
tulsi	elimination of fatigue and restoration of health
turmeric	in the treatment of skin ailments and infections

herbal bodywraps (New Age/Spa) Also, herbal wraps. Wrapping the body firmly with soft terry clothes, saturated with herbal decoctions. A weight-loss measure, the technique is also useful in the treatment of arthritis, injuries, skin conditions and sprains.

herbal formulations (Chi./Ind.) Herbal combinations whose synergy is supposed to increase the therapeutic effect multifold.

Herbal formulations are popular prescriptions in many ancient systems of medicine, including AYURVEDA, CHINESE MEDICINE, SIDDHA and UNANI.

herbal infusions (Chi./Ind.) Also, herbal teas. Various combinations of herbs are used for preparing infusions for calming the aggravation of DOSHAS, which result in ailments. The table indicates herbal combinations which can be used to tackle aggravated doshas:

Dosha aggravated	Major combination of herbs	Expected effect
vata	*Withiania somnifera, Emblica officianalis, Elettaria cardamomum, Piper longum, Ipomoea digitata, Cinnamomum zeylanicum, Cinnamomum tamala, Aegle marmelos, Ricinus communis*	a warming blend which helps in improving the digestion
pitta	*Nelumbo nucifera, Foeniculum vulgare, Rosa damascena, Coriandum sativum, Azadirachta indica, Emblica officianalis*	A cooling and gentle blend, which helps in refreshing and relaxing overheated people
kapha	*Ocimum sanctum, Adhatoda vasica, Glycyrrhiza glabra, Zingiber officinale, Piper longum, Piper nigrum, Ellettaria cardamomum, Cinnamomum zeylanicum, Hyssopus officinalis*	A stimulating blend, which simultaneously provides warmth to the entire body

herbalism (Nat.) Also, phytotherapy. The term herbalism refers to folk and traditional medicinal practices based on the intuitive use of plants and plant extracts in the treatment of common ailments.

> 'With proper usage, even a poisonous substance can turn out to be a good remedy, as a good herb, when improperly employed turns out to be a poison.'
>
> —*Charaka Samhita* (1000 BC)

herbal medicine (Nat.) An ancient worldwide system of medicine using plants to prevent and cure diseases. To the medical herbalist, a herb is any plant of medicinal value. There are at least 350,000 known species of plants.

Aesculapius, the Greek god of healing, is symbolized by a serpent, because serpents were known for their ability to seek out healing plants.

In the fifteenth century, William Caxton printed hundreds of medical textbooks, and as more and more people could read, interest in herbalism grew until the publication in 1653 of what is considered the greatest work in English on this subject, Nicholas Culpeper's *Complete Herbal*. There is enormous proliferation in the literature in the herbal medicine world, much of it from China and Russia. Research in herbal medicine is, however, difficult because herbal remedies, like homoeopathic remedies, are personalized to patients.

herbalist (Nat./New Age) 1. A person well-versed in the appearance and medicinal characteristics of herbs. 2. A dealer in medicinal plants 3. A folk- and traditional-medicine man who uses plants and plant extracts for healing.

herbology (Nat.) The study and knowledge of herbs as food and medicine. Herbs are known from ancient times for their therapeutic role. Even in modern medicine, the knowledge of herbology has found its application in the evolution of new medical formulations to fight virtually every disease and condition.

heterohypnosis (New Age) Hypnosis induced by or in another, as opposed to AUTOHYPNOSIS. A trained person, the hypnotist often aids another person, the subject, in entering into the state of hypnosis.

hexagram (Occ.) Also, shadkona yantra. A six-pointed, symmetrical figure, a MANDALA symbol, formed with two overlapping equilateral triangles of which the intersection is a regular hexagon. It symbolizes the perfect meditative state of balance achieved between man and the universe. Such six-pointed stars are found in cosmological diagrams in several religious faiths, including Hinduism, Buddhism and Jainism. In Indic symbolism, the shape is understood to consist of two triangles—one pointed upward and the other downward—locked in harmonious embrace. The two components symbolize Shiva, representing the focussed aspect of masculinity, and Shakti, the sacred embodiment of femininity, respectively. The mystical union of these two triangles thus represents Creation. The resultant hexagon from the union of these two triangles represents the six-faced Shanmukha, the mythological progeny of the divine couple.

higashi (New Age) Also, daily-life therapy. A method developed for and tested on over 3,000 autistic children in Tokyo, Japan, by Kiyo Kitahara. The approach emphasizes vigorous physical education and training for autistic students. It includes roller-skating, calisthenics, using gym equipment and performing gymnastic exercises, and is said to help in overcoming feelings of fear and anxiety associated with physiological problems in these children. According to neurologist Dr Hardy, physical exertion involved in this approach reduces the internal anxiety that autistic people feel because it causes the body to release ENDORPHINS. This might govern the behaviour of autistic people.

> 'Autism is like a dreaming state. To break this kind of unstable, weak condition, physical exercise is best.'
>
> —Kiyo Kitahara

high enema (New Age) While a regular enema washes out faecal matter from the area near the rectum, a high enema cleans out most of the colon. The colon, which sometimes assumes the consistency of a rubber tyre, is known to be an organ capable of generating many illnesses by accumulating faecal matter in its heavy mucus coating. To prevent its harbouring germs and aiding digestion, a high enema is found useful. Water at room temperature is held for 10 to 15 minutes, after which evacuation can be carried out. The process can be repeated on the same day, after some rest, or on the next day.

high self (Occ.) A spiritual consciousness in one's personality, one's higher nature which acts as a guardian angel, colleague and adviser.

higher nature, lower nature (Occ.) Expressions indicating man's refined, soulful qualities on the one hand, and his base, instinctive qualities on the other.

Hindu philosophy (Ind.) It is an inquiry into the nature of truth or reality, based on the psychic experiences of sages and seers. It shows the way to happiness.

Hippocrates (460–377 BC) (Grk.) A Greek physician, celebrated as the 'father of medicine'. He held that illness has a rational, physical explanation and that neither evil spirits nor gods were causative. He also believed that the body must be treated as a whole, not in bits and pieces. He described accurately diseases and their symptoms, and believed in the importance of rest, fresh air, nutritious diet and, above all, hygiene and cleanliness as a means to prevent and cure the diseases.

> 'Life is short, and the art long; the crises fleeting; experience perilous, and the decision difficult.'
>
> —Hippocrates

Hippocrates diet (New Age) Named after HIPPOCRATES, the 'father of medicine', this diet plan includes uncooked foods, including sprouts and wheatgrass juice, to assist in the healing process. A raw-food diet, it stresses on fruit, vegetables, sprouts, juices, and legumes in the daily menu. An essential feature of this diet is the continued cleansing and support of the organs of elimination. It has two phases: the cleansing phase and the maintenance phase; the cleansing phase aids and supports the eliminative organs and ensures eliminative functions, whereas the maintenance phase is undertaken to continue these gains and not re-create the disease-causing situation.

Hippocratic oath (Grk.) The ethical code, attributed to the Greek physician HIPPOCRATES and adopted as a conduct guide for the medical profession the world over. The oath includes (a) the obligation of the physician to students of medicine and the duties of the pupil to the teacher and (b) the pledge by the professional to prescribe only beneficial treatments according to one's ability and judgement and to refrain from causing harm or hurt and to live an exemplary personal and professional life.

hiranyagarbha (Ind.) Literally, golden germ. The first cosmological principle (TATTVA) to emerge out of the Infinite Reality; Brahma; the cosmic mind; cosmic intelligence.

Hispanic healing (Am. Ind.) Also, CURANDERISMO. The folk medicine practised by Texan Hispanics. Herbalists, midwives and masseurs are the healers (*curanderos*).Typically, the *curandero* works at three levels: the material, mental and spiritual. The physical symptoms are believed to come from supernatural causes like evil-eye (*mal de ojo*) and witchcraft (*mal puesto*). The treatment may consist of rituals, herbal remedies, potions or counter-magic, depending on what the illness is. The rituals for counter-magic include rolling the victim's photograph with that of Jesus Christ and placing it on a small altar, using prayer beads, holy pictures, rosaries and crucifixes.

hissing pranayama (Yoga) Also, hissing breath, victorious breath. A variation of PRANAYAMA, used in association with toning the throat during exhalation, to begin with, and subsequently during inhalation as well. Its practitioners claim that this method enhances concentration.

hokhmah (Heb.) Wisdom.

holding therapy (Mod.) Holding a child as a rage-reduction measure. It consists of forced holding by a therapist or parent until the child stops resisting or until a fixed time period has elapsed. Sometimes the child is not released until there is an eye contact. Although this technique was initially intended for autistic adults, it is now used for autistic children, teenagers and younger children with 'attachment disorders' and infants with 'residual birth trauma'. The use of forced holding may engender strong feelings of fear, confusion, helplessness, anger and betrayal as the child's natural attempts to break free are disregarded by those they have come to love or trust.

holism (Mod./New Age) An esoteric concept that all reality is organically one, and that every object or event has interconnections with the other. It is the idea that all the properties of a given system (biological, chemical, social, economic, mental and linguistic) cannot be determined or explained by the sum of its component parts alone. Instead, the system as a whole determines in an important way how the parts behave as there is a tendency in nature, through creative evolution, to form wholes that are greater than the sum of the parts. The concept of holism can be found in medicine too, particularly in psychosomatic medicine, especially in the 1970s. The holistic approach aims at a systemic model, where multiple factors (for example, biological, psychological and social levels) are seen as inter-connected to each other, as a disturbance at any level—somatic, psychic or social—will radiate to other levels. In alternative medicine, a holistic approach to healing recognizes that the emotional, mental, spiritual and physical elements comprise a human system, and therefore attempts are made to treat the whole person, instead of the symptoms.

> 'The whole is more than the sum of its parts.'
>
> —Aristotle

holism in science (Mod.) Also, holistic science. An approach to scientific research that emphasizes the study of complex systems. The two central aspects are:

1. the approach on whole to parts, which focusses on observation of the specimen within its ecosystem before undertaking a study of its parts, and

2. the concept that the scientist is not a passive observer and that there is no objective truth, and that the observer's contribution to the process of knowledge is equally valid and valuable.

This practice is obviously in contrast to a purely analytic tradition (sometimes called reductionism) which understands systems by dividing them into their smallest possible or discernible elements and understanding their elemental properties alone. The dichotomy in holism/reductionism is often evident in conflicting interpretations regarding experimental findings and in setting priorities for future research.

The term holistic science has been used in a multi-disciplinary sense. It is concerned with the behaviour of complex systems, recognizing the feedback within the system as a crucial element for understanding its behaviour. In other words, commitment to a multi-disciplinary approach and an emphasis on the study of problems that involve complex interactions among their constituent parts are the two dominant characteristics in holistic scientific research. Many scientific disciplines have been in recent years affected by the holistic paradigm. While some of these are being accepted as part of mainstream science (e.g., quantum physics, which has an idea of the universe as an undivided whole, any division of which—e.g., the observer and the observed—could be only arbitrary), others are often considered as proto-scientific or pseudoscientific.

holistic aromatherapy (Occ.) A variation of AROMATHERAPY, which incorporates four main concepts of HOLISM: that each person exists on many levels; that he is unique; that he needs to be part of the decision-making process; and that he has self-healing potential. In this approach, the therapist and the essential oils act as catalysts for change.

holistic medicine (New Age) A system of heath care which addresses the whole person, rather than an isolated organ or function, as the target for treatment, taking into account multiple factors such as physical, nutritional, environmental, emotional, social, spiritual and lifestyle values, and freely avails itself every mode of diagnosis and treatment. The patient is made responsible to achieve balance and well-being through his personal efforts and indulgences.

> 'As it is not proper to cure the eyes without the head, nor the head without the body, so neither is it proper to cure the body without the soul.'
>
> —Socrates

holistic nursing (New Age) A holistic approach in nursing methods. The speciality is based on practice that recognizes the body–mind–spirit connection of persons, and demands its practitioners integrate self-care and self-responsibility into their own lives. Holistic nurses are often trained in the practices of complementary/ alternative modalities. The American Holistic Nurses Association (AHNA) is committed to bringing holism, compassion, science, and creativity to an otherwise routine nursing practice. The holistic nursing involves treatment to the body (including BODYWORK, BIOFEEDBACK, ENERGY HEALING, MASSAGE and THERAPEUTIC TOUCH), mind (including HUMOUR THERAPY, IMAGERY, MEDITATION and MUSIC) and soul (PRAYER), with enhanced interpersonal interactions.

holistic psychiatry (New Age) An approach to psychiatry, incorporating techniques such as BODYWORK, BIOFEEDBACK, ENERGY HEALING and HOMOEOPATHY. The approach insists on a comprehensive individualized evaluation and treatment for people of all ages with the best of modern medicine and psychiatry, integrated with time-tested natural approaches from ancient cultures.

holistic psychotherapy (New Age) A holistic approach to healing, as promoted by Russian-born reiki practitioner Katya Salkinder, aimed at releasing energy blocks caused by emotional traumas and conflicts.

> 'My goal for you is to become indestructibly happy from within to realize your creative potential, increase your ability to function harmoniously in the world, improve the quality of all your relationships, and to do what you want to do when you tune into your innermost sense of self and purpose. My philosophy is that every obstacle is an opportunity to grow and learn.'
>
> —Katya Salkinder

holistic spa (Spa) A spa with facilities for alternative and complementary methods for body–mind–soul healing.

holoenergetic healing (Occ.) Also, holoenergetics. Healing with the energy of the whole. An approach to psycho-therapy, based on the concepts and practices of energy healing, as developed by Stanford-trained physician and author of *Healing with Love* (Harper, 1992), Leonard Laskow. Laskow identified the following four crucial phases: (a) the recognition phase, wherein the illness is identified; (b) the resonance phase, wherein the patient comes to terms with the source; (c) the release phase, wherein the disharmonious energetic pattern associated with the source is released by the patient; and (d) the reformation phase, wherein the patient replaces the dysfunctional pattern with an image symbolizing the positive life-force.

The holoenergetic principles in a nutshell are: (a) separation is illusory (b) maintenance of this illusion requires energy (c) often, physical or mental illness or stress is symptomatic of such consumption of energy (d) releasing oneself from the illusion of separation liberates tremendous energy (e) healing is the gradual elimination of the illusion of separation.

holotropic breathwork (Occ.) The word holotropic has Greek roots, and means moving toward wholeness; an approach to induce a 'non-ordinary' state of CONSCIOUSNESS through BREATHING, evocative music, MANDALA and focussed BODYWORK. Aimed at personal transformation and healing, the method was developed by Stanislav and Christina Grof in the 1970s.

holy basil (Ind.) *Ocimum tenuiflorum, Ocimum sanctum.* Also, bajiru (Japanese), bazilikum (Hebrew), gau chahng taap (Chinese), habaq (Arabic), reyhan (Turkish) tulasi (Sanskirt). Tulasi is venerated by Hindus as a mother for its role in human welfare and health. Its darker version, Krishna tulasi, is more commonly used for worship, as it possesses greater medicinal value. Its extracts are used in ayurvedic remedies for common colds, headaches, stomach disorders, inflammation, heart disease, various forms of poisoning and malaria.

> 'Tulasi, like ambrosia, rose from the churning of the ocean and like ambrosia, it is to be sought after and cherished.'
>
> —The Puranas

Holy Grail (Eur.) A symbolic TALISMAN around which innumerable legends were built. In the Christian tradition, the Holy Grail was the dish, plate or cup used by Jesus Christ at the Last Supper.

homa (Ind.) The Sanskrit term homa means fire offering, a sacred ceremony in which the gods are offered oblations through the medium of fire in a sanctified square-shaped fire pit, homakunda, usually made of earthen bricks. Homa rites are enjoined in the Vedas, Agamas and Dharma and Grihya Shastras. Many domestic rites are occasions for homa, including sacred thread ceremony (upanayana) and marriage (vivaha). Major worships in temples are often preceded by a homa. While the smoke arising from homa is believed to neutralize the harmful effects of radiation and microbes in the atmosphere, the residual ash collected from the fire-pit is used as a potent medicine for removing negative energies. The sacred fire, created by burning cow-dung cakes, grasses and wood chips along with ghee, rice, honey, etc., to the accompaniment of CHANTS, is intended to purify one's consciousness in three levels: egoic, sensual and material.

home remedies (Nat.) Domestic stock of simple ingredients, plant parts, spices and condiments used for the prevention and cure of common temporary ailments.

homeovitics (Occ.) A contemporary approach to homoeopathy, as developed in 1979 by Allen Morgan Kratz, incorporating the intensification of the body's healing energies through vitalization. Vitalization, it is believed, increases the vital energy of a substance by a stepwise series of dilutions with succussions (vigorous shaking). The energy from this vitalized substance can then be transferred to activate a less energetic one. This transfer of energy is known as resonance. It occurs when the vitalized substance (vitic) is similar or identical (homeo) to the less energetic one.

homoeo-acupuncture (New Age) An approach to healing by injecting selected homoeopathic remedies in the form of solutions into ACUPOINTs, following the standard ACUPUNCTURE procedure.

homoeo-botanical therapy (New Age) An approach to healing in which the botanical tinctures are used on the basis of principles of HOMOEOPATHY.

homoeopathy (Hom./Vib.) Also, homeopathy, homeotherapeutics. (From the Greek *homoeo*, meaning same, and *pathy*, meaning illness). A popular system of VIBRATIONAL MEDICINE, based on the principle 'like cures like'. Using natural substances (that cause symptoms much like those of the disease) in very tiny doses, HAHNEMANN, the founder of this system, attempted to stimulate the body to heal itself. The underlying idea in homoeopathy is that the drug, by closely mimicking the symptoms of the disease, obviates it.

homoeopathic posology (Hom.) The study of infinitesimal dose of homeopathic medicine. The study includes preparation, application and repetition of such doses in a systematic manner. Homoeopaths use two different dilution scales: (a) The decimal scale, in which the dilution is one in ten, or 1:10. In other words, for every drop of the tincture, nine drops of an alcohol/water mixture are added. The abbreviation X is used to indicate a remedy made using the decimal scale. (b) The centesimal scale, in which the dilution is one in 100, or 1:100. Here, for every drop of the tincture, 99 drops of an alcohol/water mixture are added. The abbreviation C is used to indicate that the centesimal scale was used. After the required dilution, the mixture is shaken vigorously (succussed). Then one drop of the mixture is added to the next dilution (again either decimal or centesimal), and the mixture is succussed again. The remedies are diluted at least for three times. The number of dilutions and the scale used are written on the label after the remedy's name. So a label that reads, for example, Aconite 3C would mean that the remedy Aconite has been diluted and succussed three times. The usual remedy strengths for home use are 6C and 12C, while the professionals use the most potent strength, 30C.

homoeostasis (Misc.) 1. The ability in an organism to automatically maintain its internal environment, including normal body temperature and chemical balance, within itself. 2. The self-regulating mechanism in the living body. 3. The inherent tendency of the body (and the mind) to gravitate towards a state of EQUILIBRIUM.

homoeovitics (Hom./Mod.) An approach to HOMOEOPATHY, in which homoeopathically vitalized nutraceuticals, complex, pluralistic formulations, are used in the treatment of chronic diseases. They are basically used to support cellular detoxification, a normal function of the body to maintain homoeostasis. Cellular toxicity is a primary contributing factor in chronic diseases such as arthritis, diabetes and hypertension.

homuncular acupuncture (Chi.) A type of ACUPUNCTURE which focusses on any group of ACUPOINTS that represents a 'homunculus', the miniature human. Such groups of acupoints are traced to the nose, face, auricle, hands and feet.

honey (Nat.) A natural source of instant energy, B vitamins and various other minerals, with mild antibacterial action. In traditional and folk practices, unprocessed raw honey, (which is neither filtered nor heat-treated) is recognized for its medicinal value. Some laboratory studies confirm that raw honey can suppress bacterial growth, particularly in open wounds. However, there is a danger of the presence of infection-causing fungus in raw honey.

ho'oponopono (Haw.) An ancient Hawaiian approach to healing. The approach recognizes the fact that people are the sum total of their experiences, often burdened by their pasts and that the emotions tied to their memories cause stress and trauma. The release of emotional blocks that cause imbalance is the major goal of this healing practice. The method involves establishing a connectivity with the Divine within, on a moment-to-moment basis, and seeks cleansing, erasure or correction of disturbing memories and thought forms.

This system does not seek to analyze, solve, manage or cope with problems. Since Divinity is responsible for all creation, the victim directly asks for correction and cleansing. Every stress, imbalance or illness can thus be corrected just by working on oneself.

hopi ear-candle treatment (Am. Ind.) An ancient method of healing, as prevalent in Asia and North America, to treat ear problems. Named after the native American tribe which first introduced this gentle therapy to the West, the Hopi candle is actually a hollow tube, made of cotton flax, honey and herb oils (e.g., chamomile, sage, St John's Wort). The candle is placed over the ear orifice and ignited so that it produces a gentle local heat which softens the ear wax inside, drawing it into the base of

the candle for easy removal.

horary astrology (Num.) An ancient, specialized astrological application using a horary chart, the basis of which is the time at which a question is posed to the astrologer and not details of horoscope of the poser of the question.

hormone (Mod.) A regulatory substance produced in an organism and distributed in tissue fluids such as blood or sap to stimulate cells and tissues into action such as growth, metabolism, reproduction and the functioning of various organs.

horoscope (Num.) An important aid in astrology, used to interpret the character or destiny of an individual.

horseradish (Am. Ind./Chi./Eur./Isl./Jap.) *Armoracia rusticana, Cochlearia armoracia*. Also, seiyôwasabi (Japanese). A plant native to south-eastern Europe and western Asia, but now popular around the world. The large, white and tapering roots of this plant and its leaves are used traditionally as a medicine and condiment in Denmark and Germany. The roots are used to treat urinary tract infections, bronchitis and coughs. Before chillies were brought from the New World, horseradish, black pepper and mustard were the only 'sharp' spices known to India and Europe.

horseshoe, significance of (Grk.) The significance of the horseshoe has been recognized from ancient times, and dates back to fourth-century-BC Greece. In medieval days, used horseshoes were nailed on doors to prevent witches from entering houses and barns. Horseshoes were hung, with heel pointing upwards, over fireplaces for luck.

hoshino therapy (New Age) A system of BODYWORK, relating to the bio-mechanical functions of the body, developed by Tomezo Hoshino, a Japanese acupuncturist. It includes a manual form of ACUPRESSURE that uses 250 ACUPOINTS.

hot bath (Nat.) A common method in HYDROPATHY, aimed at inducing perspiration, a hot bath is recommended for chronic health problems as it accelerates the elimination of toxins from the body. It works as a stimulant and aids in relaxation.

hot foot-bath (Nat.) A simple procedure of soaking the feet in a tub of hot water. This commonly used method in HYDROPATHY recommended for afflictions including gout, insomnia, pain, neuralgic and muscular cramps and sore throats.

hot hand-bath (Nat.) A simple procedure in HYDROPATHY, involving soaking the hands in a tub of hot water, beneficial for asthma, inflammation of nail, skin ailments and writer's cramp.

hotpack (Nat.) A method in HYDROPATHY, usually aimed at relieving pain.

hot-stone massage (Spa) The application of dark, smooth stones, either heated in hot water or cooled in various ways, over the body. The treatment is aimed at bringing relief to stiff and sore muscles. Sometimes stones are just placed on the body or gently stroked with light pressure on areas of the body such as back, palms or between the toes.

hot-water bottle (Nat.)A common method in HYDROPATHY, often recommended for relieving menstrual cramps, pain and sinusitis. It increases perspiration, warmth and comfort, and works as a sedative and relaxant.

hot yoga (New Age) Also, Bikram yoga. A version of YOGA in which the ASANAS are designed to stretch muscles and tendons with the thermostat set at 38°C. The system prescribes twenty-six selected asanas. The heat is said to help in more efficient and enhanced stretching of muscles.

hridaya (Ind.) Heart; from the Sanskrit hrid, meaning centre, and ayam, meaning this. The heart is considered the seat of consciousness in Hindu philosophy.

> 'Just as there is a cosmic centre from which the whole universe arises and has its being and functions with the power of the directing energy emanating therefrom, so also is there a centre within the frame of the physical body wherein we have our being. This centre in the human body is in no way different from the cosmic centre. It is this centre in us that is called the hridaya, the seat of Pure Consciousness, realized as Existence, Knowledge and Bliss. This is really what we call the seat of God in us.'
>
> —Bhagwan Sri Ramana

hridayakasha (Yoga) The psychic heart-space, often visualized in the centre of the chest.

hug therapy (New Age) It is well-known that stimulation by touch enhances physical as well as emotional wellbeing. Therapeutic touch, recognized as an essential tool for healing, is now part of nurses' training in several large medical centres. Touch is used to help relieve pain, depression and anxiety, bolster a patient's will to live, and help premature babies, who are deprived of touch in incubators, grow and thrive. Hugging dispels loneliness, tension, fear and inhibition and opens doors to positive feelings, confidence and self-esteem and imparts, above all, feelings of belonging.

> 'Don't turn away from the elderly, disabled, terminally ill or long-term care residents because their needs seem beyond your ability to give. The one thing they need the most is the most simple, yet profound gift you have to give. Your kind hand holding theirs and a hug from your heart. The gift of touch is the most powerful healing you can offer another, and it is the most powerful healing you can give yourself. Give generously and watch yourself grow rich in what matters the most.'
>
> —Kathleen Keating Schloessinger

huichol shamanism (Am. Ind.) A variety of SHAMANISM, practised by the Huichols, an ancient Indian tribe living in central western Mexico.

human body (Misc.) The human body can be viewed as an electrical system, consisting of two types of electro-magnetic fields. While the internal organs such as the brain, nervous system and heart emit low-frequency electrical impulses of the AC category, the outer shell (skin) exhibits a higher-frequency energy field. Recent studies indicate that the entire universe at the quantum level consists of a conglomeration of electro-magnetic fields at various frequencies.

> 'In each human heart are a tiger, a pig, an ass and a nightingale. Diversity of character is due to their unequal activity.'
>
> —Ambrose Bierce

human dermal filler (New Age) Derived from human tissue, bio-absorbable human temporary fillers are used by cosmetologists to fill fine or deep lines, smooth out creases and wrinkles, and for re-contouring and re-shaping lips, cheeks, noses and chins.

Human Energetic Assessment and Restorative Technic (HEART) (Occ.) A system of ENERGY FIELDWORK, developed by George M. Delalio, based on the notion that lifestyle and mental processes often disrupt the etheric pathways of healing energy produced by the brain.

human energy field and aura (New Age) As the energy field surrounding living things cannot be measured using conventional scientific techniques or equipment, there is little scientific data on human energy field and aura. Though energy does not emanate or reflect from a person, the energy itself is the person, the core. This understanding helps in maintaining one's energy field and body in harmony. As the body itself is nothing but a manifestation of human energy, dis-harmony in the energy field will cause dis-ease in the body. In other words, if the human energy field is out of balance, it can be presumed that the body too will be out of balance.

human potential movement (New Age) A movement, attributed to George Leonard, which was triggered in the mid-twentieth century to promote the cultivation of the extraordinary potential humans are endowed with and was believed to be largely untapped. By developing such potential, it was believed that humans would experience an exceptional quality of life filled with happiness, creativity and fulfillment. It was believed that the net effect of individuals cultivating such potential would automatically bring about positive changes in the world. The movement stemmed from the understanding relating to humanism and existentialism. Its formation was also strongly linked with the development of concepts relating to HUMANISTIC PSYCHOLOGY. The movement saw Abraham Maslow's idea of SELF ACTUALIZATION as the supreme expression of a human's life.

humanistic psychology (New Age) A school of psychology that emerged in mid-twentieth century which stresses on man's essential goodness and unlimited potential. It is explicitly concerned with the human dimension of psychology and the human context for the development of psychological theory. These matters are often summarized by the five postulates of humanistic psychology as given by James Bugental (1964): a) that people cannot be reduced to component parts; b) that people have in them a uniquely human context; c) that human consciousness includes an awareness of oneself in the context of other people; d) that human beings have choices and responsibilities; and e) that people are intentional, they seek meaning, value and creativity. The discipline of humanistic psychology opts for qualitative research methods as it views the usage of quantitative methods in the study of the human mind and behaviour as misguided. See also, HUMAN POTENTIAL MOVEMENT.

'It is easier to love humanity as a whole than to love one's neighbours.'
—Eric Hoffer

humanistic psychotherapy (New Age) A form of PSYCHOTHERAPY which lays emphasis on personal feelings, well-being and the response of the immediate environment than on science or sociology. It is based on the view that every human being has an innate tendency for goodness.

'A man is ethical only when life, as such, is sacred to him, that of plants and animals as well as that of his fellowman, and when he devotes himself helpfully to all life that is in need of help.'
—Albert Schweitzer

humour therapy (New Age) Laughter as a therapeutic practice. Recent studies indicate that laughing, which is a contagious emotion, can lower blood pressure, reduce stress hormones, increase muscle flexion, and boost immune function. It is also said to trigger the release of endorphins, the body's natural painkillers, and produce a general sense of wellbeing. Socially, it brings people together by breaking down the communication barriers. In view of its positive impact on health, laughter therapy programmes are incorporated in hospitals and nursing homes as part of their therapeutic regimens. In India, participants gather in the early morning everyday just to laugh out.

huna (Haw.) Hawaiian, for secret. The ancient Hawaiian esoteric wisdom based on seven basic principles, which enable a person to connect to one's highest wisdom within. The seven principles are:

Principle	Meaning
ike	the world is what you think it is
kala	there are no limits, everything is possible
makia	energy flows where attention goes
manawa	now is the moment of power
aloha	to love is to be happy with
mana	all power comes from within
pono	effectiveness is the measure of truth

huna kane (Hom.) A system of BODY-WORK, based on the ancient Hawaiian HUNA wisdom. It consists of a clothes-on body massage aimed at physical and emotional healing (akin to getting a massage along with counselling). The masseur is said to suggest to the client's unconscious mind and invite the client to release negative thoughts and emotional trauma accumu-lated in his body.

hydration facial (Spa) A mask of paraffin and essential oils, applied to re-hydrate and revitalize the skin. It is also said to help in increasing the natural fluids in the skin.

hydrochromopathy (New Age) A method of COLOUR THERAPY, in which spring water or distilled water is filled in a coloured glass bottle (or, in a clear glass bottle, wrapped in coloured gel) before placing it in direct sunlight (or artificial light) for a couple of hours at a stretch. Drinking the colour-charged water is believed to be therapeutic. While blue-charged water is used in treating fevers, green-charged is considered as tonic, and the red-charged, for fitness and health.

hydromancy (Occ.) A method of DIVINATION using water, standing or running. See also SCRYING.

hydropathy (Nat./Spa) Also, hydrotherapy. The therapeutic application of water, particularly to aid relaxation by a variety of methods, including hot and cold showers, water-jets and mineral baths. THALASSO-THERAPY, using seawater for hydrotherapy, is also popular in spas. The following table indicates the intended benefits of some simple ways of water application:

Nature of treatment	Expected benefits
drinking plenty of water (4 to 6 glasses) in the early morning, on an empty stomach	relieves athletic cramps, arthritis, common cold, constipation, diabetes, fevers, gallstones, indigestion, oedema and rheumatism
drinking plenty of water, at regular intervals, throughout the day	the elimination of toxins caused by tobacco, alcohol and drugs
hot baths/compresses	pain relief
cold baths	soothes inflammation due to injury
alternating hot and cold baths /compresses	improves blood circulation
steam	stimulates perspiration, decongests chest, minimizes pain
warm showers and herbal baths at bedtime	sedative

hyperdimensional healing (Occ.) A system of healing, as advanced by Rev. M. Glen Pruitt, which includes auric revitalization and the ATLANTEAN MEDITATION, involv-ing frantic breathing.

hypno-aesthetics (New Age) The application of HYPNOSIS to establish and maintain intimacy between one's subconscious and biochemical processes. Based on the notion that the subconscious energy is usable for physiological processes, it is believed that this therapy enhances harmony and balance.

hypno-analgesia (New Age) Lowering the perception of pain through HYPNOSIS.

hypno-anesthesia (New Age) Pain management with the help of HYPNOSIS, used in the past for the treatment of minor traumas in both adults and children.

hypnoidal (New Age) Of or resembling HYPNOSIS or SLEEP.

The hypnoidal state refers to a state with some qualities of sleep and similar to light hypnosis. It is characterized by some detachment as well as physical and mental relaxation.

hypno-meditation (New Age) An approach to healing, developed by Donald Burton Schnell, integrating the concepts, techniques and spiritual traditions borrowed from the East and the West.

hypnosis (New Age) A term coined in the 1840s by Scottish surgeon James Braid who discovered that a hypnotic trance could be achieved by merely staring at a bright light or by suggestion alone. Later, Sigmund Freud observed that through hypnosis, a person's repressed thoughts and desires could be revealed. Hypnosis and relaxation exercises form part of many alternative treatments.

hypno-therapist (New Age) A trained, and often licensed, professional who utilizes the therapeutic technique of hypnosis as part of a treatment regimen and helps people with self-improvement.

hypnotherapy (New Age) The use of hypnosis for self-improvement and/or for therapeutic purposes.

hypnotic state (New Age) A state where an individual becomes hyper-suggestible. This state is characterized by the production of a neuro-chemical, endorphin, in the blood and lowering of the level of the hormone hydrocortisone, produced by the adrenal or suprarenal glands. This bio-chemical change leads to relaxation in the body and tranquility of mind.

hypothalamus (Misc.) A small chamber, situated at the base of the brain.

hypothalamus–pituitary–adrenal axis (Misc.) A system of nerves and hormones controlling the stress response.

hyssop (Am. Ind./Chi./Eur./Jap./Kor.) *Hyssopus officinalis.* Also, hasop (Korean); jufa (Sanskrit), niu xi cao (Chinese) Hyssop's fragrant flowers and leaves are used as medicine in the treatment of asthma, colic, common cold and cough.

Ibn Sina See AVICENNA

Icho (Jap.) See GINKGO BILOBA.

I Ching (Chi.) Also called 'Book of Changes', the oldest of the written Chinese classic texts, describing the cosmology and philosophy of Chinese cultural beliefs. The philosophy is based on the notion that there exists a dynamic balance of opposites and the acceptance of the inevitability of change in life. Some regard it simply as a system of DIVINATION.

'These [*I Ching*] are not books, lumps of lifeless papers, but *minds* alive on the shelves. From each of them goes out its own voice .... and just as the touch of a button on our set will fill the room with music, so by taking down one of these volumes, and opening it, one can call into range the voice of a man far distant in time and space, and hear him speaking to us, mind to mind, heart to heart.'

—Gilbert Highet

'*I Ching*, a means to accessing the subconscious through meditation upon the symbols.'

—Carl Jung

Ice bag (Nat.) Synonymous with ice pack. A waterproof bag filled with ice, used as a therapeutic application to the body, especially the head. Such application can help reduce high fevers, swellings, pain and bleeding.

Ice therapy (Nat.) The treatment of exercise- or sports-bruises and injuries, with ice.

The immediate application of ice to the area of injuries can avoid heat, pain, redness, swelling and loss of mobility. It helps in minimizing tissue damage and promotes healing bruised areas with a wet towel and by placing a plastic bag filled with ice. Commercially available cold packs may be handy as they can be stored in refrigerators and used whenever needed. Bags containing frozen peas or corn can also be used to similar effect. Ice massage is also common. This can be applied to a bruised area, such as a tennis elbow, with slow circular strokes. While treating an injury with ice, one should ensure that ice does not come in direct contact with the skin. Ice should also not be put on open cuts and sores. Prolonged use is also reported to damage the nerves in the elbow or knee.

Ice turban (Nat.) The application of a long piece of cloth or a large towel soaked in ice-cold water as a head wrap, aimed at reducing depression and mental fatigue.

Ice-water immersion (Nat.) The immediate immersion of body-parts affected by minor burns in ice-cold water, as a first-aid method.

Ida (Yoga) Skr. for comfort. A NADI or psychic nerve associated with lunar energy.

Idea therapy (Occ.) A method of IMAGINEERING, in which AFFIRMATION of a desired belief is made repeatedly. The constant repetition of affirmations is said to help people in distress overcome their unfortunate situations.

Ideal self (New Age) Personality characteristics, modes of behaviour, emotions, and thoughts to which a person aspires or dreams about. As the gap between 'what you are' and 'what you want to be' can create disharmony, for psychological well-being and contentment it is essential that one accepts one's situation as it is, by making a list of 'plus points' or favourable circumstances with which one is endowed and thanking God for them.

ignatia (Hom.) Used to treat headaches, cramps and tremors.

i liq ch'uan (Chi.) An approach to healing, referred to as an internal martial art, I Liq Ch'uan is a way to align one's body and harmonize one's energy. The techniques of TAI CHI and ZEN also form part of this approach.

Illuminati (New Age) A group of people aspiring for enlightenment. More prominently, the term refers specifically to the Bavarian illuminati, a secret enlightenment society. The term is also used to refer to any shadow organization engaged in controlling world affairs covertly.

Illusion (Ind./Misc.) A set of beliefs, opinions or observations which may appear real, but in actuality, in accord with the facts, truth or true values, may be an illusion created by a magician. Certain schools of Indian philosophy question the illusory nature of our lives.

> 'Man's beliefs are self-serving illusions and the value system is an artificial construct.'
>
> —Jean-Paul Sartre

Imagery (Mod.) A set of mental pictures or images; the use of vivid or figurative language and expressive or evocative images in art, literature or music. Representative images, icons and statues used in art and religion help reveal latent or personal imagery. In therapeutic settings, imagery comes in handy to those who suffer from fear, anxiety and over-arousal; as a technique in behaviour therapy, patients are conditioned to use pleasant fantasies, often to the accompaniment of music, to relax and overcome adverse circumstances.

Imagery, however, is said to work best in a relaxed mental state. In its therapeutic context, the term refers to the use of imagination to fantasize or remember pleasant events and people. In the context of sports, imagery has been used as a technique that can help a student athlete picture his ideal or desired performance level. The technique can be used as a powerful tool to enhance performance and often acts as a corrective technique, energizer, practical aid, problem solver and controller of physiological response. (Davies and West, 1991).

> 'Logicians may reason about abstractions. But the great mass of men must have images. The strong tendency of the multitude in all ages and nations to idolatry can be explained on no other principle.'
>
> —Thomas B. Macaulay

Imaginal aura (Occ.) The medium through which one creates (and overturns) one's circumstances. Imaginal aura, it is believed, can be developed as a function of perception and creativity. Intention, positive self-image, visual learning, visualization and healing, manifestation and success are said to be generated and reflected at this auric level.

Imagination (Misc.) The process of forming a mental image of something, which is neither perceived as real nor can be subject to the senses. Imagination is the process which enables the human intellect to travel beyond the sensory range. It paves the way to an abstract world.

> 'Love is the triumph of imagination over intelligence.'
>
> —H.L.Mencken

Imagineering (New Age) The art and science of using IMAGINATION to make practical applications from knowledge or information. Imagineering is based on intuitively applying the laws of the physical world to an abstract, imaginary world in a consistent manner. It refers to the use of imagination in creating, or attempting to create, an imagined reality.

Immune system (Mod.) The system associated with the living body, which guards the body against the continuous onslaught of microbes, toxins, cancer cells and foreign bodies which threaten to destroy it during its lifetime. Immune system disorders occur when the immune response becomes abnormal—either excessive or inadequate. Though the immune system is normally capable of differentiating 'self' from 'non-self' tissues, at times, some immune system cells, called lymphocytes, become sensitized against 'self' tissue cells, resulting in what is called autoimmune disorder which destroys normal body tissues.

immuno-stimulant (Mod.) An agent that is capable of stimulating the IMMUNE SYSTEM to ensure the efficacy of immune response.

immuno-suppression (Mod.) An act or an agent that reduces the activation or efficacy of the IMMUNE SYSTEM. It has been found that some portions of the immune system itself have immuno-suppressive effects on other parts of the immune system, and immuno-suppression may occur as an adverse reaction to the treatment. In organ transplants, the immune system is most likely to recognize the foreign tissue and attack it swiftly. To overcome this situation, immunosuppressant drugs like cortisone find their relevance.

impressionist music therapy (New Age) The therapeutic application of impressionist music, a western style of the late-nineteenth and early-twentieth centuries, using somewhat vague harmony and rhythm to evoke mood, place and natural phenomena. The music composed by Debussy, Ravel and a host of others during this period helped evoke dream-like images, helping listeners unlock their creative and healing potentials, and paving the way towards a healing CONSCIOUSNESS.

incense (Ind.) Also, dhupa. A substance, usually made from organic derivatives such as tree resin, that gives off a pleasant aroma when burned. The burning of incense with its resultant aroma is said to purify the atmosphere both outside and inside the body, enabling one to reach higher levels of CONSCIOUSNESS. See also, AROMATHERAPY.

Indian maddar (Chi./Ind.) *Rubia cordifolia* Also, MANJISTHA (Ayur.), manchitti (Sid.), qian cao (Chi.). The powdered root of this plant finds cosmetic and therapeutic applications. The roots are considered useful in the treatment of blood clots, oedema and jaundice.

Indian system of medicine (Ind.) Medical concepts and practices which originated and developed in the Indian subcontinent, including AYURVEDA, SIDDHA, UNANI and YOGA with their respective regional variations.

indigo (Chi.) *Indigofera tinctoria* Also, natural indigo, qing dai (Chi.). TRADITIONAL CHINESE MEDICINE uses the plant in the treatment of anthrax, swellings, high fevers, eczema, gum inflammation, sore throat and boils. It is also used in the treatment of insect- and snakebites.

indigo-colour therapy (Occ.) According to some colour therapists, indigo and the deeper shades of blue are dynamic healing colours, which work both on the spiritual and physical planes of human existence.

indirect moxibustion (Chi.) A form of MOXIBUSTION in which MOXA cones are burnt not directly on the skin but on another intermediate material, such as a slice of garlic, ginger, or just a layer of salt.

individual soul (Misc.) A term used to describe the soul as a unique entity, though its interconnectedness with the cosmic soul is speculated in many philosophical treatises and religious literature.

indo-allopathy (New Age) An integrated system of medicine, which combines the concepts and practices of the INDIAN SYSTEM OF MEDICINE with those of ALLOPATHY. The hybrid system usually depends much on the sophisticated diagnostic techniques of allopathy, while opting for treatments from alternative medicine.

induction (New Age) Also, hypnosis induction. A technique in HYPNOSIS that facilitates the smooth induction of a person into a hypnotic state. It is often considered that the right set of words, which are fast and powerful, are conducive to quick induction into a hypnotic state.

infantile tuina therapy (Chi./New Age) The adaptation of TUINA THERAPY to meet the special needs of infants and young children (younger than five years). Luan Changye has authored a book on this subject.

infinitesimal dose, law of (Hom.) In HOMOEOPATHY, it is believed that the electro-magnetic energy of the original substance is retained in infinitesimal dose of dilution, while the toxic side-effects of the remedy get eliminated. HAHNEMANN claimed that as he diluted his remedies with water and alcohol and succussed, the remedies actually worked more effectively.

information therapy (Mod.) The timely availability and prescription of evidence-based health information to meet specific needs with regard to diagnosis and the treatment schedule. With the spread of the internet, information therapy promises to transform health profiles in a significant way. Alternative and complementary therapies also have an immense role to play along with mainstream medicine in alleviating suffering of the body, mind and spirit.

infratonic therapy (New Age) A therapeutic MASSAGE in which very low sound frequencies are applied through a massaging device. The method is said to increase the circulation of the blood and the lymph and also the activity of the nervous system.

inhalation therapy (New Age) The application of steam vapour, aimed at improving respiratory function. Sometimes the vapour is mixed with a selected herb or its extract (e.g., chamomile, eucalyptus, tulsi) in spas, along with essential oils to cure pulmonary and other sinus-related ailments. See also AROMATHERAPY.

initial sensitizing event (Mod.) Also, ISE. An emotional event in the client's life which triggered the problem. For example, being locked up in a toilet at, say, the age of three can trigger claustrophobia.

initiation (Yoga) 1. Expansion or transformation of one's CONSCIOUSNESS. 2. Admission as a member to an occult group or system. Hinduism considers initiation from a qualified preceptor or guru as the essential event in one's spiritual voyage.

'Where mysticism has prevailed for long, initiation has always been regarded as being most sacred. Divine knowledge has never been taught in words, nor will it ever be done so. The work of a mystic is not to teach with words but to tune those who are open to that which is offered, so that the seeker becomes an instrument of God.'

—Courtesy: *adishakti.org*

inner adult (New Age) The development of an inner adult personality at some point of time in one's life. Though it is expected to develop around the age of twenty-one years, for most it happens only when one works for it. Some never choose to have an inner adult, remaining INNER ADOLESCENTs.

inner advancement (Occ.) Also, inner unfoldment. The spritual progress of a person.

inner bodies (Yoga) The subtle sheaths within the mind–body complex of a human organism. 2. Bodies of a person within the gross, physical body.

inner bonding (Occ.) A psycho-spiritual approach, aimed at creating a powerful IN-NER ADULT, capable of curing various kinds of addictions.

inner child (Mod./New Age) Also, divine child, wonder child, child within, and true self. The inner child, which represents the emotional self, with feelings, stands created with the help of parents and other elders in one's childhood; it refers to the part of a person which experiences joy, sadness, anger, fear or affection. The frustrations, disappointments and other wounds received by the inner child continue to haunt till they are addressed with the help of religio-spiritual techniques such as QI GONG and PRANAYAMA. These techniques are believed to help in developing a wise, loving, self-affirming and nurturing Self, which instead of spanking the inner child, makes it relax through love and compassion.

inner-child cards (Occ.) A method of DIVINATION, as developed by Isha and Mark Lerner, aimed at re-awakening the child within. A seventy-eight-card TAROT deck, which illumines the mystical meaning of fairy tales.

inner childwork (Occ.) Also, Inner-child therapy. A form of PSYCHOTHERAPY, aimed at resolving childhood issues that affect adults. See also INNER CHILD.

inner enemies (Yoga) According to Vedanta, anger, delusion, desire, envy, greed and pride are the six inner enemies which cause suffering.

inner garden (Occ.) Imagining one's own state of mind as a garden, well-tended, watered and made to bloom is believed to promote well-being.

Inner healing (Occ.) An approach to healing, aimed at releasing deep-rooted energy blockages, having a link to the Freudian and Jungian theories. The approach is based on the theory that healing comes through the uprooting of negative memories or 'hurts', caused by others in early childhood, lying buried in the subconscious from where they tend to dictate our behavior without awareness on our part.

Inner life (Occ.) The life an individual leads in his or her emotional, mental and spiritual mental depths, and which is distinguishable from one's outward life and lifestyle statements.

> 'What fools indeed we mortals are, To lavish care upon a car, With ne'er a bit of time to see, About our own machinery!'
>
> —John Kendrick Bangs

Inner light (Occ.) A glow within one's IN-NER BODIES. It is believed that a moonlight-like glow is visualized inside one's head or within the whole body so as to quieten all mental fluctuations (vritti).

Inner mind (Occ.) The mind in its deeper realms, capable of performing its intuitive functions. 2. The sub-superconscious and superconscious mind.

Inner planes (Occ.) Inner states or stages in one's existence.

Inner self (Occ.) Also, 'Real Self'. 1. The essence of one's very existence. 2. The divine nature, believed to be found in all human beings, without exception.

Inner-self healing process (Occ.) An approach to healing as developed by a clinical psychologist, Swami Ajaya, based on the concept that one has two forms of inner self: a 'true self', an active, radiant, core energy, the source of abundant joy, unconditional love, vitality and wisdom, and a 'false self', a false image resulting from the shabby treatments one receives from his surroundings. The process, it is believed, lies on the rediscovery of one's true self, through experiential PSYCHOTHERAPY, ATTUNEMENT and MEDITATION.

Inner sky (Occ.) An area of the mind which is a crystal-clear inner space, free of every conceivable mental image, feeling, or identifications.

Inner smile (Occ.) A relaxation method, wherein practitioners are taught to 'smile inwardly' at organs and glands, believed to result in increased flow of QI energy. The method involves creating a source of 'smiling energy', up to three feet, in front of the practitioner. The source could be formed by creating an image of one's own smiling face or a memory of a time in which one felt deeply happy and at peace. In the next step, the abundant smiling energy so created is imagined to be drawn into the midpoint between the two eyebrows, called the third eye, from where the smiling energy is allowed to flow down through one's face, relaxing the cheeks, nose, mouth and all the facial muscles. The energy is imagined to be taken down to the thymus gland, from there to the heart and then to lungs, liver, pancreas, spleen, kidneys, genitals, etc., radiating everywhere the abundant love trapped in a smile. Smiling energy, if found in excess, is stored in the navel, to be retrieved as and when needed.

Inner tuning (Occ.) An approach to healing based on the notion that the human vocal sounds can release blocked energy.

Insight (Mod.) 1. The ability to see clearly and intuitively into the nature of a complex subject, person, situation or event. 2. Intellectual discernment 3. An increased awareness of a connective idea between different thoughts, which paves way for a new thought.

Instinct (Mod.) 1. A natural form of behaviour, which is not learned. 2. A pre-programmed course of action in behaviour. An instinct doesn't only instruct us on what to do at a certain time, but also on how to do it. While the behaviour of animals is natural, based on instincts, human social behaviour is unnatural and complicated.

Integral Yoga (Occ.) An approach to YOGA, based on the philosophy of Sri Aurobindo (1872–1950), synthesizing various traditions towards evolving an integrated approach working towards a higher state of CONSCIOUSNESS.

Integral Yoga has eight main goals: 1.

physical health and strength, 2. control over all senses, 3. clear, calm and well-disciplined mind, 4. higher level of intellect, 5. strong and pliable will, 6. love and compassion, 7. purer ego, and, 8. ultimate peace and joy.

> 'Man's highest aspiration—his seeking for perfection, his longing for freedom and mastery, his search after pure truth and unmixed delight —is in flagrant contradiction with his present existence and normal experience. Such contradiction is part of Nature's general method; it is a sign that she is working towards a greater harmony. The reconciliation is achieved by an evolutionary progress...'
>
> Sri Aurobindo

integrative manual therapy (New Age) A form of healing as developed by Sharon Weiselfish, derived from CRANIOSACRAL THERAPY.

integrative massage (New Age) A MASSAGE technique, which combines other forms of massage: BODY-READING, BREATHWORK, PROCESS-ORIENTED PSYCHOLOGY, and SWEDISH-ESALEN. It is aimed at moving energy from the head down and out through hands and feet, using not only smooth and gentle forms, but also combining with deep breathwork. It also focuses on the release of emotional blockages in the body.

integrative medicine (New Age) A system of medicine which views the patient as the key member in the medical team and applies all safe and effective therapies without being subservient to any particular medical thought or dogma. Thus, the clinical practice of integrative medicine blends the disciplines of conventional medicine and complementary and alternative medicine. The system is based on medical principles that emphasize a functional orientation to health and healing, the importance of empirical observation, and a reciprocal doctor–"patient relationship. It also includes therapeutic strategies capable of reaching all levels of human existence: physical, mental, spiritual.

> 'In love, one and one are one'
>
> —Jean-Paul Sartre

Integrative Yoga Therapy (IYT) (New Age) An approach to healing, incorporating GUIDED IMAGERY, PRANAYAMA and YOGA.

intellect (Mod.) The ability to think, reason and understand, and to use the mind creatively. 2. The faculty of knowing, reasoning and understanding.

> 'Intellect ... is the critical, creative and contemplative side of the mind ... intelligence seeks to grasp, manipulate, re-order, adjust; intellect examines, ponders, wonders, theorizes, criticizes, imagines...'
>
> —Richard Hofstadter

> 'Intellect distinguishes between the possible and the impossible; reason distinguishes between the sensible and the senseless. Even the possible can be senseless.'
>
> —Max Born

intercessory prayer (New Age) A type of PRAYER wherein the person who prays is never the intended beneficiary. Intercessory prayer is believed to be much more potent than prayer undertaken for one's own healing or salvation.

interconnectedness (New Age) A concept emphasizing the oneness and essential unity among all things in the universe.

It is increasingly realized that everything is made up of energies which are in constant transformation. The dividing line between the observer and the observed blurs out at the level of sentient beings. Mystics see this as 'all in one, and one in all'. Reality is viewed as an interdependent and interconnected phenomenon, not in isolation.

internal medicine See KAYA CHIKITSA.

internal reality (New Age) All images, fantasies, feelings and thoughts, which are imagined to occupy a space inside the subject.

internal visualization (New Age) An approach to healing, imagining complete relaxation of muscles or brain, forming a clear picture of a part of the body that is in need of healing and visualizing that healing processes are already taking place there quite actively and rapidly.

interpretative divination (Occ.) An

approach to healing through the reading of omens, portents or prodigies. The ultimate purpose in divination is the legitimation for arriving at a problematic question and not exactly the rationally correct conclusion. See also, DIVINATION.

interval training (Mod.) In the context of athletic training routines, interval training usually consists of a combination of high energy alternating short, fast bursts of intensive exercise, followed by a period of slow easy ones. In recent years, however, this has become a specialized field as trainers have designed interval programmes that are specifically suited to individual athletes. It facilitates an increase in training intensity without getting burnt-out.

intuition (Misc.) 1. Direct cognition or immediate understanding, bypassing the process of reasoning. 2. Immediate insight. Intuition is made possible through (silent) awareness, without the mind getting a chance to explain and state a reason. It is considered a far superior source of knowing than reason, but it never contradicts reason. Though it does not explain itself, it guides the one who is able to surrender to conscious spontaneous action—no matter what happens, and no matter how one is understood. Intuition plays an essential role in alternative and complementary systems of medicine.

'Science is nothing but trained and organized common sense.'

—Thomas Huxley

intuitionalism (Misc.) 1. The doctrine that one perceives truth by INTUITION. 2. An understanding that the recognition of primary truth is intuitive, or direct and immediate.

intuitive aura-reading (Occ.) A method of INTUITIVE DIAGNOSIS, aimed at reading subtle energy fields in persons and places.

invitational healing (Occ.) An approach to self-healing with TONING.

ipecac (Hom.) A remedy used to treat vomiting.

iridology (Occ.) The diagnosis of the colour and texture of the iris to detect physical and mental disorders. An examination of warning signs appearing in the iris is said to be useful in preventing the onset of disease.

iron shirt (Chi.) A series of tough exercises, aimed at reinforcing the structural strength of the body so that it can withstand the onslaught of physical attacks. The system also uses body movements conducive to cause the body's natural energy (QI) to toughen parts of the body exposed to attack.

iron shirt chi kung (Chi.) A system of BREATHWORK movements and postures, aimed at directing QI energy into vital organs.

Iroquois medical botany (Am. Ind.) Herbal medicine, as practised by the six native American communities that constitute the League of Iroquois. Herbs are considered endowed with supernatural powers and are believed not only to stall bad luck but help conquer the fear of death.

'You should try, by constant practise, to
lose your individuality, your ego, and realize that your actions are nothing but a
manifestation of the supreme consciousness.'

—Swami Satyananda Saraswati

ISPA (Spa) International Spa Association. A professional organization representing all aspects of the spa industry: club spas, cruise ship spas, day spas, destination spas, resort/hotel spas, medical spas, and mineral spring spas.

Iyengar Yoga (New Age) A system of HATHA YOGA, popularized by B.K.S. Iyengar, a yoga teacher. Iyengar's style is known for attention to detail and the scrupulous alignment of postures. He also popularized the use of yoga props such as straps, blankets, wooden blocks, chairs, blocks and belts. Each pose is held for a longer duration than in other yoga styles.

J

Jacuzzi (Spa.) The trademark name of a free-standing whirlpool bath, named after its creator. The whirlpooling action of warm water is attributed to three components: a pump, piping and water jets fitted into the tub. Water jets permit the flow of bath water and air at the same time. The bath enhances blood circulation by stimulating the nerve–endings below the skin.

jade (Gem) Also, nephrite, yu, nephrite jade. A medium-dark, green, semi-precious stone, long been considered a stone of good luck and prosperity. Worn as far back as 4000 BC, it is believed to be the concentrated essence of love, promoting self-reliance and courage in its wearer.

jaggery (Ind.) The dried, unprocessed brown-coloured sugar, extracted from sugar-cane. A traditional accompaniment to Indian meals, jaggery is helpful in cleansing the blood, guarding the lungs against air pollution, and regulating the liver function.

jala basti (Ind.) From the Sankrit jala, meaning water, and basti meaning lower abdomen. An ancient colon-cleansing process, serving the function of an enema, in which water is drawn up through the anus.

jala saurabhya utpadanam (Ind.) An ancient formulation for scented water for bathing, hair-cleansing and gargling. Apart from additives like common salt and powdered spices like nutmeg, selected herbs and plant parts were also selectively added to soften and cleanse the skin. Ginger, turmeric, neem, tulsi and sandalwood paste, and flowers such as champaka and jasmine were some commonly used ingredients.

jalandhara bandha (Yoga) One of the three BANDHAs known in YOGA, performed by bending the head downwards so that the chin touches the chest and thereby contracts the neck. This posture is believed to pave the way for PRANA to reach into the hole of SUSHUMNA. Engaging in jalandhara bandha is said to be useful in alleviating throat-related problems.

jalauka (Ind.) From the Sanskrit jalauka, meaning leech. Also, leech application. In AYURVEDA, leeches were bred to remove the impure blood and pus from morbid parts of the body, including the eyes. The leeches were applied on the selected area to enable them to suck the blood from the patient's body. As they complete this operation, they detach their bodies themselves from the patient's body. The area of the body treated with leeches was smeared with honey to hasten the process of healing.

jal neti (Yoga) Nasal irrigation with luke-warm saline water poured into one nostril, and drawn out from the other. An ancient yogic technique, jal neti is said to be of help in the prevention and cure of all diseases related to the eyes, nose, throat and brain.

Jamaican pepper See ALLSPICE.

japa (Yoga) Also, Japa Yoga. A centralizing regulation of MANTRA done through a rhythmic repetition, often in accordance with one's breathing pattern. It is considered an adjunct for MEDITATION. A simple Hindu method of japa involves using a name (nama) with an identified form (rupa), wherein a picture or idol of a deity is envisioned while repeating its name. Japa can be performed in four different ways as indicated in the following table:

Type of japa	Characteristics
Vaikhari	recited loudly
Upamsu	murmured softly
Manasika	meditated upon in complete silence
Likhita	written repeatedly on a piece of paper or in a note book

Japa is recommended as a preventive measure to curtail the generation of negative thoughts and feelings which congests the free flow of energy in the body and mind. See also CHANTS.

> 'The syllable ja in japa destroys the birth and death cycle and pa destroys all the sins.'
>
> —*Agni Purana*

Japanese enzyme bath (Jap.) Originated in Japan several years ago. The bathing ritual takes 2 to 2 ½ hours to complete and a session comprises three stages:

Stage	Description	Remarks
One	enzyme tea	After slipping into a Japanese robe (*yukata*), a herbal tea mixture containing twenty-five herbs, including peppermint, red clover and yarrow, is consumed in a tea ceremony in a garden.
Two	enzyme bath	A soak in a wooden tub filled with fibrous material (such as woodchips) and plant extracts (enzymes), a process referred to as fermentation.
Three	massage	Deep massage session for 75 minutes. A blanket wrap with selected music is an option.

The enzyme bath is said to boost circulation and metabolism, while relaxing and energizing the body.

Japanese facial (Jap.) A Japanese facial massage which is an ancient art form, aimed at restoring beauty, health and vitality. The massage combines traditional Japanese facial massage movements, lymphatic drainage and deep tissue work.

jasper (Gem) A variety of quartz, believed to bring love, joy and happiness for the wearer.

jatharagni (Ind.) The digestive fire located in the gastro-intestinal tract, which is considered essential for good health. See also, SAMAGNI.

> 'The digestive fire is the root of all fires in the body. As it causes the increase or decrease of the elemental and tissue digestive fires it should be treated with great care.'
>
> —*Ashtanga Hridaya Samhita*

Jenny, Hans (1904–72) (Mod.) A Swiss medical doctor and natural scientist who pioneered the study of CYMATICS, the study of wave phenomena. Following a meticulous methodology, he offered profound insights into both the physical sciences and esoteric philosophies. The cymatic images documented by him are awe-inspiring, not only for their visual aesthetics, but also for their message that matter is responsive to sound energy and its patterns.

Jensen, Bernard (1908–2001) (Mod./New Age) An American holistic nutritionist and iridologist for over six decades, Bernard Jensen believed that nutrition was the greatest single therapy to be applied in holistic healing.

Jesuit's barle See CINCHONA.

Jew's apple See AUBERGINE.

Jewish meditation (Heb.) A technique of MEDITATION, practised for over 5,000 years, aimed at transforming the intellectual process into a spiritual process.

Jin shin acutouch (New age) Also, Jin shin do. Described as a touch through which the Compassionate Spirit penetrates, Jin shin acutouch is a hands-on work involving gentle touching and cradling rather than massage strokes. According to the theory, there are twenty-six energy points located on either side of the body in which stagnation and blockage easily occur. Two such points are simultaneously and gently touched with a view to release tension.

Jin shin jyutsu (Jap.) An ancient Japanese art, rather than a technique, for energy healing, rediscovered in 1900 by Master Jiro Murai. It aims at balancing the energy flow in the body, besides awakening the awareness of complete harmony within oneself and the universe to which one belongs. The gentle method consists of little or no physical manipulation of tissues as it uses minimal pressure. In this method, a combination of ACUPOINTS, called safety energy locks, are held with the fingers for a minute or more in an effort to harmonize the body, mind and spirit.

jing (Chi.) From the Chinese *jing*, meaning semen or essence. Jin, semen, is considered one of 'three treasures', the other two being QI and SHEN. Considered to be the material basis for the body, jing nourishes, fuels and cools the body and hence is highly regarded in the internal martial arts. The Chinese tradition classifies semen into pre-natal semen (which one is born with) and post-natal semen (which is acquired during a lifetime from food and various forms of stimulation like QIGONG and MEDITATION).

jing gong (Chi) One of the two varieties of QIGONG (CHI KUNG), jing gong deals with meditative aspects, in contrast to DONG GONG, which focusses on dynamic techniques involved in body movements.

jingluo (Chi) The channel carrying QI energy.

jiva (Yoga) Also, atma. The immortal essence of a living being. Jiva refers to the living part of any living being, which can transcend death. Hinduism believes that at the time of death, jiva takes a brand-new physical body, depending on its desires and KARMA.

jivatman (Yoga) Individual consciousness; the Self.

jnana mudra (Yoga) A MUDRA formed by bending the index fingers of both the hands, so that their tips touch the inside of the thumbs, keeping the remaining three fingers straight. This mudra is performed in the same way as CHIN MUDRA, except that the palms of both the hands face downwards. It is believed to influence healing of several psychological and psychosomatic disorders.

Jnana Yoga (Yoga) Jnana is Sanskrit for knowledge, and is often interpreted to mean knowledge of the true self. Jnana Yoga is one of the four basic paths in YOGA, the other three being BHAKTI YOGA, RAJA YOGA and KARMA YOGA. Jnana Yoga refers to the unitive discipline of discriminating wisdom and not mere information. It is said to be the yoga for a thinker who desires to transcend the visible, material reality.

> 'When your last breath arrives, the knowledge of grammar cannot come to your aid.'
>
> —Adi Shankara

jnanendriya (Yoga) The faculty and organ of sense which helps in mental sense of perception.

journaling (Occ.) A technique for reducing stress, comprising writing about successful events in one's life.

juice fast (New Age) A short-term diet regimen comprising only of juices made from greens, fruits or vegetables. The treatment is aimed at detoxifying the body.

juice therapy (New Age) The use of the juices of greens, fruits and vegetables to cure particular ailments. Juices preferred for certain disorders are indicated in the following table:

Disorders	Preferred juices made of
allergies	apricot, carrot, grapes
anaemia	apricot, beetroot, carrot, parsley, prune, spinach, strawberry
arthritis	apple, beetroot, carrot, celery, cherry, cucumber, lemon, grapefruit, watercress
asthma	carrot, celery, grapes, lemon, orange, radish
colds	carrot, grapefruit, lemon, onion, orange, pineapple
constipation	apricot, beetroot, carrot, orange, pear, plum, prune, spinach, watercress

diarrhoea	apple, carrot, celery
gallstones	apricot, beetroot, carrot, grapefruit, lemon, parsley
haemorrhoids	beetroot, carrot, grapes, orange, plum
halitosis	apple, carrot, celery, grapefruit, lemon, pineapple, spinach, tomato
headache	beetroot, carrot, grapes, lemon, parsley, tomato
high blood pressure	cucumber, beetroot, lemon, orange, parsley, pear, pineapple
low blood pressure	apricot, carrot, grapes
overweight	beetroot, cabbage, carrot, grapes, lemon, lettuce, orange, spinach, strawberry, watercress
varicose veins	beetroot, carrot, grapes, orange, plum, tomato, watercress

jujube (Chi./Ind./Isl./Jap.) *Zizyphus jujuba*. Also, soubira (in Sanskrit), Chinese dates, da zao. Regarded as one of the five 'great fruits' in China, the fruit of jujube, rich in carotene, is used in Indian folk-medicine, along with honey, in the treatment of fever, bronchitis and other pectoral complaints. Practically the whole plant—leaf, buds, leaves, bark, fruits, root bark and stem—is known for its medicinal use in AYURVEDA. Both in China and in India, the fruit is known for its calming effect on the central nervous system. An Indian folk remedy for mental retardation prescribes the boiled fruit extract, administered along with honey, at bed-time. TRADITIONAL CHINESE MEDICINE acknowledges the value of the fruits in improvement of muscle-strength and liver-protection. The seeds are also used in insomnia. In UNANI, the fruits are used as blood-purifiers.

Jung, Carl J. (1875–1961) (Mod.) A Swiss psychiatrist and founder of ANALYTICAL PSY-CHOLOGY, whose experience in India led him to develop key concepts of his ideology, including integrating spirituality into everyday life and appreciation of the UNCONSCIOUS. Jung's approach emphasized understanding the PSYCHE through exploring the worlds of art, dreams, mythology, philosophy and religion. Though he was a practising clinician, he was drawn to exploring other areas such as alchemy, astrology, soci-

ology, arts and literature. He firmly believed that modern man, who heavily relies on science and logic, would increasingly benefit from incorporating spirituality and appreciating the unconscious realm.

> 'Every form of addiction is bad, no matter whether the narcotic be alcohol, morphine or idealism.'
>
> —Carl Jung

Jungian psychology (Mod.) A body of knowledge on ANALYTICAL PSYCHOLOGY, developed by CARL JUNG.

> 'Everything that irritates us about others can lead us to a better understanding of ourselves.'
>
> —Carl Jung

jyotisha (Occ.) From the Sanskrit jyoti, meaning light; literally, the science of lights (or stars). A profound and mathematically advanced science of ancient astrology which originated from the Vedic tradition of India. It explains how planetary patterns at the time and place of birth can help in evaluating one's strengths and weaknesses. In its study of horoscopes, jyotisha uses the sidereal (fixed-star) system, whereas Western astrology uses the tropical (fixed-date) method.

jyotisha shastri (Occ.) 1. A person well versed in the science of jyotisha 2. Astrologer.

ka (Egy.) An Egyptian term for LIFE FORCE, which is responsible for distinguishing a living organism from a dead one. It was believed in Egypt that ka could be passed on from one generation into another by males through their sperm. It was also believed that ka could be nurtured through food and drink. Ka came to be represented in Egyptian iconography as a second image of the individual portrayed.

kabbalah (Heb.) From the Hebrew *kabbalah*, meaning reception, a 2000-year-old Jewish philosophy concerning mainly God and scriptures. In its therapeutic aspects, the philosophy deals with the TREE OF LIFE which represents various aspects of one's PSYCHE. By working on creating relationships and by MINDFULNESS or focus, it is believed that therapeutic levels of consciousness can be reached.

kadidhara (Ind.) Also, kanjika amla dhara. A pain-relieving technique in AYURVEDA, in which kadi, a warm liquid extract of cooked fermented grains and herbal decoctions is continuously dripped through a nozzle in a pitcher onto the client's body. The treatment is often prescribed for rheumatic complaints.

kadivasthi (Ind.) A special treatment in which hot medicated oil is made to remain over the lower back (lumbar region) of a patient for a specified period of time, by pouring it in a bund prepared with wheat flour. This procedure is said to be beneficial for lumbar spondylitis and lumbago (low-back ache).

kahuna (Haw.) A Hawaiian witch-doctor. The term was originally the title for a Hawaiian priest.

kahuna healing (Haw.) An ancient health system, prevalent in Hawaii, with specialized disciplines. Kahuna healers are believed to possess spiritual powers (*mana*). As in modern medical establishments, the healers specialize in exclusive discipline as shown in the table:

doctor	specialized discipline of healing
kahuna haihai iwi	bone-setting
kahuna haha	diagnostics (using fingers)
kahuna hoohanau keiki	mid-wifery
kahuna hoohapai keiki	fertility
kahuna laau lapaau	herbalism
kahuna lomilomi	physical therapy and massage
kahuna paaoao	paediatrics
kahuna aloha	induction of love and feel-good factors
kahuna anaana	praying for death and witchcraft

Since the system believes that the body, mind and spirit are one, various methods involving psychic, spiritual and natural treatments are adopted as a cure for a specific problem.

kaivalya (Yoga) The term used by PATANJALI to name the goal and fulfillment of YOGA, to refer to the perfectly transcendental state, the highest condition resulting from the ultimate realization.

kalari chikitsa (Ind.) Also, marma chikitsa. The ancient system of healing orthopaedic disorders and neuro-muscular conditions. Massaging the affected area with oil, made with selected herbs, is said to be helpful in flushing out toxins from the body. The massage creates friction, causing dilation of hair follicles, thereby helping the medicated oil penetrate the layers of epidermis. The system is believed to be derived from AYURVEDA, SIDDHA and regional tribal practices.

kaleshwar mudra (Occ.) A MUDRA, formed by joining the tips of the middle fingers of both the hands, folding the other fingers, and joining the tips of the thumbs of both hands. This mudra is believed to facilitate a change in one's attitude and behaviour, and hence finds a place in de-addiction and rehabilitation programmes.

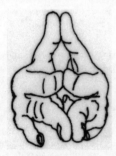

Kaleshwar mudra

kali bichromicum (Hom.) Also, potassium bichromate; used in the treatment of localized pain.

kalkarnika mudra (Yoga) A MUDRA formed by keeping the thumbs erect and folding other fingers inside the palm, and joining the knuckles. The mudra is believed to strengthen the musculo-skeletal system.

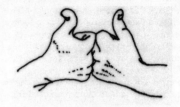

Kalkarnika mudra

kalka (Ind.) The lump of paste made by kneading the herbs along with their sap.

kanchnara (Ind.) *Bauhinia variegata*. The bark of this tree is given in a decoction, on an empty stomach, to treat goitre. Alternatively, kachnara guggula, which contains this drug as an important ingredient, is given in tablet form, to be followed by milk or warm water.

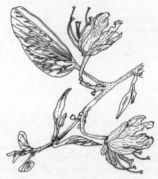

Kanchnara

kapalbhati (Yoga) From the Sanskrit, kapal meaning skull, and bhat, meaning splendour, perception of knowledge. One of the six major KRIYAs, kapalbhati refers to a rapid breathing exercise, aimed particularly at activating the mental faculties. Breathing in kapalbhati is similar to the action of bellows; exhalation is emphasized over inhalation. As a result, inhalation is done by forcing the air into the system. Normal breathing is characterized by the active contraction of only the inspiratory muscles, such as the diaphragm and external intercostals; exhalation, as a result, occurs passively on the cessation of this contraction of the internal intercostals. Kapalbhati reverses this process; exhalation is active while inhalation is passive. This induces a reversal in the flow of the nerve impulses to and from the brain, bringing about stimulation and awakening of the brain centres. Kapalbhati may aid in expelling more carbon dioxide and other waste gases from the human system than in normal breathing.

The exercise also helps relieve lung congestion, while stimulating the brain and the spinal cord. While doing this exercise, however, caution has to be exercised not to increase the speed of breathing beyond one's capacity.

> 'Kapalbhati destroys all mucus disorders.'
> —*Hatha Yoga Pradipika*

kapha (Ind.) From the Sanskrit for kapha, meaning biological water. One of the three bodily humors (THREE DOSHAS), kapha exhibits the principle of cohesion. It is an essential humor in ensuring the construction and stability of the physical body. Besides lubrication, this humor helps in healing and bestowing immunity. However, its deficiency causes a number of bodily symptoms, including sensation of dryness or internal burning, feeling of void in the stomach, looseness of joints, thirst, fatigue and insomnia. Excess kapha causes excessive sleep or drowsiness, heaviness of limbs, looseness of joints and white complexion. Various types of kapha, their location in the body and their impact are summarized in the following table:

Kapha type	Location in the body	Activities	Ailments caused by variation
Kledaka	Stomach and small intestines	Aiding digestion of food articles by moistening them	Digestive disorders
Avalambaka	Heart	Energizing the limbs	Lethargy
Bodhaka	Tongue and taste buds	Assigning taste to the food material	Tastelessness
Tarpaka	Heart	Sharpening the sense-perceptions	Impairment of sense-organs and loss of memory
Shleshaka	Joints	Lubricating the joints	Impaired joints

kapha prakriti (Ind.) The constitution of an individual dominated by KAPHA. It is characterized by three qualities: slowness, coldness and clarity. The quality of slowness manifests itself in slow but steady movements, whereas the quality of coldness renders low body temperature and poor appetite. The quality of clarity manifests itself in a pleasant appearance and behaviour. Though people with a kapha prakriti are emotionally mild, they exhibit perseverance and a strong sexual urge.

kapha churna A mixture of selected spices (CHURNA), used in AYURVEDA to stimulate digestion. Some herbs used commonly in various combinations are AJMODA, ANISEED, black pepper, CINNAMON, CLOVE, CORIAN-DER, CUMIN, dill, FENNEL, FENUGREEK, GARLIC, ginger, gurmar, hing, MUSTARD, NUTMEG, PIPPALI, red chillies, TURMERIC and tejpat.

karana chitta (Occ.) Also, karana sharira. The word derives from the Sanskrit for causal mind, and is the intuitive-superconscious mind of the soul which corresponds to ANANDA MAYA KOSHA, the 'bliss sheath'.

Karga puja (Tib.) Also Karga healing ritual. A shamanic ritual of healing performed by the Tamangs, also known as Murmis, an ethnic group of Tibeto-Burmese Buddhist horse-traders, settled in Nepal. The ritual, which is said to evoke experiences analogous to rites of passage, is believed to work as a remedy for those whose souls are possessed by the spirit, a condition a clinical pathologist would refer as dissociative trans disorder or somatoform disorder.

karma (Occ.) From the Sanskrit for action or deed. A celebrated law of consequence, one of the fundamental tenets both in Hindu and Buddhist philosophies, karma refers to an act or deed, whose consequence, or fruit of action (karmaphala) or after-effect (uttaraphala), is believed invariably to return to the doer. It is based on the principle of cause and effect. Karma is considered a neutral, self-perpetuating law of the inner cosmos, similar to gravity or magnetism being an impersonal law of the outer cosmos.

karma yoga (Yoga) Also, buddhi yoga; discipline of action. One of the four pillars of the ancient system of YOGA, Karma yoga refers to the pathway adopted for unattached performance, but carried out with total mindfulness. It is described as a way of thinking, talking and doing, in harmony and accordance with one's duty (DHARMA), without the consideration of selfish desires, or personal likes and dislikes. Action performed in such a background is without being attached to the fruits of such action (karmaphala). It is said that the practice of Karma Yoga in daily life, through action, meditation and devotion, sharpens reasoning and develops the intuitive power of acquiring knowledge to transcend the mind itself.

'When the individual no longer considers himself the doer, but merely as the instrument, the work becomes spiritualized.'

—Swami Satyananda Saraswati

karma basti An enema regimen in AYURVEDA, which usually lasts for four weeks, aimed at curing neurological and nervous disorders caused by the vitiation of VATA.

Karma Yoga (Yoga) A system of YOGA, based on the action principle, which demands consecration of every action and its fruits to the Lord. It refers to a lifestyle in which an individual performs every action while remaining connected with the Divine, thus removing attachment, staying in bal-

ance and disregarding success or failure. The practice of Karma Yoga is believed to help the practitioner gain knowledge of the Self (SELF-REALIZATION).

karuna (Occ.) Sanskrit, for compassion. The term refers to an attitude of universal sympathy, which generates a positive outlook and feelings. The attitude is said to pave the way for developing a healthy INNER GARDEN.

'There is no dharma (virtue) in heaven or earth, which can equal compassion towards one's fellow-beings.'

—A Sanskrit saying

'Be kind for everyone you meet is fighting a hard battle.'

—Plato

karuna reiki (Occ.) A type of REIKI, as developed in the last decade of the twentieth century by William Lee Rand, an American reiki master. The method aims at developing endless compassion (KARUNA) through symbols, which help as healing tools with strong vibrations. The method is taught to those who are already USUKI reiki masters.

'... I was floating on waves of energy. I was so very much at one with the currents of energy. I had no form; my spiritual essence was being transported. I began to feel an intense magnetic sensation drawing me closer to an unknown destination. I was drawn into a brilliant golden light by this mysterious force. I merged completely with this light, and instantly felt total and absolute peace. This was soul-level peace. And I was finally home.'

—Laurelle Shanti Gaia

kashrut (Heb.) From the Hebrew *kaf-shin-resh*, meaning proper. Also, kosher. The regulation prescribed under Jewish law on what is to be eaten by humans. The regulation also deals with the method of preparation of such foodstuff and the manner of their consumption. Certain animals, like camel and rabbit, are prohibited from being eaten. Birds and mammals allowed to be eaten must be killed in accordance with Jewish law and their blood should be drained out from the meat. No meat should be eaten with dairy and even the utensils for dairy cannot be used for cooking the meat.

katti basti (Ind.) The application of ayurvedic medicated oil around the lumbosacral area, as the patient is made to sleep in a prone position (i.e., on his chest). The method involves making a ring, two inches high, with the wet flour of black gram, and fitting it on the back on the affected vertebra, like a container, and pouring medicated oil in, which is retained there for fifteen to thirty minutes. This technique is said to benefit people suffering from rigid lower spine and muscle spasms in and around this area.

kayachikitsa (Ind.) Also, general medicine. From the Sanskrit kaya meaning body and chikitsa meaning treatment. An ayurvedic fitness plan which covers both the internal organs and exterior parts of the body. This holistic treatment involves change in food, clothing, residence and lifestyle, as per climatic needs. Exertion (ayam), exercise (vyayam), yoga practices (yogasadhana) and movements (gati) are included in the plan.

kaya kalpa (Ind.) The term kaya kalpa is interpreted in three ways: a) 'cushioning' against the process of AGEING; b) remaining rejuvenated and youthful and c) delaying death. An anti-ageing ayurvedic and SIDDHA intervention, kaya kalpa is a holistic approach towards physical and mental wellbeing and youthfulness, prescribing a regimen of diet, massage and exercises. The treatment helps in toning up the skin and rejuvenating tissues and organs.

Achieving longevity has been the main concern of SIDDHA MEDICINE and it has built up considerable literature dealing with kaya kalpa. PRANAYAMA is considered to influence the basal metabolic rate directly, thereby increasing longevity.

> 'The body is a sacred instrument to contain the soul and therefore must be nurtured well to safeguard the life.'
>
> —Thirumular

kelp therapy (New Age) The therapeutic use of the seaweed kelp, in ailments such as bronchitis, colitis, constipation, goitre, indigestion, obesity, rheumatism, skin problems, ulcers and urino-genital disorders. The far smaller incidence of breast cancer among the Japanese women, as compared to Americans, is sometimes attributed to the frequency of consumption of kelp. It is also known for its iodine content and helps in improving thyroid functioning. See also, SEAWEED THERAPY.

Keshav Dev, Acharya (Occ.) An exponent of the ancient wisdom of MUDRA, an essential aspect of Tattva Yoga, the yoga of elements. According to the acharya, mudra can provide instantaneous relief from common maladies and even assist with more serious ailments such as heart conditions. The FIVE ELEMENTS are said to be represented by the five fingers: the thumb represents agni or fire, the forefinger vayu or air, the middle finger akash or ether, the ring finger prithvi or earth, and the little finger jal or water. According to this theory, through appropriate hand gestures one can regulate the elemental control of the body.

keshyam (Ind.) Natural herbs and substances that strengthen hair and the hair root. Some examples are AMALAKI, FENUGREEK, horsetail, ivy, BURDOCK, sage and thyme.

kevala kumbhaka (Yoga) One of the two forms of KUMBHAKA, kevala kumbhaka refers to the spontaneous cessation of breath, which occurs due to the non-stimulation of respiratory system/organ, particularly after vigorous breathing practices. Kevala kumbhaka is believed to pave the way for the arousal of KUNDALINI.

> 'When after giving up inhalation and exhalation, one holds his breath with ease.'
>
> —Vasishtha Samhita

khechari mudra (Yoga) 'Space-walking seal'. An ancient Tantrik practice of curling the tongue back against the upper palate in order to seal the life-energy (PRANA) with what is called the 'attitude of flying upwards'. A mastery in this MUDRA is considered essential for practicing KUNDALINI YOGA.

khichri (Ind.) A mixture of boiled rice and split mung lentils, to be taken during treatments in AYURVEDA, such as PANCHAKARMA.

ki (Jap.) From the Japanese ki meaning universal energy. Japanese has over 11,442 known usages of ki as a compound, representing syllables associated with the mind, the heart, feeling, the atmosphere and flavour. The spiritual concept also finds its links with martial arts, such as Aikido. Usage is also with regard to REIKI, the understanding of ki and its development.

ki breathing (New Age/Vib.) From the Japanese *ki*, meaning universal energy. A method of BREATHWORK, combining MASSAGE and prescribed exercises, ki breathing refers to the belief that by breathing, the vital force in a person's body intermingles with that of the universe and hence becomes refreshed. Ki breathing manifests in the following three ways:

Nature of breathing	Method
External breathing (lung breathing)	drawing air into and expelling from the lungs through the nose or mouth.
Internal breathing	the process by which oxygen is taken from the air and carbon dioxide is released, through the circulation of blood in the vascular system.
Skin breathing	the process in which skin takes in oxygen, giving away carbon dioxide. Skin also regulates the body temperature by allowing heat to escape.

Correct ki breathing is said to help develop excellent coordination of the mind and body. The exercise incorporates a powerful imagination, with the practitioner imagining that the breath is drawn out completely, down to his or her toes, and the breath is inhaled from toes upwards, through one's legs, abdomen and chest, for about fifteen seconds. Ki breathing is considered an invisible practice, compared to the way roots develop in a tree under the soil. Through slow, invisible and consistent practice, ki breathing is said to help in the creation of one's own roots.

ki energetics (Jap./Vib.) From the Japanese *ki* meaning universal energy. An energy management technique, based on a sublime understanding of energy transmission. The technique consists of simple exercises to help achieve stability ('groundedness') and calmness. AIKIDO, the Japanese martial art, which uses the energy of the opponent to gain control over him, also makes use of this technique.

kickboxing (New Age) A self-defence technique believed to help the body with an intense aerobic and body-toning workout. The technique includes boxing, basic kicks, and martial-art moves.

Kilner, Walter (1847–1920) (Mod.) A British physician, who invented a special glass to enable one to view the human AURA.

He claimed that his discovery was not based on occult concepts relating to aura, but was physical. According to him, the human aura is quite sensitive to magnetism and electric currents.

kinesiology (Mod.) The study of movement in human beings. Being a multi-disciplinary approach, kinesiology necessitates the study of anatomy, biochemistry, biomechanics, neuroscience, physiology, psychology and sociology of sport. Kinesiology finds use in athletic coaching, CHIROPRACTIC, ergonomics, exercise physiology, KINESIOTHERAPY, MASSAGE THERAPY, OCCUPATONAL THERAPY, OSTEOPATHY, PHYSICAL EDUCATION and PHYSICAL THERAPY.

kinesiotherapy (Mod.) Also, kinesiatrics. The evaluation and treatment of individuals with disabilities through progressive exercise, BODYWORK and MASSAGE and passive and active movements of different parts of the body. The technique also includes education to assist clients to reach their maximum physical, social and psychological potentials. The treatment aims at maximizing the strength and flexibility of the affected muscle groups and motivates individuals to continue to improve overall functions.

kinesthetic awareness (New Age) Also, kinesthetic sense. A self-awareness programme which aims at creating a sensitivity on the movement of one's body through space. Kinesthetic awareness is said to help the body quicken its response.

kinhin (Jap.) A Japanese method which trains people to synchronize the pace of walking with breathing.

Kirlian diagnosis (Occ.) AURA ANALYSIS, based on KIRLIAN PHOTOGRAPHY.

Kirlian photography (Mod.) Also corona discharge photography, electrography, electrophotography, Kirlian. A form of photography named after Semyon Kirlian who accidentally discovered it in 1939. It is based on his finding that if an object is subjected to a strong electric field, an image can be created on the photographic plate. One of the salient aspects of Kirlian photography is its reputed ability to illuminate the ACUPUNCTURE points of the human body.

kirtana (New Age) From the Sanskrit kirtana, meaning praising. Devotional singing and dancing in praise of GURU and gods. An important form of congregational worship in many Hindu sects. Religious and meditative music plays an important role in allaying human suffering.

kledan kapha (Ind.) A form of KAPHA, located in the stomach. It is said to support, lubricate and nourish the vital parts including the joints.

kleshas (Yoga) The cause of human misery. According to Indian philosophy, ignorance, ego, attraction, repulsion and fear of death, either individually or collectively, contribute towards human misery. A wise person alone can avoid them by rigorous education and training.

> 'It is impossible to remove kleshas completely until one attains self-realization. The best that one can do is to slowly and systematically reduce them.'
>
> —Swami Satyananda Saraswati

knee-chest position (Misc.) Also, genupectoral position; a position in which a person rests on the knees and upper part of the chest, assumed for gynaecological or rectal examination. It is also the position usually adopted in the administration of ENEMA to allow more efficient irrigation of the colon as compared to sitting or a lying.

Kneipp baths (Nat.) Also, Kneipp cure. A form of HYDROTHERAPY, founded in Germany by Father Sebastian Kneipp (1821–97), a Bavarian priest. Kneipp baths involve the application of water through various methods, temperatures and pressures. Kneipp was a founder of the naturopathic medicine movement and a proponent of an entire system of healing which also involves HERBALISM, physical exercise, NUTRITION (with an emphasis on a wholesome diet of whole grains, fruit and vegetables with limited meat) and SPIRITUALITY.

knife massage (New Age) Also, cleaver cure, dow leo. A Taiwanese MASSAGE done with the help of a somewhat heavy, ten-inch-long meat cleaver, especially on patients suffering from chronic pain. The knife massage consists of deft patting, chopping or tapping motions, carefully performed, and causing no bleeding nor injury to the patient. While some patients scream at the sight of the cleaver, others are reported to even close their eyes and fall asleep during the treatment sessions. According to George Pan, a practitioner. 'As the knife touches the skin of the patient, the "negatron" from the metallic edge interacts with the "positron" released from his or her problematic (painful) spot and the patient feels a slightly piercing sensation and thereafter the pain is gone.' According to him, knife massage is akin to acupuncture and in place of needles, a knife blade performs the same function without actually piercing the skin. As patients are required to remain still, this technique is not considered suitable for children.

According to the legend, knife treatment was common among the monks in the Han dynasty (206 BC–AD 226) and Tang (AD 618–907) in China and this technique was passed on to neighbouring Japan. Originally, Samurai swords were used in pain management by ancient Chinese practitioners.

> '[Knife massage] is more effective than acupuncture at releasing the body's stored energy, washing out toxins and increasing blood flow.'
>
> —George Pan

kombucha (Chi.) A health-promoting natural beverage and folk remedy, made by fermenting tea in a mushroom culture. The culture is usually placed in sweetened black or green tea, which helps in the production of a number of valuable nutraceuticals such as glucuronic acid, glucon acid, acetic acid, lactic acid, vitamins, amino acids, antibiotic substances, and other nutrients. The kombucha culture maintained perpetually in a flask is often compared with a miniature biochemical factory affordable in every household.

Korean medicine (Kor.) Inspired by the two giant medicinal systems of Asia, AYURVEDA and TRADITIONAL CHINESE MEDICINE, Korean medicine has over the years evolved its own identity by developing its own techniques and native texts (e.g., *Hyangyak Gugeupbang*, published in 1245). The theoretical aspects of the Korean medicine derived from the Chinese (Ming dynasty), but its practise relied on the native knowledge of Korean herbal medicine (Joseon dynasty). In the early nineteenth century, Lee Jae-ma authored a book *Sasang Typology*, classifying human beings into four main types, based on the emotional traits that dominated their constitution, and developed exclusive treatments for each type. In the early-twentieth century, however, the colonization of Korea by Japan greatly affected native medicinal concepts and practices. The indigenous system of Korean medicine has now given way to the Western methods of medical intervention.

Korsakovian method of attenuation (Hom.) One of the two principal methods for manufacturing homoeopathic liquid pharmaceuticals (the other is the HAHNEMANN METHOD). The Korsakovian method uses the same container for each ATTENUATION. It requires emptying the container so that one part of the previous homoeopathic potency adhering to the wall of the container, is diluted by adding ninety-nine parts of diluent.

The next serial 1:100 dilution is thus created for SUCCUSSION. Homeopathic drug products manufactured by this method use the letter K in the potency designation, e.g. 3CK. See also, HAHNEMANNIAN METHOD OF ATTENUATION.

kosha (Yoga) Sheath, vessel, container, layer or body. According to Indian philosophy a human being is composed of FIVE SHEATHS: physical, energy, mind, wisdom and bliss bodies. The soul is believed to work at various planes simultaneously, through the sheaths.

koumarabrutya (Ind.) Paediatrics.

Krauter bath (Spa) A strong aromatic herbal bath, based on German natural remedy.

kripalu (New Age) A new version of the ancient system of YOGA, oriented towards the needs of Western or Westernized-Indian followers. Called the yoga of consciousness, kripalu emphasizes the mechanics of yoga, proper alignment ('alignment follows awareness') and the coordination of breath and movement, besides 'honouring the wisdom of the body'. The version is also characterized by 'meditation in motion', in which movement from one posture to another is reached unconsciously and spontaneously. Named after Swami Kripalvanandji, the Indian master in KUNDALINI YOGA, the version was developed in recent years by Yogi Amrit Desai.

kriya (Yoga) From the Sanskrit word, meaning action. In religious rites and ceremonies, the term kriya refers to doing of any kind. In yogic parlance, however, it has come to refer to a technique of regulated breathing. It also means involuntary physical movements, caused by the arousal of KUNDALINI. The objectives behind the six major kriyas known to YOGA are summarized in the following table:

Name of kriya	Anticipated result
Kapalabhati	Stimulation of the brain
Neti	Cleansing of the nose
Dhauti	Cleansing of the intestine
Nauli	Strengthening the muscles of the anus
Trataka	Steady gaze. This practice is said to correct eye-related defects including near-sightedness, besides developing the power of concentration.
Viparita karani	Inverted stimulation

Kriyas, like BANDHAs, help in getting rid of toxins and AMA from the body, and help in activating its endocrine functions.

Kriya Yoga (Yoga) A system of YOGA, rediscovered by Indian mystic Lahiri Mahasaya (1828–1895), and popularized in the West by Paramahansa Yogananda (1893–1952). The system consists of a number of yogic techniques which assist in achieving a profound state of tranquility and peace.

ksepana mudra (Occ.) A MUDRA formed by interlocking all the fingers of the hands except the index fingers which are kept erect and joined as shown in the illustration. This mudra is believed to benefit the large intestine and hence helps in elimination.

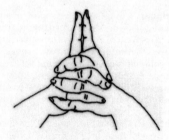

Ksepana mudra

kshira basti (Ind.) A milk medicated with herbal extracts, administered as enema (BASTI) through the anus, for providing nourishment to the body tissues, DHATUS.

kshira paka (Ind.) An ayurvedic method of preparation of medicinal decoction in milk. The preparation, as a rule has the following proportions: herbs (one part), milk (eight parts) and water (thirty-two parts). The mixture is thoroughly boiled till all the traces of water get evaporated, leaving behind the milky medicinal residue.

Kubera kolam (Occ.) Named after the god of wealth Kubera, Kubera kolam refers to the floor painting Indian housewives make in front of their homes to usher in prosperity and happiness. The kolam of the painting is in the form of a magic square of order three. It is essentially the same as the Lo Shu square, but with nineteen added to each number, giving a magic constant of seventy-two.

23	28	21
22	24	26
27	20	25

Kubera mudra (Occ.) From the Sanskrit Kubera, the god of wealth. This MUDRA is formed by touching the tip of the thumb with that of the index and middle fingers, while the tips of the remaining two fingers touch the base of the thumb. This mudra is recommended for countering congestion in the nose, from cold and infections.

kumbhaka (Yoga) From the Sanskrit word for pot-like. The practice of retaining the breath either inside one's body (ANTARANGA KUMBHAKA) or outside it (BAHIRANGA KUMBHAKA) as one undertakes PRANAYAMA exercises. Kumbhaka is an important component of pranayama.

To retain the breath, the practitioner does not close the throat or nostril but creates an extra space (or 'empty pot') within his or her body in which the breath remains suspended and motionless, like air in an empty pot. As kumbhaka is performed, the body is in a position to absorb the energy of the breath, which percolates inside. It also imparts an experience of one's awareness, focussed and concentrated within one's being. As the breath is retained outside after exhalation, a unique experience of emptiness, silence and broadened awareness is experienced by the practitioner. What one really achieves here is a state of equipoise in meditation, undisturbed by the fluctuations of one's mind. The repetition kumbhaka over time helps expand one's awareness and broaden one's outlook, set towards health and well-being. It is essential that the practice of kumbhaka be smooth and natural and should not be prolonged until breaking-point.

> 'No strength in the world is comparable to what one derives from kumbhaka.'
>
> —*Shiva Samhita*

kum nye relaxation (Tib.) From the Tibetan kum nye, meaning subtle body. A self-healing and confidence-improving technique, as developed by Tarthang Tulku, a Tibetan master, which includes breathing exercises, self-massage, slow movements and VISUALIZATION. In an exercise called 'flying', there is the following instruction: 'Extend the arms very slowly out from the side up to stretching above the head and then equally slowly back down again.' One such cycle may take between two and ten minutes. The practise of breathing in and out of both the nose and mouth at the same time is recommended while doing this exercise. While doing it, it is essential to focus one's awareness on the subtleties of sensations and the quality of experience one faces as the movement progresses. The whole exercise thus gives an avenue for linking body and mind in the presence of awareness given to the sensations.

Kum Nye has in recent years gained popularity in the West through publications by Tarthang Tulku and Ngakpa Chogyam.

kundalini (Yoga) From the Sanskrit word, meaning coiled energy. Also, kundalini shakti. The primal energy in the living human body, which is visualized by psychics as a serpent lying coiled and asleep in potential form at the lowest psycho-energetic centre of the body, MULADHARA. By focussing one's awareness intensely on this dormant energy, it is believed to be awakened for eventually being lifted up through a channel for reaching its ultimate destination (SAHASRARA) of supreme bliss, enlightenment and unconditional love. It is here that kundalini unites with Lord Shiva, who is believed to reside there. TANTRA considers this union of kundalini with Shiva as the ultimate goal for any worship. See also, KUNDALINI YOGA.

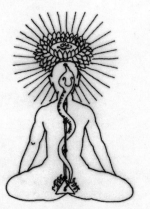

Kundalini

kundalini pranayama (Yoga) A form of PRANAYAMA, which includes the technique of VISUALIZATION along with prescribed breathing exercises.

> 'In kundalini pranayama, the bhavana is more important than the ratio between puraka, kumbhaka and rechaka.'
>
> —Swami Sivananda

kundalini yoga (Yoga) The technique of awakening and uplifting KUNDALINI through CHANTING, BREATHING and YOGA exercises. When awakened, the kundalini stretches forth through the psychic centres located in the vertebral column right from one end to the other, with its head at the centre of SAHASRARA and the tail at MULADHARA. The awakening of the kundalini is believed to result in the acquisition of super-normal powers.

> 'The kingdom of God is within you.'
>
> —Jesus Christ

kur kur (Spa) A course of spa treatments, which typically include ALGOTHERAPY, HERBS, mineral water and MUD BATH.

kutaki churna (Ind.) An ayurvedic formulation containing powdered rootstock of *Picrorhiza kurroa*.

kutir (Ind.) The living quarters, especially of a yogi.

kvatha (Ind.) In AYURVEDA, the term refers to a herbal decoction.

kyo and jitsu (Jap.) From the Japanese *kyo*, meaning emptiness or desiring a need; *jitsu* means fulfillment or compensating for the need. The concepts of kyo and jitsu go to show that like YIN AND YANG, both co-exist in the body–mind complex and they are the means by which one can exist. According to this concept, hunger, thirst, sex-needs and various wants, both biological and psychological, are governed by the presence (or absence) of one of the two. The body–mind complex makes a continuous attempt to keep these two forces in balance for its very survival. A harmony or balance achieved in their operation alone leads to health and happiness in life. In the body a kyo condition is felt as weakness or looseness, and a jitsu condition as strength or stiffness—both affect the smooth flow of QI energy and hence balancing them both in the physical and mental planes is considered vital for good health.

Kyo–jitsu has its application in SHIATSU, a system adopted for unblocking the congestion of QI energy in the MERIDIANS. According to the concept, while there is nothing wrong with desiring the fulfillment of a want, it should not become a pattern. It also differentiates between need-based desires and greed-based ones; the latter causes sickness at the individual level as well as an unhealthy society.

lastone therapy (Spa) A MASSAGE technique used in several spas, aimed at evoking a sedative and reenergizing respose in the body. The massage uses heated and frozen stones, applied on the body. See also HOT-STONE MASSAGE.

labyrinth walking (New Age) A technique of using a labyrinth for the purpose of focussing and calming the mind. The labyrinth is traditionally believed to be related to wholeness. The labyrinth is believed to symbolize a journey to our own centre and back again out into the world. Labyrinth walking has long been used as a MEDITATON and PRAYER method.

lachesis (Hom.) A remedy in HOMOEOPATHY, derived from the venom of the bushmaster snake. It is used to treat conditions that cause the same symptom as the venom itself causes; the physical complaints of one needing lachesis also mirror the physical haemorrhagic destruction of poisoning from the bushmaster snake.

Lao Tzu (Chi.) Literally, old sage in Chinese. The Chinese philosopher who lived in the sixth century BC and advocated that humans must make themselves an integral part of a harmonious universe by learning to be flexible. He was also said to be saddened and disillusioned that men were unwilling to follow the path to natural goodness. His teachings were composed in 5000 characters, the *Tao Te Ching* (The Way and its Power).

> 'A man is born gentle and tender
> On his death, he's hard and stiff
> Herbs are tender and filled with juice
> On their death, they are shrunk and dry
> So the tough and unbending is the pupil of Death
> The gentle and flexible is the disciple of Life
> Thus an army without flexibility never wins a battle
> A tree that is unbending is easily sawn
> The hard and strong will fall
> The soft and supple will survive.'
> —Lao Tzu

langhana (Ind.) Abstinence from food. According to AYURVEDA, langhana provides rest to the gastro-intestinal tract, thereby enabling the digestion of accumulated toxins in the digestive tract, particularly in the colon. This technique also relives constipation and flatulence. See also FASTING.

> Fasting is the first principle of medicine.'
> —Mevlana Rumi

laconium (Spa) Also Finnish sauna. A dry, gentle sauna which warms up the body and induces intensive perspiration. It helps in stimulating the circulation while accelerating the elimination of toxic wastes from the body. It is said that over a period, regular perspiration in laconium could help fight stress and stress-related disorders. Several spas around the world combine laconium with a cold plunge and showers. Laconium is believed to stimulate the heartbeat and regulate blood pressure and infuse a feeling of freshness and well-being. Experts suggest the duration of stay should be not more than fifteen to twenty minutes, twice or thrice weekly. Laconium should be followed by twenty to thirty minutes of rest.

laughter therapy (New Age) A method of healing which encourages people, particularly the elderly, to laugh in every conceivable interaction with their fellow-humans. According to some psychologists, laughter helps especially the elderly in the release of negative emotions such as anger, fear and boredom. By making laughter a routine, it is expected that seniors will come to grips with seemingly unsolvable problems in such a way that they can simply laugh them away. It is suggested that laughter is not necessarily an outcome of happiness but happiness could result from laughter.

Laughter is also said to be nature's way of helping us survive odds. It is also recommended in pain management as patients who opt for it are found to move through their pain more quickly than those who don't.

> 'The human race has only one really effective weapon, and that's laughter.'
>
> —Mark Twain

lavender (Eur./Isl./New Age) *Lavandula angustifolia* Also, common lavender, khuzaama in Arabic, rabandin in Korean, rabenda in Japanese, xun yi cao in Chinese. A flowering plant native to the Mediterranean region, especially the Pyrenees. It is used as an ornamental plant, and the flowers and leaves are used in folk medicine, either in the form of lavender oil or as TISANE. Diluted with a carrier oil, lavender oil is used as a relaxant in MASSAGE.

law of attraction (Occ.) According to this law, humans attract situations, people and events in their lives, in accordance with their own thoughts, feelings and attitude. This would mean that by consciously re-orienting one's thoughts, feelings and attitudes, humans can mould their overall circumstances.

laxative food (Misc.) Foods which have a mild laxative effect. Honey, fresh fruits and vegetables such as apple, banana, fig, grape, plum, peach, pineapple, pomegranate, prunes, raisin, cabbage, greens, lettuce, onion, senna leaf and spinach are laxative.

laya (Yoga) From the Sankrit word meaning 'a time span which has no beginning nor end'. In Indian music, the term refers to the inherent rhythm in a melody or a raga, which can be felt but not measured.

In the system of YOGA, laya refers to the stream of consciousness with which a yogi is attuned, and which has no beginning nor end. In both yoga and music the term thus refers to the passage of time which is a continuum. Laya also means a deep concentration in which one's ego is erased.

Leadbeater, Rev. Charles Webster (1847–1934) (Occ.) An English clergyman and a member of the Theosophical Society, Leadbeater conducted several investigations on super-physical realms and wrote prolifically on occult matters.

> 'The modern occult revival owes more to him [Leadbeater] than to anyone else; his concepts and ideas, his popularizing of occult and Theosophical terms and principles run through all modern works on these subjects. . .'
>
> —Gregory Tillett

lecanomancy (Occ.) A method of DIVINATION in which stones are dropped in a basin containing water and the sound emanating and the ripples formed in water are interpreted. Sometimes, instead of stones, oil is poured into the water and the shapes and outlines of oil on the water are interpreted.

ledebouriella root (Chi.) *Saposhnikovia divaricata*. Also, fang feng. The root of this plant is traditionally used in China in pain management. Known also for its antibiotic and antiviral properties, the root has its use in the treatment of expelling 'wind' and relieving headaches and body aches.

ledum (Hom.) Also, marsh tea. A remedy used in HOMOEOPATHY in the treatment of animal stings and bites.

leech application (Ind.) Also, jalaukavacharan. From the Sanskrit jalauka, meaning leech. An ancient AYURVEDIC method of drawing out pus and blood from infected areas with the help of leeches.

Leeches were grown to remove impure blood and pus from morbid parts of the body, including the eyes. Called rakta mokshana or blood-letting, this method (jalaukavacharan) is said to be useful in the treatment of the abscesses, bald patches, leucoderma and other skin ailments, and painful oedema. A day before jalauka is scheduled, oleation and fomentation are performed on the area of the body where leeches are to be introduced. The leeches are applied on the selected area to enable them to suck blood from the patient's body. As they complete this operation, they detach their bodies themselves from the patient's body. At this point, powdered turmeric is applied to the mouth of the leeches by squeezing them lightly so as to enable them to vomit out the blood. After seven days' rest, they are used again for sucking blood. The area of the body treated with leeches is smeared with honey to quicken the process of healing.

L-field (Occ.) Also, life-fields. A phenomenon considered common to all forms of life. According to Harold Saxton Burr who worked at Yale, all living organisms are encompassed by their own energy fields which he called life-fields or L-fields. In the 1930s he set up several experiments which showed that changes in environmental electromagnetic fields, caused by such things as the phases of the moon, sunspot activity, and thunderstorms, substantially affected the L-field. He found he could detect a specific field of energy in a frog's egg, and that the nervous system would later develop precisely within that field, suggesting that the L-field was the organizing matrix for the body. His student and colleague Leonard Ravitz focussed especially on the human dimension, beginning with a demonstration of the effects of the lunar cycle on the human L-field, reaching peak activity at full moon.

lekhana basti (Ind.) From the Sanskrit lekhana, meaning strong and penetrating. An ayurvedic enema, known for its strong and penetrative action in alleviating KAPHA-related disorders.

lekhaprartha havana (Occ.) An ancient practice of writing prayers on a piece of paper and burning them in sacred fire in a temple. Prayers can be written in any language, but should be clearly legible, in black ink on white paper. Writing prayers is considered to involve the mind more deeply and help in wholehearted concentration.

lemonade diet (Mod./New Age) A system or diet of citrus, lemon and lime, intended to effectively cleanse of the whole body and facilitate weight-loss, as formulated by Stanley Burroughs.

lemon grass (Chi./Eur./Heb./Isl./Nat./New Age) *Cymbopogon*. Also, chou geung in Chinese, citronella grass, essef limon in Hebrew, fever grass, hashisha al-limun in Arabic, karpurapul (Siddha), remonsô in Japanese. A plant genus of about fifty-five species of tall perennial grasses, native to warmer parts of the Old World. Lemon grass is widely used in Asian (particularly Khmer, Thai, Lao, Sri Lankan, Vietnamese) and Caribbean cooking. East-Indian lemon grass (*Cymbopogon flexuosus*), also called Cochin grass or Malabar Grass, is native to India, while the West-Indian lemon grass (*Cymbopogon citratus*) traces its origin to Malaysia. While both can be used interchangeably, *C. citratus* is more suited for cooking. In India *C. citratus* is used as a medicinal herb. It is also used in AROMATHERAPY for its calming effect.

lepidolite (Gem) A stone traditionally worn to promote love, peace and protection and whose metaphysical attributes have been identified by psychics as hope and transition, it is recommended for those who suffer from lack of expression or tension.

Lepore technique (New Age) A holistic healing technique, developed in 1980s by Donald J. LePore, a pioneer in nutritional research, based on BIOKINESIOLOGY and NUTRITIONAL THERAPY. The prescriptions include BALNEOTHERAPY, FLOWER REMEDIES, HERBS and MUSCLE TESTING.

ley lines (New Age) A theory which refers to the alignment of a powerful earth energy, through connectivity with various geographical sites on the earth, attributed with mystical and religious importance. According to this theory, places of worship, such as churches, mosques, synagogues, temples and places of natural and spiritual importance, such as caves, groves and wells, are located in this trail. These places are believed to be linked with people's health and well-being.

life (Misc.) A characteristic state of living organisms. Terrestrial organisms are characterized by cellular, carbon-and-water-based, complex organization, and have a metabolism, capacity to grow, respond to stimuli, ability to reproduce and, through natural selection, adaptability. A wider definition of life includes viruses too which, though cellular, do not metabolize.

life extension (Mod.) A movement, which originated in the 1980s, the goal of which is to extend one's life through intervention. The movement is based on the footing that an extension of life can be achieved by retarding, or even reversing, the process of AGEING by minimizing the chances for accidents, infections and diseases, particularly age-related afflictions such as cancer and cardio-vascular diseases and by following a good diet and exercise regimen (calorie restriction with adequate nutrient supplementation and a schedule of rejuvenating exercises, both on the physical and mental plane).

life force (Occ.) The soul, spirit or vital energy without which an organism becomes dead. Variously referred to in different cultures as breath, etheric body, CHI, QI, PRANA and PSYCHE, thymos, and later pneuma, in Greece, life force is a hypothetical force as it can neither be physical nor chemical. In YOGA, breathing has been a central theme for all ideas concerning life force. Breath energy has been acknowledged from ancient times as an animator of all earthly forms of life.

> 'Life engenders life. Energy creates energy. It is by spending oneself that one becomes rich.'
>
> —Sarah Bernhardt

life enhancement (New Age) A plan for good health and well-being, offered in health-spas which usually employ a team of health professionals such as physiotherapists, food experts, nurses, music therapists, health advisers, psychotherapists, personal trainers and yoga gurus to help their clients build their confidence level.

lifestyle (Misc.) Specific attitudes, habits or behaviour traits (likes and dislikes, tastes and preferences), associated with a person. Unhealthy or unnatural acquired lifestyles can generate metabolic and psychosomatic ailments.

> 'The greatest discovery of my generation is that a human being can alter his life by altering his attitudes of mind.'
>
> —William James (1842–1910)

light (Misc.) A form of energy which makes physical objects visible to the eyes. As a spiritual reference, however, light refers to that which illumines inner objects and is perceived by closing the eyes in MEDITATION.

light therapy (New Age) Also, phototherapy. Therapeutic exposure to prescribed wavelengths of light. Apart from natural sunlight, equipment like dichroic lamps, fluorescent lamps, lasers and LEDs are also used, particularly in problems related to skin, such as acne vulgaris and psoriasis.

limbic system (Mod.) From the Latin *limbus*, meaning arc. A system in the brain, responsible for emotional expression. The system includes the structures in the human brain involved in emotion, motivation, and emotional association with memory and is considered to play an active role in an individual's health and well-being.

linga mudra (Occ.) A MUDRA formed by keeping the folded fingers of the right hand with the thumb kept erect on the open palm of the left hand. The mudra is believed to impart mental strength.

liniment (Ind.) A warming rub containing oil infusion of aromatic herbs, especially CAMPHOR, CAPSICUM, deodar, eucalyptus, ginger or wintergreen often used to relieve muscular aches. As one rubs the affected part, the liniment causes mild irritation, which enhances circulation of blood in the area of its application.

lip diagnosis (Ind.) Also, ostha. An ayurvedic method of diagnosis made by examining the patient's lips. Some conclusions that can be reached by studying the lips are summarized below:

Lips	Probable conclusion
Yellow-tinged lips	jaundice
Blue-tinged lips	heart ailments
Dry and coarse lips	dehydration
Pale lips	anaemia
Multiple pale brown spots on lips	worms in the colon
Repeatedly occurring inflammatory patches along the lip margin	herpes

liposuction (Mod.) Also, lipoplasty, suction lipectomy. A procedure which helps in sculpting the body by removing unwanted fat accumulated in specific areas of the body such as the abdomen, buttocks, cheeks, chin, hips, knees, neck, thighs and upper arms. Though this technique is not a substitute for dieting and exercising, it can be helpful in addressing stubborn areas of fat that don't respond to traditional methods of weight loss.

liquorice (Chi./Eur./Ind./Jap.) *Glycyrrhiza glabra*. Also, atimadhuram (Siddha), gan cao in Chinese, kan zo in Japanese, sweet wood, yastimadhu in Sanskrit. Liquorice is used as an expectorant in AYURVEDA and also finds its application in the preparation of tooth powder. It is also known for its healing qualities in mouth and peptic ulcers. According to TRADITIONAL CHINESE MEDICINE, liquorice tones the spleen, enhances the flow of QI energy, eliminates toxins, expels phlegm and soothes coughs. In European folk-medicine it is used to treat gastric ulcers. In SIDDHA MEDICINE it is used to soothe irritated tissues in asthma patients. Recent reports from UNANI researchers suggest that it could be of use in treating AIDS.

listening diagnosis (Chi.) A method of diagnosis in TRADITIONAL CHINESE MEDICINE. Careful listening to the respiration and voice. In addition to more precise diagnostic methods such as PULSE and TONGUE diagnosis, listening provides valuable inputs in locating problems or disease. While a strong voice indicates a healthy QI flow, a weak voice is interpreted as a sign of qi deficiency in the system. Whether one speaks smoothly or not also reflects heart or liver conditions. Shouting, laughing, singing, crying and groaning are said to help in balancing the body.

liver cleansing diet (New Age) A dietary regimen which avoids foods such as meat, poultry, eggs, sugars and sugary foods, dairy products, nuts, coffee, tea, chocolate, oily or fried foods and alcohol is considered to help damaged livers.

living foods lifestyle (New Age) A dietetic regimen, popularized by Ann Wigmore (1904–94), which recommends eating 'living' or uncooked foods, such as fruits, vegetables, sprouts, fresh juices, nuts and seeds and fermented food (e.g., sauerkraut and miso) and unfiltered honey.

lochak pitta (Ind.) A form of PITTA, located the eyes and eye cavities. All ophthalmic problems are related to its aggravation.

Lok Hop Ba Fa (Chi.) Also, *Liu Ho Pa Fa, water-boxing*. An esoteric martial art from China, developed by a Taoist priest Chen Bok over a thousand years ago, the system prescribes selected movements, all of which resemble the course a river takes as it meanders down mountains—from flowing with no effort on its part, around every obstacle in its way, sometimes slowing down to the stillness of a lake, and at other times, assuming a powerful force when it falls from dizzy heights. The system, which is counted among the softer versions of martial arts, relies on inner strength over muscle power. It attempts to harmonize the six facets of humans, viz., body, MIND, CHI, idea, spirit and movement, which can be achieved through eight methods:

Method	Notes
chi or breath	controlling breathing by focussing one's attention on breathing
ku or bone	mustering force within one's bones
hsing or shape	mimicking various animate and inanimate objects, like an innovative dancer

hsui or following	merging with the moves of the opponent
ti or lift	feeling that one is made to hang on the head
huan or return	balancing one's movements and posture
le or reserve	maintenance of peace and calm
fu or conceal	refraining from revealing one's intentions

lomilomi (Haw.) From the Hawaiian *lomi*, meaning to rub, press, squeeze, massage. A popular, revitalizing MASSSAGE of Hawaii, practised by KAHUNA. The practitioner uses his fingers and palms as well as elbows, feet, forearms, knuckles, even stones and sticks. It is also referred to as massage with loving hands because of its gentle, continuously flowing short strokes. Lomilomi is performed along with prayer.

longevity (Misc.) Long life or the length of a person's life. Various factors contributing to an individual's longevity include diet, exercise, hygiene, nutrition and lifestyle. In recent years, several organizations have been exploring ways and means to prevent ageing and age-related disorders.

lotus (Chi./Ind.) *Nelumbo nucifera*. Also, Chinese waterlily, he ye (Chi), kamala in Sanskrit, sacred lotus, thamarai in Tamil; an aquatic herb with elegant and sweet-scented flowers, known for its medicinal use in ancient Chinese and Indian systems of medicine to treat fevers and diarrhoea.

> 'Cooling and antidotal.'
>
> —*Priya Nighantu*, referring to the lotus

low-impact aerobics (Mod.) A form of aerobics which minimizes jumping to exclude impact-related injuries. The workouts include arm and leg movements with each session starting with a warm-up and gentle stretching.

lu e mei (Chi./Jap./Kor.) *Prunus mume*. Also, maesil in Korean, ume in Japanese, Japanese apricot. Native to China, the tree is also grown in Korea and Japan. In Chinese medicine, it is used for relieving stomach aches caused by dominant liver QI. Bainiku-ekisu, a juice concentrate of Japanese apricot, is a traditional Japanese folk remedy for the treatment of dyspepsia.

luffa (Afr./Chi.) Also, Chinese okra, loofah scrub, ridge gourd. The cucurbit fruit (*Luffa acutangula*), grown in Africa and Asia, usually harvested before ripening and is used as a vegetable. Sometimes the fruit is allowed to mature on the plant, where it withers, losing all its sap and shape. The resultant skeleton luffa is used in kitchens and spas in Asia and Europe for the effective removal of dead skin (EXFOLIATION) and for stimulating circulation in the body.

lulur (New Age) Also, Javanese lulur. Described as the queen of body treatments, the traditional Javanese lulur treatment starts with a version of DEEP TISSUE MASSAGE, which traces its roots to ancient Bali. The style is distinguished by long strokes, aimed at greater energy flow. The massage is followed by a turmeric cold yogurt scrub to help nourish the skin. The body is then polished with a paste of rice, peanuts and scented woods like agar and sandalwood. Finally, a hot shower, with scented flowers, is given. This body treatment was popular with Javanese royalty in the seventeenth century.

lycopene (Mod.) A bright-red carotenoid pigment found in red-coloured fruits such as grapefruits, papayas, rosehips, tomatoes and water melon. It is an antioxidant, preventing diseases of AGEING, including some forms of cancer (colon, mouth, oesophageal and prostate) and heart disease. Lycopene also reduce the risk of diabetes, male infertility and osteoporosis.

lycopodium (Amer./Chi./Eur./Hom.) *Lycopodium clavatum*. Also, common clubmoss, running clubmoss, shen jin cao in Chinese. An evergreen plant, found in Great Britain, northern Europe and North America, used in folk medicine to induce appetite. The pale yellow pollen collected from the spores of this plant is used in making a homoeopathic remedy, also known as lycopodium. Homoeopaths prescribe this for ailments such as earaches, sore throats, and digestive disorders.

lymph-system massage (New Age) A technique that massages lymph nodes and the lymph system. The method uses gentle strokes, as developed in the 1930s by Hans Vodder, a Danish doctor. It was introduced in the US in 1982. One characteristic of this massage is that the strokes are always with the muscle fibres rather than cross fibres, as the lymph system runs in the direction of the muscle fibres. The massage is aimed at improving the function of the lymph system, which is designed to eliminate toxins from the body. It is said to be useful in the treatment of acne, arthritis, burns and swellings.

lymphodrainage (New Age) A non-invasive anti-ageing massage which uses a delicate pumping technique to drain trapped toxins and purge smaller tissues from the face and neck.

macrobiotic lifestyle (New Age) From the Greek *macrobios*, literally big life or longevity; a lifestyle aimed at acknowledging a consciousness of the polar principles that govern the universe. The idea is based on the ancient Chinese and Indian philosophy that the manifested world can be understood in terms of the two antagonistic but complementary cosmic principles YIN and YANG. Macrobiotic lifestyle is based on the understanding that nothing is entirely either yin or yang; a given object or condition is yin or yang in relation with another object or condition. According to some critics, the relationship between the concept of macrobiotics and the Chinese ying–yang theory is vague, since macrobiotics distinguishes yin and yang according to structure while the Chinese theory distinguishes them by function. To illustrate, while macrobiotics classifies the earth ('compact') as yang and heaven ('diffuse') as yin, yin–yang theory does just the opposite.

macrobiotics (New Age) A holistic dietary concept, advocated by Yukikazu Sakurazawa (1893–1966), also known as George Ohsawa, in his *Zen Macrobiotics*, published in mimeographed form in 1960. It includes a dietary prescription, a system of medicine, and a philosophy which encourages an exercise plan and social interactions, but does not claim to be a form of therapy or medicine.

The dietary prescription classifies foodstuffs in accordance with their energetic characteristics (see table), grouped into cold and hot, expansion and contraction, outward and inward, up and down, purple and red, light and heavy, and water and fire, illustrating the concepts of yin and yang. Oshawa considered whole grains, particularly brown rice, as falling near the midpoint between yin and yang. He also classified food in terms of climate (hot-yielding yin foods, cold-yielding yang foods), pH (acid or alkaline), taste (sweet or salty), colour (purple or red), and water content (perishable or dry). However, an orange (despite its yang color) was considered yin because of its being grown in tropical and subtropical regions, and its acidic, sweet, and succulent characteristics. Orange juice is more yin because of its greater water content. Both foods were considered undesirable from a macrobiotic standpoint, particularly for persons living in temperate or colder regions, because they are too yin relative to whole grains. The diet recommends whole grains, non-dairy vegetarian food regimen with a small allowance for fish.

A typical macrobiotic diet comprises half whole grains, a quarter selected vegetables, 10 per cent proteins and the rest fruits, nuts and seeds, in addition to liquid.

Yin food (expansive energetic characteristics)	Yang food (contractive energetic characteristics)	Foods that balance yin and yang (ideal foods)
Alcohol	Cheeses (hardened)	Beans

Cream	Fish	Brown rice
Milk	Meat	Fruits
Fruit juices	Poultry	Nuts
Sugar		Vegetables
		Whole grains

madhyama (Ind.) From the Sanskrit for middle, average or neutral; the middle path celebrated in religion. In Indian music, it refers to the middle note of the musical octave.

magic (Occ.) Also, real magick. 1. An act aimed at causing deliberate change. 2. The ancient art of invoking supernatural powers for controlling natural events, including the spread of diseases. The practice of using charms, spells or rituals to attempt to halt infectious diseases with religious fervour has been an ancient custom in many parts of the world.

'To me magic is an effect, which is inexplicable. The method might be trickery, or the method might be what you call paranormal. But I think the easiest way to define magic is in terms of the effect.'

—Peter Lamont

magic square (Occ.) A square array of numbers such that when the numbers in any row, column or main diagonal are added the sum is the same.

The constant sum is regarded as the magic sum or magic constant and such magic squares have been popular in ancient times in many cultures around the world. As they were believed to have divinatory qualities, they were used in various manners, including in TALISMANs to be worn as protection against evil influences of spirits and to ensure longevity.

magnetic therapy (New Age) The application of magnets for therapeutic purposes. The technique is based on the belief that subjecting some parts of the body to the energy fields of magnets will help balance the energy flow within the body. Bracelets, jewellery, shoe insoles, blankets and mattresses containing magnets are currently marketed. The latest addition to the array of products is magnetized water.

'Symptoms of cardiac arthrosclerosis and brain arthrosclerosis have been observed to disappear after six to eight weeks of nightly exposure to a negative static magnetic field.'

—William H. Philpott

magnetobiology (New Age) Also, electromagnetic therapy, magnetic-field therapy. An approach to healing employing electromagnetic energy. The energy devices used could be electrical, magnetic, microwave or infrared. According to the American Cancer Society, relying only on such measures and avoiding conventional medical care could result in adverse health consequences.

mahabali mudra (Occ.) A MUDRA formed by joining the tips of the thumb and the middle finger of one hand with those of the other and touching the tips of the index finger and ring finger of one with those of the other hand. This mudra is believed to activate the MULADHARA.

mahabhringaraj oil (Ind.) An ayurvedic hair-care oil made from several medicinal herbs including BHRINGARAJ, MANJISHTA, raktachandana, BALA, TURMERIC, BARBERRY, horsegram and LOTUS, steeped in sesame or coconut oil. It is massaged into the hair to control dandruff and premature graying, and to induce sleep. It is also used as a balm to reduce swelling and painful conditions.

mahanarayana oil (Ind.) A medicated oil, celebrated in the classical texts of AYURVEDA and known for its role in pacifying aggravated KAPHA. It contains extracts of fifty-six herbs, processed with sesame oil and milk on a low fire for several hours. Mahanarayana oil is used for external application (BAHYA SNEHANA) during PURVAKARMA. Massaging with this oil is said to result in improved circulation around the joints. It is also known for its analgesic qualities and its anti-inflammatory effect.

Maharishi Mahesh Yogi (Yoga) (b.1917) Born Mahesh Prasad Varma, the maharishi is a leader of the TRANSCENDENTAL MEDITATION movement, founded in 1957 in

India as the 'spiritual regeneration movement', based on the tenets of the science of MANTRA. The maharishi taught his meditation techniques to millions around the world and encouraged the scientific scrutiny of the YOGA.

mahasirs mudra (Occ.) A MUDRA, formed by joining the tip of the thumb with the tip of index finger and middle finger, and the tip of the ring finger with the base of the thumb. This mudra is believed to aid digestion.

maha yoga (Yoga) Literally, great yoga; a term used to refer to KUNDALINI YOGA. As the awakening of KUNDALINI, the serpent power, is believed to acquire the state of SUPER CONSCIOUSNESS, the system came to be referred to as the maha yoga.

ma huang (Chi./Jap.) *Ephedra sinica*. Also, joint fir, desert tea. Native to China, the dried aerial parts of this plant are used in the treatment of asthma and colds, and as a general stimulant which induces sweating.

makarasana (Yoga) Literally, the crocodile posture. Practising this asana is considered helpful in overcoming insomnia.

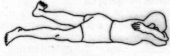

Makarasana

makko-ho exercises (New Age) Developed as a way to rejuvenate the limbs, properly align the hips and spine, stimulate blood circulation, sensitize the nerves and increase flexibility of muscles, this set of four to six daily exercises, though physical, make psychological demands on practitioners. However, while these exercise demand persistence, patience and a willingness to withstand minor pain, they are helpful when done over a period of time.

Makko-ho is to be practised every day, each pose being held for just a minute. Its practise is believed to help relieve stress by enhancing energy flow within the body.

The following are the four exercise positions considered ideal.

First exercise: Sit erect with heels together and soles turned upward. Then lean forward to the floor, while keeping spine straight.

Second exercise: Sit erect with legs extended in front, feet together. Keeping spine straight, lean forward and rest the chest on legs.

Third exercise: Sit erect with legs extended toward sides and the feet angled backward. Keeping spine straight, lean forward and rest the chest on the floor.

Fourth exercise: Kneel on the floor, toes pointed straight backward, and sit on the floor between the two feet. Keeping the spine straight, lie behind and keep the back flat on the floor.

While practising makko-ho exercises what matters is the action of commencing a stretch, not how far one actually stretches.

mala Also, malam. From the Sanskrit for toxins and waste; waste products arising due to catabolism such as sweat, urine and faeces. Mala constitutes one of the eight diagnostic approaches in several systems of medicine.

manas (Yoga) From the Sanskrit for mind. 1. The 'lower' mind, said to be bound with one's senses. 2. A means to experience pleasure, pain, hunger, want, etc. See also, BUDDHI.

> 'If an animal does something, we call it instinct; if we do the same thing, for the same reason, we call it intelligence.'
>
> —Will Cuppy

Manchurian tea (New Age) Also, Kargasok tea. A tea prepared from the Kombucha mushroom. It is made with a 'starter culture' that is added to black tea and sugar. See also KOMBUCHA.

mandagni (Ind.) From the Sanskrit mand, meaning slow, and agni, meaning fire; the slow digestion. According to AYURVEDA, when agni digests little food and takes long, it can cause respiratory problems, nausea, excessive salivation and fatigue in an individual. See also SAMAGNI.

mandala (Yoga) A circular and mystical diagram, which symbolizes the cosmic law, with neither beginning nor end. There has been an age-old belief that placing such mandalas in one's habitation enhances greater energy exchanges, thus ushering greater harmony in homes and in religious places of worship. While constructing a mandala, Buddhist monks chant and meditate to invoke the divine energies of the deities to be occupied in them.

'Mandala, a universally occurring pattern, is associated with the mythological representation of the self.'

—Carl Jung

mandrake (Chi.) *Podophyllum emodi.* Also, bankakri (Urdu), gui jiu (Chinese). TRADITIONAL CHINESE MEDICINE recognizes the medicinal use of the root-stock (rhizome) of this herb, used as a hepatic stimulant. Its antibiotic and anti-cancer properties are also being exploited.

manduki kriya (Occ.) From the Sanskrit, for 'the frog attitude'. An ancient practice in TANTRISM, wherein a practitioner attunes himself or herself to smell the fragrance of one's astral body, imagined to emit the aroma of CHANDANA.

mango–ginger (Ind.) *Curcuma amada.* Also, amba haldi. A member of the ginger family, whose rhizome smells like fresh mangoes. It is used in Indian folk medicine for treating bronchitis, flatulence, halitosis, hiccups and indigestion. The crushed rhizome is also applied externally on sprains and wounds.

manipulative and body-based methods (New Age) An official classification for alternative treatments that are based on manipulation and/or movement of one or more parts of the human body. ACUPRESSURE, BODY WORK, BOWEN TECHNIQUE, CHIROPRACTIC, MARTIAL ARTS, MASSAGE THERAPY, MEDICAL ACUPUNCTURE, METAMORPHIC TECHNIQUE, MYOFASCIAL RELEASE, OSTEOPATHY, ROLFING, SHIATSU, TAIJIQUAN and TUI NA are some examples.

manipuraka (Yoga) Also, manipura, solar plexus chakra, third chakra. One of the seven major chakras, located in the solar-plexus area and affecting the functions of the adrenal glands and pancreas. It is symbolically represented by a lotus flower within petals and a red triangle. One's willpower and wisdom are attributed to the functions of this chakra.

manjishta (Ind.) *Rubia cordifolia.* In AYURVEDA, the red root of this plant finds its use primarily in clearing the aggravation of PITTA. It is also used for removing tumours.

mantra (Yoga) From the Sanskrit man, meaning to think, and tra, meaning tool. A syllable, word or verse, considered sacred or powerful, especially when chanted or recited with concentration and devotion. Initially it is chanted loudly and eventually in silence. It is said to help change one's consciousness level taking it to a more stable position.

Mantra is chanted with various aims, including conquering fear, overcoming dangerous situations, accumulating wealth and conquering enemies and adversaries. According to experts, the sound vibrations in mantra help cope with situations through a healthy re-patterning which paves way for peace and success.

Besides all Eastern religions, some Jewish meditation techniques include mantras, though they are not known by this name. In the Islamic Sufi tradition, chanting the ninety-nine names of Allah and the Prophet are popular. In Christianity, repetitive prayer, using rosaries and chants are not uncommon.

A mantra is believed to enhance one's protective consciousness, through the transmission of vibrations. Some mantras used by Hindus, and believed to be curative are shown in the table below:

Health issue	Associated mantra
For digestion	1. *Agastyam Kumbha Karanam Cha Shamincha Vaada Vaanalam Bhojanam Pachanaarthaaya Smaredabhyaam Cha Panchakam*
For good health	1. *Aum Aim Hrim Shrim Namah Sarvadharaaya Bhagavatey Asya Mama Sarva Roga Vinashaya Jvala Jvala Enam Dirghaayusham Kuru Kuru Svaahaa*

2. *Achyutam Chaamritam Chaiva Japedushadhakarmaani*
3. *Aum Namo Paramaatmaney Parabrahma Mama Sharirey Paahi Paahi Kuru Kuru Svaahaa*
4. *Maam Mayaat Sarvato Raksha Shriyam Vardhaya Sarvada Sharira Rogyam Me Dehi Deva Deva Namostutey*

To counter diseases and discomfort

1. *Aum Hrim Hansah*
2. *Aum Shrim Hrim Klim Aim Indrakshyai Namah*
3. *Aum Sam Saam Sim Sum Soom Sem Saim Sam Saha Vam Vaam Saha Amrita Varech Svaahaa*

To counter fevers

1. *Aum Namo Bhagavatey Rudraaya Namah Krodeshwaraaya Namah, Jyot Patangaaya Namop Namah, Siddhi Rudra Ajaapayati Svaahaa*
2. *Aum Namo Maha Uchchishta Yogini Prakirna Dranshtaa Khaadati Tharvati Nashyati Bhakshyati Aum Thah Thah Thah*
3. *Aum Vindhya Vaanana Hum Fat Svaahaa*

For sound sleep

1. *Aum Namo Bhagavatey Chhandi Chhandi Amukasya Jvarasya Shara Prajvilita Parashupaaniye Parashaaya Fat Aum Agasti…Shaayinah*

'Through the repetition of the mantra Om and meditation on its meaning, knowledge of the atman and the destruction of obstacles to that knowledge is obtained.'

—Sage Patanjali

mantra japa (Yoga) An ancient Vedic concept which involves the recitation MANTRA as one of the main procedures in prayer rituals (PUJA). It involves the repetition of mantras, using beads (RUDRAKSHA), 108 or 1008 times. It is believed that one achieves one-pointedness by such recitations.

mantra yoga (Yoga) An approach to MEDITATION with selected MANTRA. It is an acknowledged fact that the continuous repetition of sacred syllables and verses helps in achieving higher levels of consciousness. For a believer, the divine form inherent in the mantra becomes manifest through continuous repetition.

'Mantra itself acts as a pathway between normal states of consciousness and super consciousness.'

—Swami Satyandanda Saraswati

man tuo luo (Chi./Jap.) Also, Datura metel L. The flowers of this plant have been traditionally used as an anaesthetic and to induce sleep, the leaves are used in the treatment of rheumatoid arthritis and the seeds are considered helpful in promoting blood circulation and thereby relieving pain.

manual lymph drainage (New Age) A gentle technique in MASSAGE, using the hands and fingers to simulate wave-like movements through rhythmic strokes. By stimulating the lymph glands, which play a crucial function as part of the body's defence mechanism against infections and diseases, the blockage of lymph is addressed and its flow is taken care of. This anti-ageing technique is said to be useful not only in detoxifying the body, but also in draining fluids and regenerating the tissues. The expected results include a reduction in lymphodemas and odemas, relief in fatigue or chronic pain and deep relaxation. See also, LYMPHODRAINAGE.

manual therapy (New Age) An ancient healing method in which the hands are employed for alleviating pain. The therapist or masseur develops over a period of time the expertise to scan with his hands areas which are blocked or dysfunctional. After locating the structures responsible for pain, he or she uses various methods such as soft-tissue mobilization, connective tissue techniques, MYOFASCIAL RELEASE THERAPY, mobilization of the joints, mobilization of the spinal segments, mobilization of neural tissue, visceral mobilization, strain and counter-strain. Such techniques have also been found useful in alleviating the symptoms relating to neuro-musculoskeletal pain syndromes, such as low-back pain.

Marichyasana (Yoga) Named after a legendary sage, Marich, this ASANA is aimed at increasing energy levels while reducing the accumulated fat around the waist.

marma points (Ind.) Also, lethal spots, marmasthana. Sensitive points in the body in which VITAL FORCE is concentrated. SUSHRUTA (sixth century BC) who compiled *Sushruta Samhita*, identified 107 marma points in the body and cautioned that direct injury to these vital spots should be avoided as hurt to them could be fatal. As marma points are Located at vital meeting-points of two major systems such as veins and blood vessels, nerves and bones, muscles and bones, ligaments and joints.

When they are affected or ruptured, the organs linked to them through energy channels are not supplied with energy and as a result get diseased, depending on the amount of PRANA they are deprived of.

Marma points are believed to bridge the gap between the physical and astral body of an individual, and understood as energy-carriers between the mind and the body's various organs and tissues. When these points are traumatized, due to a blockage of energy, the health of an individual can be severely affected. Marma points are distributed all over the human body as indicated in the following table:

Marma points in the human body	Number of Points
upper extremities of the body	22
lower extremities of the body	22
thorax	09
stomach and abdomen	03
back of the trunk	14
head region including the neck	37
in musculature	11
in blood vessels	41
in tendons and ligaments	27
in bones	08
in the joints	20

Sushruta also identified marma points on the basis of prognostic evaluation as indicated in the table below:

Name of marma group	Effect after injury	Number of marma points
Sadhya pranahar marma	causing instant death, when there is injury to the marma point	19
Kalantar pranahar marma	causing death after a while	33
Vishalyaghan marma	causing death after a lapse of time	03
Vaiakalyakar marma	causing debility after the injury to marma points	44
Rujakar marma	causing pain after the injury to marma points	14

Marma points are considered important for gauging the DOSHAS, their degree of accumulation and their vitiation, more particularly with reference to the diagnosis of VATA disorders which are associated with trauma.

marma massage (Ind.) Also marma-point massage. A form of MASSAGE, aimed at helping the release of blocked energy in the MARMA POINT. Aromatic oils and herbal decoctions are also used. For example, to remove congestion in the head region, camphor, eucalyptus and methol are used near the nostrils, whereas sandalwood oil is preferred for treating headaches and applied near the area of the THIRD EYE. The technique used is gentle and soft flowing.

marma therapy (Ind.) Also, marma puncture. A therapeutic procedure in Ayurveda. Akin to acupuncture, marma therapy comprises pressure being applied on marma points. The treatment also includes MASSAGE with oils. The treatment is reported to be useful for people suffering from stress and trauma. Other ailments such as chronic fatigue, frozen shoulder and migraine are also said to respond favourably to this treatment.

martial arts therapy (Chi.) The application of martial arts in the treatment of a mental or physical disorders. Applications include promoting kinesthetic balance in the elderly or impaired, as undertaken in TAI CHI CH'UAN, or reducing aggressiveness through appropriate exercises. Children with low self-esteem also benefit from self-defense skills.

massage (New Age) Also, massage therapy. A non-invasive, holistic treatment, massage is perhaps the most widely practised alternative therapy. Massages aim at inducing relaxation, pain relief, improved circulation and enhanced functioning of the immune mechanism. Massage therapists use not only their fingers and palms but occasionally also their elbows, feet, forearms and knees, depending on the requirement of the client. Seventy-five methods of massage have been identified of which some important ones are ABHYANGA, DEEP TISSUE MASSAGE, MANUAL LYMPH DRAINAGE, NEUROMUSCULAR MASSAGE and SWEDISH/ESALEN MASAGE. It comprises five basic modes: effleurage or stroking, rubbing or friction, petrissage or kneading, tapotement or percussion, and vibration or shaking the muscles and other soft tissues.

Massage therapists are also referred to as bodyworkers. See also BODYWORK.

> 'The object of massage is to disperse the effete matters found in the muscles and not expelled by exercise.'
>
> —Avicenna

massage aromatherapy (New Age) Massaging with an oil mixture, consisting of both essential and non-essential oils. See also, ABHYANGA.

massage chair (New Age) Also, shiatsu-massage chair. A chair designed to simulate the human touch for the person who sits on it. Many massage chairs are designed to be used in the treatment of common ailments such as headaches, indigestion and back pain. It is designed as a substitute for a manual massage. The client can choose different options by pressing the appropriate buttons. The options include EFFLEURAGE, FRICTION, PETRISSAGE, TAPOTEMENT and VIBRATION.

Materia Medica (Misc.) Latin, meaning medical matters. A body of collected references on the therapeutic characteristics of substances employed for healing. The term was coined by Dioscorides, the Greek pharmaco-botanist (first century BC) who used this as the title of his pioneering work relating to the details on about 600 phyto-medicines and a number of animal and mineral products of medicinal value. In recent times the term is used less, as the term pharmacology has come to substitute it.

Materia Medica and Formulary of Ayurvedic Drugs (Ind.) The MATERIA MEDICA of AYURVEDA consists of detailed references on natural drugs, derived from various plant, animal and mineral sources, both terrestrial and aquatic. The drug extracts are administered in various forms—crushed materials, juice extracts, decoctions, infusions, distillates, powders, tablets, pills, jams, syrups, fermented liquids, medicated oil and bhasmas. *Ayurvedic Formulary of India* published by the Government of India, contains valuable information on ayurvedic formulations respectively.

materialism A doctrine which holds that reality is all that matters. The doctrine considers that thoughts and feelings are but the effect of the movement of matter. In other words, materialism acknowledges no other worlds of existence but the physical world.

matra basti (Ind.) A type of ENEMA, administered every day with oil, intended to reduce VATA-related disorders. The daily enema is prescribed for those suffering from excess physical activity, including too much exercising, walking, sex or lifting heavy objects. There is usually no dietary restriction for those who undergo this treatment which is aimed at strengthening the body.

matsyasana (Yoga) Sanskrit, for the fish posture; an ASANA, believed to benefit those suffering from asthma, diabetes or lung diseases.

maximum life span (Misc.) The maximum number of years an animal or human can live. The oldest-ever person, who lived for 122 years and 164 days was a French woman, Jeanne Calment. The maximum life span for humans has remained about 115–120, through known history, unaltered by the steady improvements in life expectancy in recent years. While path-breaking inventions in medical practices, more particularly in research regarding antibiotics, and the increased availability of adequate nutrition, have prolonged the average life span, the maximum human life span has, however, remained more or less constant.

According to gerontologists, the secret for increasing the life span lies in restricting the intake of calories, while ensuring adequate nutrition. Recent advances in biomedical molecular engineering promise to contribute towards extending the maximum life span significantly in the near future.

The following table indicates the maximum life span of humans and some animals:

Animal	Maximum life span (in years)
cat	34
dog	29
elephant	78
goldfish	49
horse	62
human	122.5
mouse	04
tortoise	188
whale	210

In the plant kingdom, the longest-living perennials are woody, stemmed trees of which a great basin bristlecone pine is estimated to be over 5000 years. See also, KAYA KALPA.

maya (Yoga) From the Sanskrit ma, meaning not, and ya meaning this; an illusion.

According to the Vedas, maya is pure illusion, unreal. The captivating nature of maya is acknowledged by the Upanishads. According to Indian philosophy, making a distinction between one's consciousness and one's physical body, and between one's body and mind is a consequence of ignorance (AVIDYA). According to it, maya shrouds the true nature of one's self, as it differentiates between one's self and the rest of the world.

Mayan medicine (Am. Ind.) The indigenous, traditional medicine of the Mayas. The system was based on the philosophy that the body, mind and spirit are components of a whole and that harmonizing them with each other and with other elements in nature alone brings health and well-being.

Midwives in Central America are depositories of knowledge, passed down orally from one generation to another; their knowledge of paediatrics, gynaecology and obstetrics is vast.

meda (Ind.) Sanskrit, for fat. According to AYURVEDA, fatty substances constitute one of the seven bodily tissues or DHATUs. Though once it was held that obesity was a mere aesthetic problem, it has now been linked with coronary heart disease, strokes, diabetes and osteoarthritis. Once a lifestyle disease of the industrialized West, obesity has now invaded many parts of the developing world as well. There are several factors which contribute to obesity including excessive eating, lack of physical exercises, endocrine abnormalities and genetic or family traits.

medical acupuncture (New Age) A modern interpretation of ACUPUNCTURE, developed for Western practitioners such as osteopaths, physicians, and physiotherapists who have no formal training in TRADITIONAL CHINESE MEDICINE.

The significant difference between traditional acupuncture and Western medical acupuncture is that while the former is rooted in insight from over thousands of years, often described with Taoist metaphor, the latter is based on current concepts of pathology and incorporates an understanding of anatomy, endocrinology, neurology and physiology.

medical spa (Spa) Also, medi-spa. A SPA, which offers comprehensive medical services—naturopathic, traditional or complementary—under the expert supervision of qualified medical and para-medical professionals. Some spas have specializations including cosmetic procedures, diagnostic testing, preventive care, or a combination, under one roof.

medicated oil (Ind.) Oil produced by steeping and straining plants and plant parts. Herbal extracts are cooked in oil for a considerable period of time before it is cooled and bottled. In AYURVEDA, sesame oil is the most widely used oil base. Clarified butter from cow milk (GHEE) is also used as a 'vehicle' for transmitting the medicinal properties of herbs to the body. Medicated oils are usually applied externally.

meditation (Yoga) An ancient awareness-training technique in the path of enquiry of knowing oneself. The process is of immense help in transforming an individual's negative thoughts and experiences into positive thoughts and feelings. It helps increase one's emotional response, thereby limiting his or her intellectual response to the minimum.

There are many methods for initiating the process of meditation, including ASANAS, by assuming suitable body postures conducive for meditation, breathing (PRANAYAMA), CHAKRA meditation, CHANTing, DANCE YOGA, KINHIN (walking meditation), MANTRA meditation, KUNDALINI meditation, satsang or congregation of the like-minded, VIPASSANA, YANTRA meditation, TRANSCENDENTAL MEDITATION, TRATAKA (object meditation) and ZAZEN. There is a general consensus among the students and scholars of meditation that a GURU plays an important role in initiating and conducting this process.

meditation, the three approaches of (Yoga) There are three approaches to meditation: through developing AWARENESS, through cultivating CONCENTRATION, and through appropriate expression. While awareness implies MINDFULNESS of thoughts, feelings and sensations as they emanate, concentration relates to the mental impact of a sound or MANTRA, diagram or YANTRA while expression could be revealed through a smile or gesture or MUDRA. Like stability and stillness, dance and soft movements are also used in experiencing the effects of meditation. The positive effects of meditation may be attributable to a rise in the levels of MELATONIN in the body.

'Meditation is neither contemplation nor concentration. It is a non-mental, no-mind living. It is to be in contact with the world with no mind in between.'

—Osho

Mediterranean-in-motion See TAI CHI CH'UAN.

Mediterranean diet (Mod.) A modern version of a diet and culinary pattern popular in countries in the Mediterranean basin, particularly Cyprus, Greece, Italy, Portugal, Spain and Turkey. The common features of the diets in these countries are a high consumption of cereals (bread), fruits and vegetables, goat cheese, olive oil and fish; most of the food eaten is rich in flavour. The diet is low in saturated fat, high in mono-unsaturated fat and dietary fibre. Red wine, an important component of the diet, is consumed in moderation, and said to hold the key to the diet's health benefits.

Although the Mediterranean population tends to consume considerable amounts of fat and olive oil, the lower rates of cardiovascular diseases make its critics give credit not only to the diet but also to other factors such as environment, genetics, lifestyle and leisure activities of the people of these regions.

medium (Occ.) A psychic or sensitive person who has the gift or talent for allowing spirits to enter his or her body, to be used as a vehicle for transmitting messages from the 'other' world. In traditional societies, belief in mediums greatly helped contain grief from bereavement, as the bereaved came to terms with a loss which would otherwise create an emotional void. By acknowledging the survival of the human soul even after death, the loss for the bereaved, however great, became bearable.

Mediums are of two types: physical and mental. In a physical medium, the spirit conveys, with the help of audible voices, raps, or materialized figures, information about themselves, their life in the spirit world and a recollection of their earthly life in the past. These are often demonstrated in private séances.

There are three forms of mental mediumship, including CLAIRVOYANCE, when mediums see the spirit, CLAIRAUDIENCE, when mediums hear the spirit, and CLAIRSENTIENCE, when mediums sense the presence of the spirit through its thoughts. Mental phenomena is more often demonstrated in public seances. Trance mediumship is a form of mental mediumship in which the medium is overshadowed by the spirit communicator and allowed to speak directly through the medium. See also, MEDIUMSHIP, PSYCHIC MEDIUM.

mediumship (Occ.) The ancient concept and practice of a person serving as a channel to facilitate communication between spirits (usually dead relatives) and living people. Such communications help people overcome the trauma caused by their loss.

megavitamin therapy (Mod.) The administration of large doses of vitamins, often several times more than what is the recommended dietary allowance (RDA). The method, devised by American Nobel laureate Dr Linus Pauling, is said to have been found beneficial to smokers, heavy drinkers and high-strung people to overcome conditions as diverse as the common cold and cancer. However, according to some nutritionists, there are side effects from the excessive intake of vitamins.

melatonin (Mod.) A hormone secreted at night by the pineal glands in the human brain. This hormone has a myriad possible health benefits and has been described as the most important molecule of the coming century.

It is reported that melatonin helps in regulating the body's circadian rhythm, an internal twenty-four-hour time-keeping system that plays an important role in our sleeping and waking patterns. Melatonin cycles have been found to get disrupted with exposure to excessive light in the night or too little during the day, as do lifestyles associated with jet lag, shift work, study needs and the exposure to low-frequency electromagnetic fields (as is common in household appliances). Sleeplessness and irregular menstrual cycles in women are attributed to such exposure.

Melatonin is also known for its antioxidant properties. Its secretion found to diminish with age. See also, AGEING.

memory (Misc.) The human ability to store, retain, and subsequently retrieve information. Traditional studies of memory relate to philosophy. However, in modern times, memory has grown into a new branch of science, combining cognitive psychology and neuroscience.

Memory is classified into sensory memory, short-term memory and long-term memory. Sensory memory often corresponds to the initial moment when an item was perceived. This basically refers to one's senses and how one remembers the touch, smell, taste, vision or hearing of a person or thing. Short-term memory comes into play when, for instance, one recalls what one had for dinner the previous night. Driving a car is related to long-term memory.

> 'One of the keys to happiness is a bad memory!'
>
> —Rita Mae Brown

> 'I have discovered a sure recipe for memory and wisdom'. 'No, Theuth', replied Thamus, '... Those who acquire it will cease to exercise their memory and will be forgetful.'
>
> —Plato, *Phaedo*

memory recall (New Age) In HYPNOSIS, a method employed for recalling minute details of past events.

Mensendieck method (New Age) A paramedical system for ensuring correct body mechanics, proper posture and appropriate muscle function. Bess Mensendieck (1861–1957), who developed this system, viewed the musculoskeletal system of the body as a remarkable machine with a capacity for adapting itself to perform perfectly the most complex movements. She prescribed movement schemes for correcting the common abuses of the body. She believed that if movements were executed correctly, it would result in a well-functioning body.

There are four major aspects in her prescription: a) proper alignment and balancing of all parts of the body during all activities; b) conscious development of body sense and muscular awareness; c) improvement in relationship between body and mind and conversely, mind and body; and d) active relaxation. The system has been in use in Europe, particularly in Denmark, the Netherlands, Norway and Sweden and is applied in dealing with problems relating to chronic back-pain, occupational stress, post-operative recovery and sports injuries. It demands no equipment, but motivation and perseverance to unlearn faulty postural habits.

mental aura (Occ.) A field of AURA, said to extend for about four to eight inches around one's physical body. Perceivers observe that this aura bears a bright shade of yellow, harbouring thoughts and mental processes. It is said to reflect one's beliefs, concepts and attitudes. It also reflects the constraints that distinguish an individual from others. One's mental conditions and illness or health can be studied by an aura reader.

mentals (Hom.) In HOMOEOPATHY, symptoms relating to the mental state, mood and ideas.

mercurius vivus (Hom.) Also, quicksilver. A remedy in HOMOEOPATHY, used to treat excessive sweat, nausea and body-shaking.

meridians In TRADITIONAL CHINESE MEDICINE, subtle and invisible pathways in the body through which vital energy (QI) flows are referred to as meridians. There are twelve main meridians, of which six are considered YIN and six YANG, besides numerous minor ones. They form a network of energy channels throughout the body, which interconnect various parts, regions, organs, nerves and blood vessels of the body. The entire body system is believed to be interconnected in such a way that energy constantly flows from one meridian to the next, thus circulating through the entire body.

When energy flows freely through the meridians, the body is said to be balanced and healthy. When there is a disruption or blockade, it is manifested as ill-health—physical, mental or emotional. Skilled practitioners are trained to detect stagnant, under-active or over- active flow of qi via palpation of the twelve specific pulses located on the patient's wrists. See also ACUPOINTS, PULSE reading.

meridian shiatsu (Chi.) An ancient method to locate and use MERIDIANS. It helps in assessing the condition of meridians and devising touch applications that assist the energy circulation in the body to maintain good health.

meridian system of healing (Chi.) An approach to healing, focussed on MERIDIANS.

Mesmer, Franz Anton (1734–1815) (Occ.) A Swiss-German physician, who founded the doctrine of ANIMAL MAGNETISM, also known as mesmerism. Mesmer's technique allowed him to produce an abnormal condition resembling sleep in another person. In this state, the mind of the individual remained passive and was subject to the will of the operator. The state of HYPNOSIS was used in healing people. The concept elaborated by Mesmer had been used earlier in the occult art of SHAMANISM.

'It (mesmerism) is a marvellous, valuable gift of God ... by means of which the strong will of a well-meaning person could infuse the vital energy upon a sick one by contact or even without it...'

—Hahnemann

mesomorph One of the three basic body types, characterized by a well-defined muscular body, with a large, prominent bone structure. Other traits typical to the mesomorph are well-defined features of the face, heavy jaw, long and broad face, developed arms and legs with muscled digits of the hand and thick skin.

mesotherapy (New Age) A popular CELLULITE treatment technique which originated in Europe in the mid-twentieth century. It directly targets deep layers of the skin for optimum therapeutic effectiveness. The treatment involves micro-injection of chemicals and vitamins, with an automatic fine-needling device in the fat layer under the skin. The treatment is aimed at reducing subcutaneous fat deposits. See also, OBESITY.

metabolism (Mod.) The rate at which the body is able to burn up its fuel and transform it into energy.

meta fitness (New Age) A modern concept of body-shaping, fitness and weight-loss, without pain and struggle, popularized by Suzy Prudden and Joan Meijer-Hirschland. The application of the power of mental and emotional energies and low-impact exercises to change one's body is the main theme in this regimen. The invigorating exercises prescribed here target every area of the body.

metamorphic technique (New Age) A gentle form of MASSAGE on reflexology ME-

RIDIANS in the legs, hand and head which correspond to the vertebral column. The massage is performed by anyone trained in foot reflexology. No specific healing results are claimed with this technique, but it is said to help the individual's own innate intelligence free deep blocks in the body's energy pattern. The technique was introduced in the 1960s by Robert St. John, a British naturopath.

metaphysics From the Greek *meta*, meaning after, and *phúsis* meaning nature. 1. A branch of philosophy aimed at explaining the nature of the world. 2. A study of being or reality. The subject makes attempts to elucidate the notions by which people understand the world.

metaphysical healing (Occ.) A method of healing, based on the belief that negative mental patterns, when left unchecked, eventually result in physical illness. It is believed that certain common negative thinking habits affect particular areas of the body. For instance, monetary worries are believed to cause lower-back pain. The healing technique therefore aims at reversing negative mental patterns, which cause diseases, into positive patterns to pave the way towards health and well-being. According to this belief, longstanding guilt, resentment, and anger aggravate sickness, while self-love, self-acceptance, and self-worth help in overcoming their negative impact.

miasm (Occ.) From the Greek, for pollution or stain. 1. An energetic concept about ailments, which transcends commonly held knowledge/belief that the causes for a disease can be logically explained. 2. In the religious concept, an inimical and invisible infectious principle, comparable to what is morally understood as sin. 3. A weakness in the VITAL FORCE in an organism.

Susceptibility or hypo-immunity leads to a miasmatic infection. The miasmatic force acts as a threat to the vital force throughout the life of an organism. SAMUEL HAHNEMANN (1755–1843), a German physician and the founder of HOMOEOPATHY, considered miasms one of the fundamental causes of disease and classified them into three categories: psoric, that which is characterized by allergies and chronic skin ailments (other than syphilitic ones); sycotic, characterized by warts and tumors, responsible for many urinary disorders and sexual diseases; and syphilitic, characterized by depression and other psychological disorders, responsible for diseases of blood, bones and nervous system.

'Psora is that most ancient, most universal, most destructive, and yet most misapprehended chronic miasmatic disease which for many thousands of years has disfigured and tortured mankind... and become the mother of all the thousands of incredibly various chronic diseases...'

—Samuel Hahnemann

microcosm–macrocosm (Yoga) A concept distinguishing a 'miniature universe' from the 'great universe'. In Hindu philosophy, the outer world or physical universe is considered to be the macrocosm of the inner world. While the inner world is attributed with qualities of the outer world, it is also considered mystically larger and more complex than the physical universe. It is believed that the inner world of CONSCIOUSNESS precedes the physical form of the outer world. The human body is viewed as a microcosm of divine creation and hence is considered divine.

micro-dermabrasion (Cos.) A popular method of painless and non-invasive EXFOLIATION, in which the top layers of skin are removed by spraying (sandblasting) with ultra-fine, sterile micro-particles of aluminium oxide, diamond or salt crystals. Apart from removing dead skin from the face, this cosmetic treatment is also said to be helpful in dealing with blackheads, minor lines, pores, scaly skin, skin discolouration and whiteheads. This process is said to stimulate collagen production and blood flow in the area of treatment.

mind (Misc.) The collective aspects of one's CONSCIOUSNESS and INTELLECT, as evident through one's perception, imagination, thoughts, emotions and will. The 'higher' intellectual mind, considered the sign of human civilization and dominated by reason and memory, can be distinguished from 'primitive' emotions (e.g., fear, hate, joy and love).

In Indian philosophy, the mind is categorized in to three forms on the basis of three predominant traits (GUNAs): pacific or pure (SATTVA), active (RAJAS) and indolent or impure (TAMAS). These three traits are believed to lead to five types of functioning one can notice in humans: dull and lethargic (mudha), distracted (ksipta), scattered (viksipta), focussed (ekagra) and organized or regulated (niruddha). According to this philosophy, regulated action is a sign of efficiency and excellence.

'For the primitive mind, everything is a miracle, or rather nothing is; and therefore, everything is credible and there's nothing either impossible or absurd.'

—Lucient Levy-Bruhl

'What is mind? No matter. What is matter? Never mind.'

—*Punch* (1855)

mind, the five constituents According to Indian philosophy, the state of mind in a person can be distinguished on the basis of five sets of characteristics as indicated in the following table:

Category	State of mind	Essential features
Conscious mind	wakeful state of consciousness (jagrat chitta)	The normal waking, thinking state of mind as perceived when one wakes up from sleep
Subconscious mind	impression mind (samskara chitta)	Considered as the layer of mind, placed 'beneath' the conscious mind. The subconscious mind is considered responsible for the storage of all the experiences of an organism, irrespective of the fact whether they are consciously remembered or not. It is believed that the subconscious mind holds all impressions from the previous lives of the individual. It is also considered as the centre of all involuntary processes in the body—psychological, physiological or neurological.
Sub-subconscious mind	subliminal mind (vasana chitta)	The portion of the subconscious mind formed by intermingling of two thoughts or experiences of similar intensity, sent into the subconscious mind at different points of time. The sub-subconscious mind is considered a vibration—distinguishable from that in the subconscious mind. It influences the external mind to react to situations in accordance with the nature of vibrations accumulated therein—positive, negative or indifferent.
Superconscious mind	the mind, illuminated with the all-knowing intelligence of the spirit (karana chitta). It is also referred to as turiya, the fourth, as it refers to a mental condition which	In Sanskrit, several terms can be found to refer to the various levels of the superconscious mind: universal state of consciousness (vishvachaitanya), non-dual state of consciousness (advaita chaitanya), spiritual state of consciousness (adhyatma chetana)

lies beyond the three states: wakefulness (jagrut), dream (svapna) and deep sleep (sushupti)

| Sub-superconscious mind | the mental state which functions through the conscious and subconscious states of mind (anukarana chitta). | This is considered a mental state which brings forth clarity, intuition and insight. |

'No one should allow his mind to be a vehicle for others to use; he who does not direct his own mind lacks mastery.'

—Hazrat Janyat Khan

mind, the three phases of the (Yoga) According to the ancient Indian perspective, the mind could be viewed as comprising three aspects as indicated in the following table:

Phase of mind	Role
Instinctive mind (manas chitta)	operating within the sensory and motor organs of the body, as can be perceived in the behaviour of animals and 'uncultured' human beings
Intellectual mind (buddhi chitta)	operates in the faculty of thought and intelligence, as expected in the behaviour of 'cultured' human beings
Superconscious mind (karana chitta)	operates in the strata of creativity, insight intuition, benevolence and spiritual sustenance. It is also the state of unconditional love and reverence to all living and non-living manifestations around one's being. It is considered as the state to be adopted to generate a healthy and sustainable way of life.

mind–body connection (New Age/ Yoga) A concept which acknowledges that psychological and social factors contribute as much towards ailments in organisms as physiological factors. Like the need for cleanliness and hygiene in one's physical surroundings, it is also considered necessary to keep one's mental and emotional faculties uncluttered in order to enjoy good health.

'As it is not proper to cure the eyes without the head, nor the head without the body, so neither is it proper to cure the body without the mind.'

—Socrates

mind–body intervention (Yoga) The procedure adopted for supporting the enhancement of one's mental capacity to induce healing in the body. There are such methods employed, especially in ALTERNATIVE MEDICINE, including ALEXANDER TECHNIQUE, AROMATHERAPY, AUTOSUGGESTION, THERAPY, BACH FLOWER REMEDIES, HATHA YOGA, MEDITATION, SELF-HYPNOSIS, VISUALIZATION and YOGA.

mind energy (Yoga) An ancient concept in Indian philosophy attributes immense power to one's mind, acknowledging its role as a great driving force. It is considered that mind energy has two poles: a thought field (e.g., an idea or a thought) and a form field (e.g., an object or an act). It has three inherent action-qualities (GUNAs): truth or light (SATTVA), desire or passion (RAJAS) and darkness or indifference (TAMAS). Of the three gunas, sattva is regarded as the highest as it brings happiness and wisdom. However, all these three qualities are relevant for tackling life-situations.

'When mental energy is allowed to follow the links of least resistance and to fall into easy channels, it is called weakness.'

—James Allen

mindfulness (New Age) A mental training, aimed at increasing one's awareness to focus on the present moment, without assigning any value judgement whatsoever. Every gesture, word or movement that arises at the moment of observation is welcomed wholeheartedly and accepted with reverence. Mindfulness is not confined only to the realms of thoughts and feelings; even a bodily function otherwise considered irreverent can assume a divinity or glory as one injects awareness into it. Buddhist schools of philosophy refer to 'right awareness' which is considered to pave the way for developing intuition and insight. By cultivating an awareness of incoming and outgoing breath, through constant practice, one can develop 'right awareness'.

'Wherever you go, there you are.'

—John Kabit Zinn

mind power (New Age/Mod./Occ.) The age-old belief that the mind can play a crucial role as the cause of a disease as well as its cure. As every thought is believed to have a counterpart in a word or sound, appropriate tones and words (MANTRA) find their application in healing. AFFIRMATIONS also help in creating self-confidence. See also, AUM.

'A strong positive mental attitude will create more miracles than any wonder drug.'

—Patricia Neal

mineral springs spa (Spa) A SPA located at the source-site of a mineral-rich thermal spring and offering various treatments connected with HYDROPATHY.

minor chakras (Occ./Yoga) The CHAKRAS or energy-centres in the body, usually associated with joints at the knee, elbow and shoulder. In addition to the eight chakra indicated in the following table, there are also other chakras associated with the palms of the hands and the soles of the feet and at the ends of the fingers and toes. Unlike major chakras, which are the spinning vortices, the minor chakras are visualized as spikes of energy exuded from the body. The systems of healing-touch such as PRANIC ENERGY and REIKI apply such rays of energy emanating from these minor chakras to stimulate the process of healing. Given below is the location and number of minor chakras along with their functions.

Location of the minor chakras	Number of the minor chakras	Representing
knee chakras	2	movement
elbow chakras	2	gait and flexibility
thigh chakras	2	stability
shoulder chakra	1	strength
genitalia	1	reproduction

minor pranas (Yoga) The sub-categories of PRANA. There are five minor pranas in the body, each of which is assigned with specific functions, as indicated in the following table:

Minor prana	Role
naga	controls salivation and hiccups
kurma	controls opening of the eyelids and blinking
krkara	causes sneezing and creates the hunger sensation
devadatta	controls sleep and yawning
dhananjaya	pervades the entire body and is said to linger in the body for quite sometime even after the death of an organism

miracle healing (New Age) From the Latin *miraculum*, meaning something wonderful; a general belief, particularly in a religious context, that miracles can cure disease. Miracles are believed to occur with divine intervention.

'There are two ways to live your life. One is as though nothing is a miracle. The other is as though everything is a miracle.'

—Albert Einstein

mitahara (Ind.) An approach to moderation in food intake. Mitahara emphasizes on wholesome SATTVIC FOOD, and the stomach only half-full. A quarter of the stomach should be filled with water and the remaining quarter left for air. According to AYURVEDA, food should be represented by all the six tastes, i.e., astringent, bitter, pungent, salty, sour and sweet. For meditating yogis, the ideal quantity of food is considered no more than what he could hold by cupping each of his hands. Moderation in diet, apart from physical exercise, is generally acknowledged as healthy.

mobile spa (Spa) A spa which can be transported to a client's home, office, or any other preferred location and which offers in the services available in the ordinary spas.

moisturizers (New Age) A complex mixtures of chemical agents specially developed to make the epidermis (external layers of the skin) softer and more pliable. Moisturizers restore the water-content (hydration) and also build a barrier against water-loss. Some moisturizers can, however, cause allergies.

moksha (Ind.) Also, mukti. From the Sanskrit for liberation or release; liberation from the cycle of birth and death. According to Hindu philosophy, it refers to a dissolution of the sense of self, transcending one's sense of CONSCIOUSNESS, of time, space, and causation (KARMA).

monism (Yoga) A metaphysical view, wherein reality is viewed as a unified whole, not as its parts. All divisions are viewed as made of one essence, principle, substance or energy. Monism is distinguished from dualism, which holds that in the ultimate analysis, there are only two kinds of substance (e.g., YIN AND YANG) and pluralism, which holds that reality lies in divisions.

monodiet (New Age) The intake of an exclusive type of food. Usually a particular variety of fruit or its juice or any selected vegetable is eaten for a whole day. The GRAPE diet is a popular monodiet, aimed not just at weight-loss, but detoxification of the body and revitalizing the senses. This restorative diet is also supposed to boost the energy levels in the body. Before undertaking a monodiet, a physician's advice is recommended to rule out underlying ailments.

moon effect The effect of the moon on the human mind and behaviour. According to ancient belief, a full moon is associated with mental illness, even crime and disaster.

Three researchers, Ivan Kelly, James Rotton and Roger Culver (1996), after examining some 100 studies on the effects of a full moon on calamities, including homicide, domestic violence, fertility, suicide and traffic accidents, concluded that there was no scientifically reliable indication of an impact of a full moon. This conclusion was corroborated by Gutiérrez-García and Tusell (1997) who studied 897 suicide deaths in Madrid and found there was no significant relationship between the phases of the moon and suicide rates. However, according to German researchers, Hall, Mittmeyer and Filipp (2000), there was a definite correlation between new and full moons and the amount of alcohol consumed. This was based on their findings that most of those with an excess of 2ml of alcohol per 100 ml of blood in their blood samples were caught driving by the German police during the five-day full-moon cycle.

'A woman is fertile, in accordance with the moon.'

—An ancient Babylonian inscription

moonstone (Gem) A colourless, white, yellow, orange or gray translucent stone with a white or blue sheen, often worn in rings and pendants. The stone reflects light in a distinctive shimmering phenomenon known as adularescence. Moonstone is found in many parts of the world, including Brazil, India, Sri Lanka and Tanzania. Wearing it is believed to control passion.

'Love, hopes and dreams
This moonstone seems
To bring in sun beams!'

—Anon

Moor-mud therapy (New Age) Also, balneo peat therapy, Moor peat bath. The application of Moor mud, an organic, therapy-grade peat from the natural decomposition of hundreds of plants, for hydration of the skin and EXFOLIATION. Moor mud is popular in the spa industry as it contains organic residues of flowers, whole plants and grasses, transformed in nature over thousands of years to form a nourishing mass easily dissolvable in water. It contains amino acids, fulvic acids, humic acids, minerals, vitamins and several trace elements which can easily be absorbed by the human skin and are therefore useful in anti-ageing treatments.

MORA therapy (New Age /Vib.) A form of treatment modality which helps in augmenting the patient's own healing power ('ultra-fine electromagnetic oscillation'). Morell and Rasch, who discovered this method in 1977, named it by using the first syllables of their names. The system is based on the belief that each individual possesses a unique spectrum of ultra-fine electromagnetic oscillations which can be electronically sensed, processed and then used as therapy and that functional disturbances occur whenever the delicate balance is upset by interfering and unnecessary (pathological) oscillations. MORA therapy aims at specifically eliminating these interfering oscillations by using their own 'mirror images' to cancel them out, thus unburdening the body and facilitating natural self-healing.

A patient is treated with a MORA device via a hand and a foot electrode. The patient's own oscillations enter and exit the MORA device via the electrodes and cables in the same way as nerve impulses are conducted into ECG or EEG devices. A MORA device is said to be even able to determine, via a physically active biological filter, which section of an individual's micro-magnetic information spectrum will provide the most beneficial therapy at a given time. The body's debilitated regulatory forces are accordingly strengthened via the optimal amplification of that spectrum.

mother tincture (Hom.) An aqueous or alcoholic extract of the original drug substance used in HOMOEOPATHY. As a source remedy, the mother tincture is further diluted to make the required therapeutic dosage.

motivational enhancement therapy (Mod./New Age) An approach to motivate clients towards identified goals. Emphasis is placed on eliciting from clients self-motivational statements of desire for and commitment to change. It is based on the belief that intrinsic motivation is necessary to bringing about change in a client's behaviour. Though planned and directed by a counsellor, it is largely a client-centred approach. The client sets his or her own goals, though the coordinator may advise in formulating them, often exploring a broader range of life goals. The client is the agent of change, with help from a coordinator.

motivational therapy (Mod./New Age) 1. An approach in which a patient is encouraged to develop a negative view of habits such as substance abuse, along with a desire to change his behaviour. A motivational therapist does not directly advise or argue with the patient, avoiding, rather than contradicting the patient. There is, however, an expression of empathy while motivating the patient. The success of this method is said to be dependent on the quality of the therapist and how far he or she is able to influence the patient in changing his addictive habits. Originally published in the form of a book by Miller and Rollnick (1991), motivational therapy has of late been transformed into a treatment strategy, which includes a variety of approaches, including the removal of guilt from the minds of the clients, adequate emotional support, reassurance and sympathy.

mouna (Yoga) From the Sanskrit word for silence. In the yoga system, remaining silent for a day or two is considered to influence one's behaviour towards others.

moxa (Chi.) From the Japanese *moera*, meaning to burn, and kusa, meaning herb. 1. A herbal preparation made of dried mugwort (*Artemesia vulgaris*), rolled like a cigar. These rolls are burnt on the end of needles and heated in MOXIBUSTION. 2. A cone of cotton-wool or other such combustible material, placed on the skin and ignited in order to produce counter-irritation.

moxibustion (Chi) From the Japanese *mogusa*, meaning herb, and the Latin *bustion*, meaning burning. Also, moxabustion; the use of MOXA for warming

ACU-POINTS. A popular technique in TRADITIONAL CHINESE MEDICINE which aims at restoring the smooth flow of QI in the MERIDIANS and helps overcome diseased conditions in the body.

Moxibustion is of two types: direct moxibustion is a traditional therapeutic technique in which a small, cone-shaped moxa is placed on top of an ACU-POINT and made to burn over the skin. Direct moxibustion may have some undesirable effects such as blisters and burn at the moxibustion site. In an attempt to prevent such skin damage, some acupuncturists use indirect moxibustion in which a medium (e.g., sliced ginger) is placed between the skin and the moxa. Sometimes the burning moxa is also extinguished a little before it reaches the skin.

Mozart effect (Misc.) A concept, which explores the broad applicability of compositions and piano sonatas by Wolfgang Amadeus Mozart (1756–91) on overcoming primary learning difficulties of children. The effect was initially described by Alfred Tomatis, a French physician, after three decades of research in his book *Pourquoi Mozart?* (1991). A paper published by Rauscher and Shaw (1993) endorsed this work by stating that a brief exposure to a Mozart's *Sonata for Two Pianos* in D major K. 448 could produce a temporary increase in spatial reasoning scores, amounting to the equivalent of 8–9 IQ points on the Stanford–Binet IQ scale. However, a paper titled 'Prelude or Requiem for the *Mozart Effect?*', published in 1999 by Chabris and Steele, challenged these findings. Bridget and Cuevas (2000) concluded that when compared to a no-music condition, listening to music by Bach or Mozart for ten minutes produced no effect on subsequent mathematical problem-solving performance. In a reply published in 1999, Rauscher, however, said that it was never claimed by them that Mozart enhanced intelligence; the effect was 'limited to spatial–temporal tasks involving mental imagery and temporal ordering.'

> 'When I am …completely myself …or during the night when I cannot sleep, it is on such occasions that my ideas flow best and most abundantly. Whence and how these come I know not nor can I force them… Nor do I hear in my imagination the parts successively, but I hear them at the same time all together.'
>
> —Wofgang Amadeus Mozart

> 'Mozart is the human incarnation of the divine force of creation.'
>
> —Johann W. von Goethe

mrigi mudra (Yoga) From the Sanskrit *mrigi*, meaning deer; a MUDRA, formed by touching the middle portions of ring and middle fingers with the front part of the thumb. The index and little fingers are kept straight, making a shape that looks like the mouth of a deer. This mudra is recommended for controlling bouts of sneezing. It is also said to stabilize the wandering mind.

mucus (Misc.) A slippery secretion in the lining of various membranes in the body, mucus contains antiseptic enzymes such as lysozymes and immunoglobulins.

Mucus acts variously in the body. It prevents foreign particles from entering the body, especially through the nostrils. It also protects the lungs, and prevents tissues from drying out. Excessive mucus production in the respiratory tract results in common cold. In the digestive system, mucus is used as a lubricant for food particles. A layer of mucus found in the inner walls of the stomach helps in protecting the stomach tissues from being corroded by the acids which aid digestion.

mucusless diet (New Age) A diet regimen developed by Arnold Ehret (1886–1922), who was a patient of a chronic ailment, Bright's disease. The diet prohibits the intake of eggs, fat, meat, milk products and starchy foods, as they form mucus in the body. Relying on the Book of Genesis, he maintained that fruits and green leaf vegetables devoid of starch were capable of cleansing and rebuilding the system and were the ideal food for mankind.

mud bath (Nat.) The application of mud, ash, peat, etc., originally intended to clean the skin before the discovery of soap. It is also a folk remedy in the treatment of arthritis and rheumatism. In the seventies, mud baths became popular to help feel rejuvenated and reduce stress.

A mud bath lasts for ten to fifteen minutes and is followed by a shower.

mud pack (Nat.) The application of mineral-rich mud to clean the skin surface and stimulate circulation.

mudra (Occ.) Also, finger-lock. A symbolic gesture, made with the hands and fingers, known for their use in conveying emotions and ideas. Considered sacred, such hand positions are said to be related to the energy flow in the body.

Mudra is commonly employed while doing ASANA. Each mudra is believed to play a specific role in developing specific attitudes in humans. For example, Indian religious icons assume ABHAYA MUDRA, executed with outward-facing open palms, believed to dispel fear from the devotee's mind and help develop an attitude of fearlessness. The hands and fingers are not always used in executing a mudra. The KHECHARI MUDRA, for instance, is done with the tongue.

Mudras in yoga are also said to be symbolic of MANTRA. Assuming the right body and hand gesture, along with the appropriate mental attitude, is considered synergetic to all practises of YOGA, including ASANA, BANDHA and PRANAYAMA. It is also believed to help achieve harmony and equilibrium of the mind and body. The ancient Indian treatises on yoga, *Gheranda Samhita, Hathayoga Pradipika* and *Shiva Samhita* identified about twenty-five different stances, including the widely practised ANJALI MUDRA, ASVINI MUDRA, DHYANA MUDRA, JALANDHARA MUDRA, JNANA MUDRA, KHECHARI MUDRA, SAMBHAVI MUDRA, and VIPARITA KARANI.

'Be obscure clearly!'

—E.B. White

mukha bhastrika (Ind.) A cleansing method in AYURVEDA, using the process of hyper-ventilation. Practising mukha bhastrika is believed to help in cleansing the lungs and reduce toxic accumulation therein.

mukhabhyanga (Ind.) A face massage offered in AYURVEDA to keep away wrinkles. While relaxing the face muscles, this massage is also said to stimulate the lymph flow, thereby promoting rejuvenation.

mukhadhavanam (Ind.) Also, mukhavasam. A traditional Indian mouthwash, with aromatic herbs and spices.

mulabandha (Yoga) One of the three BANDHAS or 'energy locks', said to be useful in the prevention and cure of mind-related illnesses.

muladhara (Yoga) Also, first chakra; root chakra. One of the seven major CHAKRAS, situated at the base of the spine, in the gonads, sacrum or ovaries. The chakra represents memory, sexual and survival instincts and is considered the foundation of existence. The primal energy in the human body, KUNDALINI, is believed to lie coiled and asleep, like a serpent, in this chakra. Through intense concentration, it is believed that the dormant energy can be aroused, to be further lifted through a series of CHAKRAS in the body. On reaching its final destination in the crown chakra (SAHASRARA), the union of the KUNDALINI with Lord Shiva, residing there, is believed to occur. TANTRISM considers this union of KUNDALINI with Shiva as the ultimate goal in worship.

multani mitti A mineral-rich, bacteriostatic clay with moisturizing effect, originating in Multan, the north-western region of the Indian subcontinent. Milk and rice bran added to this clay has been used from ancient times to improve the skin. It also helps in drawing out the toxins from the skin. Taken internally, it is believed to decrease the absorption of harmful substances. Arthritic pain caused by inflammation is also said to be reduced when treated with multani mitti. It also reduces the pain associated with burns and insect-bites. Multani mitti is used with various other ingredients, depending on the skin conditions:

Skin condition	Traditional method employed for application
Vata type	a paste of multani mitti in yoghurt, GHEE (clarified butter) and besan (chick pea flour)
Pitta type	a paste of multani mitti with rose water and besan

Kapha type a paste of multani mitti with neem leaves, apple cider, MUNG DAL flour, lemon juice and honey.

multiverse (New Age) A set of several universes; concept that humans coexist with an infinite number of baby universes.

mung dal (Ind.) *Phaseolus mungo.* Also, balatang, green gram, mongo bean, mungo. Extensively used in Indian cuisine, the sprouted bean is a good source of vitamin B. It is also used, boiled or raw, in poultices.

murchha (Yoga) Also, murchha kumbhaka. A form of PRANAYAMA, in which exhalation is done slowly. During retention of breath, JALANDHARA BANDHA is done by pressing the chin against the chest until one feels as if one is going to faint. By making the mind senseless, murchha is said to create a sense of joy.

mushti mudra (Occ.) A MUDRA formed by bending the fingers and touching the ring finger with the thumb. This mudra is believed to activate the liver and stomach.

> 'Music is your own experience, your thoughts, your wisdom. If you don't live it, it won't come out of your horn.'
> —Charlie Parker

> 'Music washes away from the soul the dust of everyday life'.
> —Red Auerbach

music of Cluny The medieval abbey in southern France, where chants and hymns were used to heal the sick and assist the dying.

> 'The singer alone does not make a song/ One man opens his throat to sing/The other sings in his mind.'
> —Rabindranath Tagore

music therapy (New Age) The therapeutic application of melodies, rhythms or Indian ragas as complementary medicine.

Music therapy finds its application in areas relating to interpersonal and social development, developing motor skills, self-awareness and cognitive development. The overall impact of different genres of music is summarized in the following table:

Musical genre	Overall impact on the listener
Gregorian chants, based on rhythms involved in natural breathing	Creation of a sense of a relaxed spaciousness and hence can be recommended for stress-reduction and meditation.
Slower baroque music (Bach, Handel, Vivaldi, Corelli)	Creation of a sense of stability, order, predictability and safety and hence can be useful in creating a mentally stimulating environment for study/work.
Classical music (Haydn, Mozart)	Creation of a sense of clarity, elegance and transparency and hence can be recommended for improvement of concentration and memory.
Romantic music (Schubert, Schumann, Tchaikovsky, Chopin, Liszt)	Creation of a sense of individualism, nationalism or mysticism. Feelings of compassion, love and sympathy could be enhanced.
Impressionist music (Debussy, Faure, Ravel), based on free-flowing musical moods and impressions	Evocation of dream-like images.
African heritage music	Creation of a sense of deep joy and sadness, wit and irony and

(jazz, the blues, Dixieland, soul, calypso, reggae)	affirmation of humanity. Can be uplifting and inspiring.
South American music (salsa, rhumba, maranga, macarena)	Creation of a sense of liveliness and movement.
Big-band, pop and top-40 and country-western	Creation of a sense of well-being. Can inspire light and moderate movements.
Rock music (Elvis Presley, the Rolling Stones, Michael Jackson)	Creation of a sense of active movement, tension and pain-relief, can stir the passions.
Ambient, attitudinal or New Age music with no dominant rhythms (Seven Halpern, Brian Eno)	Elongation of the sense of space and time. Can induce a state of relaxed alertness.
Heavy metal, punk, rap, hip hop, grunge	Can excite the nervous system, leading to dynamic behaviour and self-expression.
Religious and sacred music including shamanic drumming, church hymns, gospel music and spirituals	Creation of a sense of being grounded in the moment, leading to feelings of deep peace and spiritual awareness. Can be analgesic.

'The power of music to integrate and cure ....is quite fundamental. [It is the] profoundest non-chemical medication.'

—Oliver Sacks

'Mustard is highly useful for vitiated conditions of kapha and vata.'

—*Guna Patham*

mustard (Chi./Eur./Ind./Heb./Isl./Jap.) *Brassica nigra*. Also, asuri (Ayurveda), black mustard, gaai choi (Chinese), hardal shahor (Hebrew), hukkyeoja (Korean), khardal (Arabic), kuro-garashi (Japanese). An annual weedy plant cultivated for its seeds, which are commonly used as a spice. The plant is believed to be native to the southern Mediterranean region of Europe and has been cultivated for thousands of years. Ground seeds of the plant mixed with honey are widely used in eastern Europe as a cough suppressant.

myofascial release therapy (New Age) A form of MASSAGE, in which fascia or connective tissue that surrounds the musculatures in the body is manipulated so as to achieve greater flexibility. In this treatment, gentle pressure is applied to fascia for restoring the normal alignment and functions. According to John Barnes who developed this system in the late 1960s, myofascial release can be helpful in the treatment of neck and back pain, headaches and sports injuries which recur.

na (Ind.) Tamil, for tongue, the examination of tongue. One of the eight diagnostic procedures in SIDDHA MEDICINE. According to this system, the colour of a person's tongue can reveal which DOSHA is vitiated. Thus, if the tongue is somewhat black or blue, it indicates VATA-aggravation; if reddish, PITTA and if whitish, it can be due to KAPHA.

nada (Yoga) Sanskrit for intonation or vibration. 1. The acoustic sound, familiar to one's faculty for hearing 2. Spontaneous psychic sounds heard during advanced stages of MEDITATION. 3. Flow of consciousness, as sound is linked to one's CONSCIOUSNESS.

Nada is considered the non-material source of all matter. It is consciousness to the whole elements, that which manifests in the form of nature and which is bliss and non-dual. It is visualized as a 'thread-like' link between the material and spiritual divide in humans. In the Indian tradition sound-consciousness (dhwani) is divided into four forms as shown in the table:

Stages of sound-consciousness (dhwani)	Characteristics	Probable BRAIN WAVE pattern
PARA (the highest; the farthest). It is also referred to in various ways: rava shabda, the inner silence, the root sound, the sound potential, etc.	a transcendental state of consciousness (TURIYA). The purest and subtlest form of sound, which forms the basis of the universe. A conceptually non-vibratory condition of sound, beyond the reaches of the human senses or understanding. Because of the extreme subtleties in its frequencies, it often gets equated with silence. It represents a highly active phase of silence and it should not be linked with the inertia associated with silence; it is a silence, pregnant with sound, awaiting delivery. Para is uncaused, *sui generis* and 'unstruck' (ANAHATA), and has no limits and boundaries. The Upanishads refers to it by its symbol, AUM and its nature is visualized in the form of light (jyoti) and silence.	delta
PASHYANTI (literally, that which can be seen/visualized)	a subconscious visual state, which harbours the power of WILL (iccha shakti). A sound heard in a dream-	delta/theta

like state of consciousness. It also refers to the finest impulse of speech, intuitively connected to the object of contemplation. The seat of pashyanti is traced to the navel . region in the human body (manipura).

MADHYAMA (the intermediate)	a dream-like state (svapna) in which the subtle and psychic body (sukshma sharira) operates. It refers to finer and unexpressed sound as in whispers. It is more a mental speech, which could be distinguished from its audible counterpart. The seat of madhyama is the heart region (anahata). This state is associated with the power of knowledge (jnana shakti).	theta/alpha
VAIKHARI	a wakeful state (jagrat) in which the physical body takes charge of the control of human life, which includes its very survival and preservation. Vaikhari exhibits the power of action (kriya shakti). Audible sound frequencies (either music or noise or neutral sound waves) produced by striking two objects (AHATA) are heard through the ears and responded to physically, psychologically or neurologically in a positive, negative or neutral manner by the human beings. As the physical body operates in the wakeful state, vaikhari is manifested only in the physical realm of one's existence.	beta

'While uttering a word, the speaking desire inspires our mind to speak, after referring to the intellect.'

—Panini

nada anusandhana (Yoga) Sanskrit, for the cultivation of one's inner sound. A common practice in the system of YOGA, which makes use of sounds emanating from CHANTS and PRAYER uttered with or without the accompaniment of a musical instrument.

'Audible utterance of 'aum' produces a sense of sacredness. However, real understanding of aum is obtained only by hearing it internally and then becoming one with it in all creation.'

—Yogananda

nadabrahma meditation (Yoga) Also, Osho nadabrahma meditation. From the Sanskrit nada, meaning sound, and Brahma, meaning the omnipresent, omniscient and omnipotent God. A sitting method of MEDITATION in which an inner balance between the mind and body is sought to be created through humming and/ or hand movements. As humming creates the sensation of vibration in the body, one visualizes a hollow tube or vessel in front being filled up by such humming. It is also visualized that long after the humming is over, the vessel in front echoes the humming vibrations back to the practitioner, who then becomes just a listener to those vibrations created by him or her. While doing this meditation, one is advised to have an empty stomach and as soon as the meditation is over, the body and mind should remain inactive for at least fifteen minutes, preferably in SHAVASANA.

> 'So in nadabrahma, remember this: let the body and mind be totally together, but remember that you have to become a witness. Get out of them, easily, slowly, from the back door, with no fight, with no struggle. They are drinking—you get out, and watch from the outside...'
>
> —Osho

nadanadi shakti (Yoga) Sanskrit for the energy current of sound. AUM, evolving as PARA NADA, as experienced in deep MEDITATION. It is both visualized and heard vibrating through the nerves as a constant high-pitched hum. The quality of this sound is said to be comparable with the drone of a swarm of bees or from a tanpura.

nada upasana (Yoga) Also, nadopasana. Listening to the inner sounds as a part of contemplative exercise during MEDITATION.

> 'Yoga has a sly, clever way of short-circuiting the mental patterns that cause anxiety.'
>
> —Baxter Bell

nada yoga (Yoga) An integral part of the system of YOGA, which aims at developing a spontaneous interaction between sound and CONSCIOUSNESS. According to this system, a NADA can be grossly physical (AHATA) or sublimated to the subtle realms of the MIND. It refers to the methodologies of penetration of NADA into the deeper (higher) layers of one's consciousness, which enable one to experience the finer aspects of oneself. Thus nada yoga can pave the way for SELF-REALIZATION. This ancient system rests on the belief that the universe is a projection of mere sound vibrations and that different sound frequencies recall different levels of one's existence/experience: physical, energetic (pranic), mental, supra-mental and blissful (ananda)—from gross to subtle as one starts transcending or expanding one's awareness.

> 'In the beginning was the word and the word was with God and the word was God.'
>
> —The Bible

nadi (Ind.) From the Sanskrit word, meaning flow or channel. A subtle energy channel, through which the vital energy (PRANA) flows in the human body. According to AYURVEDA, there are 72,000 such channels, which interconnect CHAKRAs. Of these, three are major nadis: IDA, a 'lunar' channel of feminine physical–emotional energy and which flows downwards, ending on the left side of the body; PINGALA, a 'solar' channel of masculine, mental–intellectual energy and which flows upwards, ending on the right side of the body; SUSHUMNA, the major channel which passes through the spinal column from the root-chakra (MULADHARA) at the base to the crown chakra (SAHASRARA) at the top of the body and through which the KUNDALINI energy, lying dormant in the root chakra, rises when awakened and reaches SAHASRARA, the crown chakra.

Apart from carrying the vital energy in their network, nadis are believed to perform an extra-sensory function, particularly in instinctive responses of the body. According to some authors, ida and pingala represent the two hemispheres in the brain, right and left, respectively. Both these nadis are activated through the practise of alternate breathing through the left and right nostrils as in PRANAYAMA. As a consequence, both the hemispheres get stimulated and activated so as to perform their tasks in harmony with each other.

nadi shuddhi (Yoga) Also, nadi shodhana. Purification of NADIs, the energy channels in the body. The purification is done through breathing exercises, e.g., breath control and breathing with alternate nostrils. It is considered helpful for concentration (DHARANA) as well as meditation (DHYANA).

nadi sutra kriya (Yoga/Vib.) A procedure for touching MARMA POINTS, aimed at balancing energy levels in the body.

nadi swedana (Ind.) Localized, penetrating stream administered specifically to the joints and the spinal areas during the practise of PURVAKARMA.

nail diagnosis (Misc.) The examination of nails as a diagnostic tool. The following table indicates the inferences generally drawn after observing specific nail characteristics:

Condition of nails	General inference
Shell-shaped nails	neurosis, irritable, nagging and fault-finding nature
Narrow and long nails	nervousness, personality with stifled emotions
Short nails	argumentative or contradicting nature
Thin, short and brittle nails with ridges but without a moon	hyperactivity of endocrines
Shiny, long and narrow nail with a large moon	hypothyroidism
Transverse, white lines on the nail	feverishness, possibility of coronary heart diseases, toxicity
Transverse grooves on the nail	malnutrition or long-standing illness
Transverse ridges on the nail	feverishness, nervous shock, nutritional deficiencies
Longitudinal ridges on the nail	chronic skin ailments, rheumatic conditions, hyperthyroidism
Longitudinal lines on the nails	digestive problems or calcium deficiencies
Concave nails on the outer surface	nutritional deficiencies, skin ailments, syphilis, mental imbalance
Convex nails	chronic heart diseases, cirrhosis of liver, lung tumour, tuberculosis
White spots on the nail	anxiety, exhaustion and nervousness
Rough, dry and crooked nails with a tendency to break easily	predominance of VATA
Tender and soft, pinkish nails which can be bent	predominance of PITTA
Strong and shiny nails	predominance of KAPHA
Yellow nails	jaundice or delicate liver conditions
Blue nails	cardiac problems
Redness of nails	high content of red blood cells

nama sankirtana (Yoga) Group singing and chanting, usually in praise of God. The repetition of certain phrases, usually the names of God, set to simple musical notes and often accompanied by movement or dance, is believed to help people balance stress caused by materialistic living.

namah Shivaya (Occ.) Sanskrit, for homage to Lord Shiva. Also, the five-syllabled mantra, panchakshara. Each of the five syllables of the Hindu MANTRA of Shaivism represents the following:

Syllable of mantra	Esoteric meaning of the syllable	Body part represented by the syllable
Na	veiling grace of the Lord	legs
Ma	the world	abdomen
Shi	Shiva	shoulders
Va	revealing grace of the Lord	mouth
ya	soul	eyes

'Homage to the source of health and to the source of delight. Homage to the maker of health and to the maker of delight. Homage to the Auspicious, and to the more Auspicious.'

—*Krishna Yajur Veda*

naprapathy (New Age) 1. A gentle MASSAGE of the connective tissues and ligaments which encase the spinal columns, aimed at restoring optimal flow of energy within the body. 2. A holistic approach to locomotor disorders which include the study on corrective changes to be made with regard to DIET, lifestyle, movement and NUTRITION.

naraka Sanskrit, for an abode of darkness; literally, pertaining to man. 1. Hell. 2. The seven lower worlds as represented by the LOWER CHAKRAS, corresponding to the state of one's CONSCIOUSNESS.

The region of NARAKA	Corresponding (lower) chakra	Characteristics assigned to the parts of the human anatomy
Put or childless	atala, the wheel of the bottomless region	fear and lust assigned to the hips
Avichi or joyless	vitala, the wheel of negativities	anger, assigned to thighs
Samhata or abandoned	sutala, of 'great depths'	jealousy, assigned to the knees
Tamisra or darkness	talatala, the wheel of the lower region	confusion, assigned to calves
Rijisha or expelled	rasatala, the wheel of subterranean	selfishness, attributed to ankles
Kudmala or leprous	mahatala, the wheel of the great lower region	lack of conscience, attributed to feet
Kakola or black poison	patala, the wheel of the fallen	malice, attributed to soles

nasagra mudra (Occ.) A MUDRA practised during PRANAYAMA. The mudra is said to facilitate inhalation and exhalation through specific nostrils.

nasal irrigation (Yoga) Also, saline irrigation. Regularly flooding the nasal cavity with warm saline to remove the dirt and toxins accumulated. It is a personal hygiene practice, which traces its origin to NETI, and is commonly practised in Asia, the Middle East and eastern Europe. The practice helps promote good nasal health by eliminating the symptoms of chronic sinusitis: cough, halitosis, headaches, etc. It opens the sinus drainage passages up, enabling them to perform their normal function. The isotonic solution is prepared from non-iodized salt (quarter to half teaspoon), dissolved in lukewarm water, equal to or slightly warmer than the body temperature (one cup).

nasya karma (Ind.) Also, nasya. One of the PANCHAKARMAS, mentioned in AYURVEDA, in which drug is administered through the nostrils. Nasya karma is often performed in connection with diseases related to the head region. It clears clogged channels in the head region, facilitating the movement of PRANA energy, prevents premature graying of hair and keeps it from falling. It is also a preventive treatment for various KAPHA-related problems, including migraine, sinusitis, catarrh and bronchitis, and is said to be useful in mitigating ailments including cervical spondilitis, headaches, facial paralysis, mental disorders and Parkinson's. It is also believed to defer age-related disorders.

The following are the methods commonly in use in nasya karma.

Method of nasya	Administration of drug	Physical conditions addressed	Mental conditions addressed
Pradhamana or virechana	blowing dry powdered drug (e.g., brahmi) into	for the alleviation of KAPHA disorders (e.g., common cold,	attachment, greed and lust

	the nose with the help of a tube	drowsiness, epilepsy, headache, hoarseness of voice)	
Bruhan or nutrition nasya	introducing drops of GHEE, oils, salt, milk, etc., medicated with herbs (e.g., ashwagandha, shatavari, etc.) into the nose	for the alleviation of VATA disorders (e.g., dizziness, dry sinuses, heaviness of eye-lids, loss of sense of smell, migraine, nervous disorders, stiffness in the neck)	anxiety, fear, feelings of emptiness and negative approach
Shaman or sedative nasya	teas, decoctions or oils containing prescribed herbs	mainly PITTA disorders such as conjunctivitis, ringing sensation in the ears, thinning of hair, etc.	anxiety, impatience, irritability
Navana or decoction nasya	combination of oil and decoction of prescribed herbs	used in VATA–PITTA or KAPHA–PITTA disorders	hysteria
Marshya nasya	ghee or oil is used in the preparation of nasal drops	cataract, diseases of ears, eyes, nose, mouth or head	mental tension and negative thinking
Pratimarshya or daily oil nasya	simply dipping a clean (little) finger in ghee or oil and massaging the nasal passage every day	cataract, diseases of ears, eyes, nose, mouth or head	mental tension and negative thinking

Nataraj meditation (Occ.) Also, dancing meditation. An active movement-based MEDITATION, about an hour long, with special music effects. The idea is that the division between the dancer and dance blurs so that the dancer, who is the centre of the ego, is lost in dance.

Nataraj meditation is performed in three stages.

Stage	Duration (in minutes)	Procedure
first	40	eyes are closed, one is completely absorbed in the process of dance and oblivious to surroundings. One remains just a witness.
second	20	eyes are closed as one lies down, remaining motionless, silent and calm.
third	05	one dances in joy, celebrating life.

> Develop river-like generosity, sun-like bounty and earth-like hospitality.'
> —Shaykh Muinuddin Chishti

natrum muriaticum (Hom.) Also, common salt. A remedy in HOMOEOPATHY, used in the treatment of conditions that cause excessive thirst and craving for salty foods.

natural healing (Nat.) An approach to healing, based on the notion that the body can take care of itself and get cured naturally, with little or no external aid.

natural hygiene (Nat.) A variation of NATURE CURE. The procedures for hygiene relate to procedures including BATHS, ENEMA, FASTING and FOOD THERAPY.

natural urges, suppression of (Ind.) According to Charaka, the author of

CHARAKA SAMHITA, natural urges relating to urine, faeces, flatus, semen, vomiting, sneezing, eructation, yawning, hunger, thirst, tears and sleep, and breathing, caused by over-exertion, should never be suppressed, as their prolonged suppression leads to ill-health, both physical and psychological.

naturally occurring hypnosis (New Age) A heightened state of suggestibility as may occur naturally, as in daydreaming.

nature cure (Nat.) The progenitor of NATUROPATHY. The system is based on the assumption that diseases are caused by violations of laws of nature and that true healing involves a return to nature.

naturology (New Age) 1. A method of healing which comprises several approaches, including ACUPRESSURE, HERBS, HOMOEOPATHY, IRIDOLOGY, NATURAL HYGIENE and NATUROPATHY. 2. A study of the dietary, intellectual and spiritual health benefits derived from nature.

naturopathic obstetrics (Nat./New Age) A system of childbirth in a non-hospital setting. Prenatal and postnatal care using modern diagnostic techniques are however made available to the clients.

naturopathy (Nat.) Also, naturopathic medicine. A term coined by Benedict Lust, a nineteenth-century researcher, to denote a host of measures which contribute towards healing of body and mind. The three fundamental tenets that govern the system are: a) the body cures itself and every treatment should be therefore aimed at self-healing rather than being a symptomatic cure. b) symptoms in diseases are a result of the elimination of toxins from the body and hence should not be suppressed through medication; and c) any intervention to cure should be gentle and non-violent and take into account the physical, mental, emotional, spiritual and social aspects. ACUPUNCTURE, DIET, FASTING, HERBAL MEDICINE, HOMOEOPATHY, HYDROTHERAPY and MASSAGE are some widely employed natural methods.

> 'Never does Nature say one thing and Wisdom another.'
>
> —Juvenal

nauli (Yoga) One of the six major KRIYAS. A physical exercise in which the abdominal muscles are churned with the help of rectus muscle. Considerable negative pressure inside the abdominal cavity, developed through this practice is said to be of great value in keeping the body system clean and healthy.

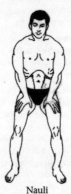

Nauli

navana nasya (Ind.) Also, 'decoction' nasya. A type of NASYA, in which drops of medicated oils and decoctions are instilled inside the nose to fight various VATA–PITTA and KAPHA–PITTA disorders.

navarakizhi (Ind.) Also, njavarakizhi, pindasweda. A MASSAGE performed with small linen bundles and a packet of navara rice cooked with herbs and cow milk. By massaging (or softly pressing the body) with such hot packets, the patient is made to sweat profusely. Navarakizhi is used to treat arthritis, rheumatism and neurological disorders.

necromancy (Grk.) From the Greek *nekros*, meaning dead, and *manteia*, meaning divination. A form of DIVINATION in which the practitioner seeks to summon the spirits of the dead to predict the future. Necromancy was popular among the peoples of ancient Babylonia, Chaldea, Greece and Persia.

needle acupuncture (Chi.) A form of ACUPUNCTURE in which needles are inserted into the skin. In ancient China, nine different types of needles were used. The most commonly used needle now is the filiform (threadlike) needle, made of stainless steel. Other types of needles are also used, including three-edged needles, plum-blossom needles or seven-star needles, intradermal needles and press needles.

Most needles used today are pre-sterilized and disposable, of different lengths and gauges. They may also be made of silver or gold. Acupuncture needles are left in from a few seconds to thirty minutes, depending on the nature of the treatment.

needle sprays (Spa) Fine jets of hot or cold water splashed softly on the body through minute apertures, to produce an invigorating effect.

neem (Ind.) *Azadirachta indica.* Also, Indian lilac, margosa, nimba (Skr.), vembu (Tam.). The flowers, leaves, bark, root, fruit, seed and oil of this tree have been known for over 4,000 years in India for their medicinal value, particularly in the treatment of infections. Its leaves, bark, twigs and the oil extracted from the seeds exhibit antimicrobial activity and are applied on boils and swellings. They are also used as an effective pesticide to protect food grain from insects. The oil is applied on arthritic joint swellings, the twigs are used to clean the teeth and gums, an extract of the bark and twigs are used to treat fevers and nausea, the leaves are used to aid digestion and stimulate the liver. Infusions of the leaves are also used to treat lung conditions and to decrease levels of glucose in the blood of diabetics. In AYURVEDA, the seed oil is used to cure leprosy.

> 'Nimba, a great medicine and a blood-purifier.'
>
> —Priya Nighantu

neem hakim 1. A herbalist 2. A quack.

negative-ion therapy (Mod.) The use of negatively charged air particles to prevent or cure diseases. Negative-ion therapy artificially introduces negative ions by the use of special apparatus to treat allergies, hay fever and respiratory conditions.

Nei Ching (Chi.) The oldest writing on ACUPUNCTURE, attributed to Huang Ti, who ruled China around 2600 BC. It contains details about specific ACUPOINTS and also refers to sedation points which reduce overactive energy.

nephomancy (Occ.) A type of DIVINATION based on the observation and interpretation of clouds—their colours, shapes and positioning in the sky.

Historically, the Celtic Druids made extensive use of nephomancy. In recent times, ever-changing cloud formations are observed as a form of MEDITATION.

neti (Ind./Yoga) One of the six major KRIYAS, used for cleansing the nose. See also, NASAL IRRIGATION.

netra basti (Ind.) Also netratharpan tharpanam. The application of medicinal preparations such as medicated ghee on closed eyelids, as a nourishment for the eyes and also to treat conjunctivitis, burning, vision problems and glaucoma. It is also helpful in easing tension in dry or tired 'computer eyes'. In the southern-style of netratharpana, a small dam-like structure is constructed with the paste of flour of black gram around each eye and medicated ghee is poured in, with the eyes closed. The ghee is kept in for about an hour, before it is washed off. This treatment is said to be helpful in overcoming eye-strain. It is also believed to improve vision in the long run.

network spinal analysis (New Age) A system of chiropractic as developed in 1983 by Donald M. Epstein, and based on the premise that a maladjustment of the spinal cord, nerves and vertebrae can cause mechanical tension in the body.

neural therapy (Vib.) A system of VIBRATIONAL MEDICINE, as developed in Germany in the early part of the twentieth century by physicians Ferdinand and Walter Huneke. It was believed that injections of local anesthetics into areas of 'energy' disturbance ('interference fields') could relieve pain, immobility, and dysfunction. Neural therapy treatments thus involves injections in scars, glands, trigger points, ACUPOINTS and the sites of old fractures or past infections.

neuro-biological explanation of emotion in human beings (Mod.) According to recent understanding of neurobiological processes, whether human emotion is considered pleasant or unpleasant is processed in the limbic system of the mammalian brain and manifests as, either in isolation or in combination, non-verbally expressed feelings such as anger, consent, cooperation, diffidence, determination, authority, disagreement, disgust, dislike, embarrassment, fear, happiness, hate, interest, irritability, liking, love, sadness, shame, surprise, and uncertainty. In emotions, it is found that neuro-chemicals, such as dopamine, noradrenalin and serotonin, either step up or step down the brain's activity level and is manifest in body movements, gestures and postures. Innate (or primary) emotions, such as fear, are said to depend on limbic system circuitry, with the amygdala and anterior cingulate gyrus the key players. Like smell, emotions are either pleasant or unpleasant, and rarely neutral and like odours, feelings defy logic.

neuromuscular techniques (New Age) The techniques of MASSAGE, employed with a view to normalizing the neuro-muscular component in all dysfunctions. Some popular techniques in use are muscle energy techniques, PNF, strain-counterstrain, TRIGGER POINT, skin rolling and stretching.

New Age (New Age) A cultural movement or lifestyle, which became popular in the 1980s and 1990s, characterized by a quasi-religious set of beliefs and philosophies, encompassing a wide variety of concepts including animal rights, astrology, environmentalism, ESP, herbalism, meditation, mysticism, naturalism, nuclear freeze, the occult, parapsychology, planetary awareness, reincarnation, spiritualism and being vegan. An implicit commitment to complementary medicine and its pseudo-scientific applications is concurrent in this movement.

Nichiren Buddhism (Jap.) A Japanese religious concept and practice named after its founder, Nichiren Daishonin (1222–82), which lays emphasis on healthy lifestyle practices. The main ritual in Nichiren Buddhism is chanting the MANTRA *Nam Myoho Renge Kyo* which is Japanese for 'I devote my life to the law (Lotus Sutra) itself'. Chanters repeat this mantra to enter into deeper levels of consciousness. Followers also recite some sections of the Lotus Sutra as part of their daily practice. The chant is performed in front of a scroll called the Gohonzon. Chanting is usually performed for about thirty minutes at night and in the morning and is believed to bring about changes in a person's life. Nichiren Buddhists firmly believe that everyone can change his or her destiny and bring about the effects they desire, which include recovery from illness.

> [To chant] means to activate the innate Buddha-nature. The activated Buddha-nature… will then appear in one's life as enforced life power and wisdom to live like a 'lotus flower in a muddy pond.'
>
> —Yukio Matsudo

nine-star ki (Chi.) Also, jiu xin, kyu sei. A system of DIRECTIONOLOGY and futuristic astrology which developed from the ancient Chinese astrology. The system is said to help in determining the best directions for travel and also the directions to be avoided on specific dates. Nine-star ki is considered as much more than astrology, as its astrological implications are connected to astronomical realities (precession cycle) and the biological condition and health of individuals.

niram (Sid.) Tamil, for colour. One of the eight kinds of diagnoses stipulated in SIDDHA MEDICINE.

Nirmala Devi, Mataji (Yoga) (b.1923)An Indian spiritual leader who discovered a process of en masse SELF-REALIZATION called SAHAJA YOGA.

nirmanu (Yoga) A method to purify NADIs, the subtle-energy channels. The nadis are purified by two processes, viz., samanu and nirmanu. The samanu is done by a mental cleansing which includes chanting of BIJA MANTRA. The nirmanu is done by physical cleansing as in SHATKARMAS.

niruha basti (Ayur.) Colonic irrigation with a herbal decoction, aimed at removing toxins and wastes.

niyama (Yoga) A set of behaviour components, advocated in PATANJALI'S YOGA SUTRAS. These include purity (shaucha; in the traditional codification, this item is listed under YAMAS), contentment (santosha), austerities (tapas; this includes the endurance of opposites such as hunger and thirst, heat and cold, and standing and sitting), self-study or the study of scriptures (svadhyaya) and self-surrender (ishvaraprani dhana; devotion to God). The observances are said to be of help in settling one's mental as well as emotional conflicts, thereby imparting calmness and tranquility to the practitioner's mind.

In numerous other ancient religious scriptures, ten niyamas are identified, including:

hri: remorse, being modest and showing shame for misdeeds;

santosha: contentment, being satisfied with the resources at hand and therefore not desiring more;

dana: giving, without thought of reward;

astiya: faith, believing firmly in the teacher, the teachings and the path to enlightenment;

ishvarapuja: worship of the Lord, the cultivation of devotion through daily worship and meditation, the return to the source;

siddhanta shravana: scriptural listening, studying the teachings and listening to the wise of one's lineage;

mati: cognition, developing a spiritual will and intellect with the guru's guidance;

vrata: sacred vows, fulfilling religious vows, rules and observances faithfully;

japa: recitation, chanting mantras daily;

tapas or austerity: the endurance of opposites such as heat and cold.

> 'What is moral is what you feel good after.'
> —Ernest Hemingway

noble silence (Yoga) The state of silence of body, speech and mind, as required to be observed by practitioners of VIPASSANA.

non-contact therapeutic touch (Vib.) In VIBRATIONAL MEDICINE, a non-physical 'touch' which could be therapeutic; in holistic medicine, several methods such as DISTANT HEALING, PRAYER, REIKI and SPIRITUAL HEALING.

non-directive hypnotherapy (New Age) In HYPNOTHERAPY, a technique in which a patient is asked to go back in time to locate the root of the problem at hand.

non-local consciousness, theory of (Mod.) A viewpoint of the universe being an ocean of energy, in which the constructs of time appear illusory. The theory, propounded by physicist David Bohm, refers to the objective world as the 'explicate order' which is actually infused with and animated by the ocean of energy or 'implicate order'. Both these realms are considered parts of an enormous flowing whole, reflecting the intense coherence within a group, called 'holo movement' by Bohm.

non naceral (Nat.) A fundamental principle in NATURAL HEALING that maintains that the cure should never be worse than the ailment.

Norse magic (Occ.) Magical traditions of western Europe, aimed at promoting physical, mental and spiritual health.

nose bath (Nat.) Sniffing up the saline water to counter chronic catarrh.

nosode (Hom.) In HOMOEOPATHY, a remedy made from a diseased source. For example, the nosode tuberculinum is made from tissues infected with tuberculosis.

nuad bo rarn (New Age) A system of BODYWORK, wherein the practitioner manipulates the subject into HATHA YOGA-like postures. It is aimed at facilitating the smooth flow of vital energy within the body. According to this system, there are 84,000 energy channels (*sen*) in the human body, of which ten can be considered vital.

numerology (Num./Occ.) In OCCULTISM, the study of meanings in numbers. Originally developed by the Chaldeans, Egyptians and Indians, the system is based on the understanding that the entire universe is mathematically constructed and that all events and situations can be explained in terms of numbers. Each number is attributed with certain characteristics, such as strong or weak, male or female, harmony or disharmony. Numerologists use the definitions in numbers in conjunction with each other to find the meaning of whatever they may be describing. Some of the characteristics of numbers as assigned in NEW AGE/Wiccan writings and in Chaldean system are summarized in the following table:

Numbers	Characteristics represented	Associated colour
0	void, infinity	black
1	activation, new beginnings, consciousness	brown
	Astrology: Sun	

2	duality, duality of physical/non-physical, duality of male/female astrology: Moon	red
3	creative, perfection in creation astrology: Jupiter	orange
4	earth-based, ego, physical solidity astrology: Uranus	yellow
5	healing, growth astrology: Mercury	green
6	new ideas, vision astrology: Venus	blue
7	perfection, creation, completion, physicality astrology: Neptune	violet
8	infinity, eternity, non-physical/angelic astrology: Saturn	silver
9	end of a cycle astrology: Mars and Pluto	gold

The numbers following the cycle of 9 in base 10 are also assigned characteristics as, for example, number 10 indicates God or the Wheel of Fortune; 11 refers to new beginnings and courage; 13, maturity or totality; 18, good luck; 144, all possibilities.

> 'I sought the Truth in measures and numbers,' said Confucius, 'but after five years I still had not found it.'
>
> —Chuara Tzu (290 bc)

numerological divination (Num./Occ.) The use of name and date of birth of an individual to analyze and define his or her characteristics and propensities. Each alphabet in English is assigned a unique number: A, J, S=1 B, K, T=2 C, L, U=3 D, M, V=4 E, N, W=5 F, O, X=6 G, P, Y=7 H, Q, Z=8 I, R=9. There, however, appears no scientific verification on the inferences arrived at by this method.

numerology in science (Occ.) Scientific theories whose primary inspiration appears to be mathematical rather than scientific. In the scientific community, numerology is often regarded as a PSEUDO-SCIENCE, but some mathematical physicists continue to be fascinated by the coincidences numerology infers.

nurse, the four qualifications of (Ind.) According to AYURVEDA, a nurse must be endowed with cleanliness, compassion, knowledge, and skill.

nut grass (Ind.) *Cyperus rotundus* The bulbous root of nut grass is considered a cure for disorders of the stomach and irritation of the bowels. Native physicians administer it in the treatment of biliousness, diarrhoea, dysentery, erysipelas, excessive thirst, fevers, leprosy, nausea, ophthalmia, pruritis, sores, ulcers and urinary concretions. The root extract of nut grass is reported to possess tranquillizing properties. Recent research has confirmed its analgesic, antipyretic and muscle relaxant properties.

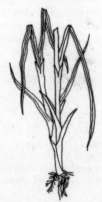

Nut grass

nutmeg (Ind.) *Myristica* spp. This tropical evergreen tree is indigenous to south-east Asia and Australasia. Nutmeg and mace are the two spices derived from the fruits of the tree. Nutmeg is composed of 10 per cent essential oils, contains myristicine, which controls stomach gases, and has a euphoric effect, though it is toxic. Arabs use nutmeg oil to combat itching, freckles and bad breath.

nutraceuticals (New Age) A food or naturally occurring food supplement held to be proactive or beneficial for health. Foods fortified with herbs, vitamins, minerals, or other supplements to promote health and prevent disease come under this category.

nutrition (Mod.) The study of balanced diets, aimed at promoting health. The ability of the body to grow or heal is attributed to the type of nutrition available to or preferred by an organism. Lack of proper nutrition is also considered to have a definitive impact on the process of thinking.

nutritional therapy (New Age) A complementary therapy which prescribes nutrition for the maintenance of good health. It also prescribes food and food supplements to trigger the process of natural healing. Fish oil, iron, vitamin C and folic acid are some commonly prescribed dietary supplements.

The differences between the role of a dietician and that of the nutritional therapist are:

Role of a dietician	Role of a nutritional therapist
A dietician is concerned with the Recommended Amounts of Nutrients (RDA), based on the amounts of various nutrients needed to prevent diseases such as beriberi and scurvy and as prescribed by the governmental regulations in this regard.	A nutritional therapist works on optimum amounts of nutrients which, according to him or her, are required to minimize health problems and promote optimum health.
A dietician is not concerned with the role of nutrition in certain health problems, such as asthma, menstrual disorders or sinusitis.	A nutritional therapist not only encourages the body to heal itself through his prescriptions, but also helps in prevention of such health problems by prescribing preventive nutrition.
A dietician is concerned with a specific disease of the client on which it focusses.	A nutritional therapist approaches in a holistic manner, rather than aiming at just prescribing a symptomatic treatment.
A dietician is generally not concerned with environmental issues.	A nutritional therapist takes into account environmental factors while prescribing the treatment.
A dietician uses scientific research.	A nutritional therapist may even use research from peer-reviewed, experiential sources, such as folk remedies and practices which have not been scientifically endorsed.

nux vomica (Hom.) A remedy in HOMOEOPATHY, nux vomica is used in the treatment of symptoms caused by the excessive consumption of food, alcohol or caffeine.

nyasa (Occ.) 'Placing'. In TANTRISM, a practice of infusing various body parts with life force or PRANA. The method adopted can be through touching or through DISTANT HEALING, by intensely concentrating on the affected parts of the client. Systems like PRANIC HEALING and REIKI reflect this idea.

O

obesity (Misc.) A body condition with excessive body weight. When food (energy) intake exceeds energy expenditure for metabolic activities, fat cells serve as energy reservoirs, helped, to a smaller extent, by muscle and liver cells. BODY MASS INDEX (BMI) is the scientific measure of obesity. A BMI of more than 30 indicates obesity. Another method to determine obesity is to assess the percentage of body fat by weighing a person under water or by taking into account the subcutaneous fat layer in a pinch of skin, through what is called the 'skinfold test'.

Men with over 25 per cent body fat and women with over 30 per cent are considered obese. According to recent clinical studies, obesity can be correlated with several ailments, more particularly with cardiovascular diseases and diabetes mellitus type 2.

The treatment for obesity hinges on an energy-limited diet, coupled with increased physical movement and exercises.

obsession (Occ.) 1. In WICCA, the unwanted interference or influence of a more powerful and aggressive spirit on a weaker one. The influence alters the normal behaviour of the subject. 2. Recurring intrusive, distressing or frightening thoughts or ideas. Traditionally, most mind-related problems are believed to be related to obsession.

occultism (Occ.) 1. A phenomenon involving the supernatural, or that which is mysterious and beyond ordinary knowledge. 2. Hidden aspects of nature.

occupational therapy (Mod.) A health-care profession, concerned with restoring useful and near-normal physical functionality following disabling accidents or sickness. Pioneered by American social worker Eleanor Clarke Slagle (1871–1942). This patient-specific therapy assists people with mental or physical disabilities to achieve the highest level of functioning as possible in their day-to-day work, play and leisure.

Occupational therapists, trained in the study of human growth and development with special reference to the physical, affective, cognitive and environmental components of injury and illness, study and identify imbalances in the patient's life and designs activities to overcome them. He aims at improving the patient's ability to perform daily activities, recommending adaptation, adaptive equipment and usage training, assessing performance skills and suggesting treatments, and also guiding caregivers and family members.

odic force (Occ.) Also, od, odyle. A hypothetical VITAL FORCE, a 'new imponderable force allied to electricity, heat and magnetism', expounded by a chemist, Baron Carl von Reichenbach (1788–1869). Akin to PRANA and CHI, odic force was also considered to permeate all living things, viz., plants, animals and humans, though no connection between BREATH and odic force was seen by its propounders. It is considered visible in complete darkness as coloured AURAS, surrounding all living things. It is also considered to have a positive and negative flux and a light and a dark side and that individuals could 'emanate' it from their hands, mouth or forehead.

It was also once thought that the concept of odic force would explain the phenomenon of HYPNOTISM. It was also believed that CRYSTALs stored odic force within themselves as 'crystalod'.

Through his concept of odic force, Von Reichenbach (1788–1869) strove to develop a scientific footing for the otherwise only perceived universal life force. He maintained that only psychically sensitive and psycho-kinetically adept individuals could visualize aura, but the concept was not generally accepted.

ojakshaya (Ind.) 1. Depletion of OJAS, the vigour and vitality in a living organism. 2. A diseased condition; loss of vigour and vitality.

ojas (Ind.) The 'essence' of tissues, the most refined product of DHATU metabolism that sustains life, by controlling the body's immune mechanism. It also refers to the semen, strength, vigour or vitality of an organism.

> '[ojas] is the last remaining conclusive material of the sapta dhatu.'
>
> —Sushruta

ojakshaya (Ind.) Depletion in OJAS has a deleterious effect in an organism, causing, for example, fear, confusion, uncertainty, anxiety and lack of interest or enthusiasm. Too much ojas, produces over-enthusiasm, assertiveness and aroused senses.

Oki-do (New Age) Also, Master Oki's way; The Okido way of living is an approach to healing, as developed by Masahiro Oki (1921–85), an expert in eastern healing methods, borrowing methods from oriental systems of healing such as CHINESE CHIKWANDO, MACROBIOTICS, TAI CHI, TIBETAN MEDICINE, YOGA and ZEN.

Okinawan karate (Jap.) Blending the traditional Okinawan martial arts with Chinese Kenpo, this modern karate was evolved in the nineteenth century. Karate develops core strength and confidence. It also improves aerobic and flexibility conditioning.

omen (Occ.) A sign, related to a future event. The falling of comets, occurrence of eclipses, dreams, howling of dogs and the hooting of owls can be interpreted to augur either good or bad fortunes.

oneiromancy (Occ.) The interpretation and assigning of meanings to dreams. In ancient Egypt and Greece, dreaming was considered a supernatural communication of a future event, good or bad. The ancient Greeks constructed temples (asclepieions) exclusively for sick people, wherein cures were believed to be affected through dreams.

Dream interpretation was a part of PSYCHO-ANALYSIS in the late-nineteenth century. The manifest part of a dream, i.e, what is perceived, was analyzed to reveal the latent meaning thereof. Sigmund Freud's *The Interpretation of Dreams* is considered a seminal works on dream interpretation. According to Calvin S. Hall (1953), dreaming is a cognitive process; a dream is simply a thought or sequence of thought that occurs during sleep and dream images are visual representations based on personal experiences.

one-pointedness of mind (Yoga) Also, ekagra. In YOGA, a state of mind wherein the mind is firmly concentrated on an object with no distraction or diversion whatsoever. Disciplined practitioners are expected to achieve such a state of mind through practice of YOGA. The real practice of yoga meditation is said to begin when the mind has attained the ability to be one-pointed.

onion (Chi./Hom./Ind.) *Allium cepa*. The onion has had a long history of medicinal use. The ancient Egyptians used onions as a diuretic, to induce perspiration, prevent colds, soothe sciatica, relieve pains and address cardiovascular problems.

onsen (Jap.) A Japanese hot spring for bathing in the traditional Japanese method. Water is changed once a day, after all the family members have bathed.

opal (Grem.) A gem, said to be endowed with the ability to cure eye ailments.

operant conditioning techniques In PSYCHOLOGY, a host of measures devised for modifying behaviour patterns such as alcoholism, aggression, delinquency, drug addiction, eating disorders and smoking. Operant conditioning is reported to have successfully provided workable avenues for many problems related to human behaviour.

optimum health balance (Mod./New Age) Also, OHB. An approach to healing, as developed by Charles Benham, an English kinesiologist, based on the principles of AP-PLIED KINESIOLOGY. This system integrates muscle response with the use of a series of cards containing what is called vibrational symbols. Each of over 400 such symbols represent a wide range of conditions in the body—structural, chemical, emotional and electro-magnetic—and facilitate what is called an 'in-depth conversation' with one's body. The purpose of OHB is to raise the patient's energy to the highest level possible at the time of balance, by using universal energy and healing icons.

oracle (Eur.) A method of DIVINATION, in which spirits or gods are consulted through a human medium.

orange-colour therapy (Occ.) Considered the colour of joy, the therapeutic value of orange colour is believed to be a useful supplement in the treatment of afflictions such as hyperthyroidism and kidney-stones. In certain parts of India, orange clothes are worn by new mothers in the belief that they will increase lactation. See COLOUR THERAPY.

oregano (Chi./Eur./Isl./Jap.) *Origanum vulgare*. Also, anrar (Arab.), hana hakka (Jap.), kekik (Turk.), ngou lahk gong (Chi.), pot marjoram. Derived from the Greek *oros*, meaning mountain, and *ganos*, meaning joy. A plant native to Europe, the Mediterranean region and southern and central Asia, Oregano is an important culinary herb, particularly so in Greek and Italian cuisines. The herb is known for its high antioxidant activity, due to its phenolic acid and flavonoid contents. It is also found to show antimicrobial activity against many foodborne pathogens.

> 'Joy of the mountains.'
>
> —Translation of the word 'oregano',
> from its Greek root

organic food (Misc.) Food, produced exclusively by using organic manure and without the use of chemicals, either as fertilizer, growth hormones or pesticides. Food with certain chemical contents have been shown to be carcinogenic; there is thus a growing awareness of the health benefits of organic food.

organization of the living system, theory of A hypothesis, propounded by Chilean neuro-scientist Humberto Maturana (b.1928), that living systems are organized in a closed, circular process that allows for evolutionary change in the way the circularity is maintained, but not for the circularity itself. They are cognitive systems, and living is a process of cognition. This statement is valid for all organisms, with or without nervous systems. According to him, reality is a consensual communal construction which appears to 'objectively' exist.

> 'When one puts objectivity in parenthesis, all views, all verses in the multiverse are equally valid. Understanding this, you lose the passion for changing the other. One of the results is that you look apathetic to people. Now, those who do not live with objectivity in parentheses have a passion for changing the other. So they have this passion and you do not. For example, at the university where I work, people may say, 'Humberto is not really interested in anything,' because I don't have the passion in the same sense that the person that has objectivity without parentheses. And I think that this is the main difficulty. To other people you may seem too tolerant. However, if the others also put objectivity in parentheses, you discover that disagreements can only be solved by entering a domain of co-inspiration, in which things are done together because the participants want to do them. With objectivity in parentheses, it is easy to do things together because one is not denying the other in the process of doing them.'
>
> —Humberto Maturana

orgone energy (Occ.) 1. The subtle, trans-dimensional energy matter of the universe. 2. The biological energy, expressed as emotions, sexual feelings, etc., in life-processes. According to Austrian–American psychiatrist and psychoanalyst Wilhelm Reich (1897–1957), who coined the term orgone energy, all life processes, including emotions and sexual feelings, constitute its expression. Any deficiency of this energy, according to him, results in mental illness. Reich was of the view that the illness could be overcome by intense love or sexual orgasm which, according to him, represented the 'fullest expression'. The concept, similar to the concepts of ANIMAL MAGNETISM, ODIC FORCE, ETHER, LIFE FORCE, PRANA and QI, faced severe criticism from the scientific community. See also, ORGONE THERAPY.

orgone therapy (Occ.) A holistic approach for treating emotional and physical ailments by eliminating or reducing barriers that block the natural expressions of emotion and healthy sexual feelings. See also, ORGONE ENERGY.

Oriental herbal medicine (New Age) The use of HERBs as medicine as widely prevalent particularly in China, India, Korea and Tibet.

Oriental medicine (New Age) A general term used to include systems of healing which originated in the East, including ACUPUNCTURE, AYURVEDA, SHIATSU and YOGA. These systems were influenced by oriental religious beliefs and philosophical outlook.

Oriental massage (New Age) A system of MASSAGE, in which care is taken to apply knowledge relating to the psychic channels in the body, viz., MERIDIANs and NADIs. Oriental massage can be applied to parts of the body or successively to the whole body, to heal injury, relieve psychological stress, manage pain and improve circulation.

original sensitizing event (Occ.) Also, initial sensitizing event. In HYPNOSIS, a term frequently used to describe memories that are replayed in the imagination in a manner that may influence our behavior and/or attitudes.

ortho-bionomy (Occ.) Greek, for the correct application of the laws of life; a gentle technique of MASSAGE, touch, dialogue and movement education as developed in 1976 by Arthur Lincoln Pauls, a British osteopath and a black belt in judo. The technique is referred to as 'the most homoeopathic' of BODYWORK, since homoeopathy moves towards the direction that the illness takes and uses its own energy to overcome it. It is also somewhat akin to the way a martial artist

uses his opponent's energy to defeat him. In ortho-bionomy, a client is placed in a comfortable position that helps alleviate the pain, then works from there to release it. The approach has been used in the treatment of arthritis, imbalanced posture, muscle pain and spasms.

orthodox medicine The conventional system of medicine. See also, ALLOPATHY.

orthomolecular medicine (New Age) An approach to health based on the notion that many diseases and abnormalities results from chemical imbalances in the body and can be prevented or cured by achieving optimal levels of chemicals such as AMINO ACIDs, ANTIOXIDANTs, dietary minerals, VITAMINs, etc., from various natural sources. The orthomolecular field is based on research in biochemistry, medicine, nutrition and pharmaceuticals, combined with the clinical trials. See also, MEGAVITAMIN THERAPY.

orthomolecular psychiatry (New Age) The use of ORTHOMOLECULAR MEDICINE to treat psychiatric problems. It is believed in this system that specific dietary supplements and measures may be effective in treating mental illness. Specific techniques commonly employed include individual biochemical workup, dietary measures, juice fasting, nutritional supplements, etc. Megadoses of vitamins, for example, are administered in the treatment of AGEING, alcoholism, drug addiction, anxiety, autism, depression and hyperactivity. The system has been in vogue since 1950s when psychiatric physician-biochemists Abram Hoffer and Humphrey Osmond came to work as pioneers.

osteopathy (Mod.) An approach to healing founded on the assumption that any skeletal deformation could interfere with normal functions of the nerves and blood-vessels, causing most diseases. Osteopaths adopt a holistic approach as the philosophy requires addressing the whole person.

osteoporosis (Misc.) Literally, porous bones. A progressive disease in which bones become fragile and weak. The disease most commonly affects post-menopausal women.

ouija (Occ.) Also, planchette, spirit board, talking board. A board and a pointer used for

DIVINATION. Sometimes, the finger of the participant is placed on the planchette containing numbers, letters or symbols so as to spell out the communications from the world of spirits.

The ouija board has been known since the time of the Roman emperors. It was also in popular use in China and Greece long before the Christian era. According to some parapsychologists, ouija is a useful tool to tap into the subconscious. Some criticize it as it may tinker with potentially mischievous occult forces or spirits.

outer healing (Occ.) A system of healing, aimed at detoxification and rebuilding through techniques such as BODYWORK, BREATHWORK, DIET, FENG SHUI, HERBS and LYMPHATIC THERAPY.

out-of-body experience (Occ.) An experience in which one has the sensation of floating outside one's body. Sometimes, one experiences looking at one's own body from a place outside it. Some people are said to have experienced this phenomenon when in danger or near-death experiences, or in dream-like states. Some are said to have induced such a state during MEDITATION. An explanation often suggested is that CONSCIOUSNESS is a separate entity from the body and can exist without the support of the latter. It is also believed that the disembodied consciousness can see, hear, feel, taste or smell.

oxygen facial (Cos.) A SPA treatment which uses oxygen and other nutrients, applied or sprayed onto the face. The treatment, aimed at relaxing and rejuvenating the body, is said to reduce signs of AGEING, such as wrinkles on the face. The deep-cleansing effect of the facial, followed by the application of pure oxygen, also improves the tone, texture and elasticity of the skin.

oxygen therapy (Mod.) The application of oxygen in the treatment of certain lung diseases such as emphysema and sarcoidosis which affect the lung function so severely that supplemental oxygen is needed to continue one's normal bodily function.

pachak pitta (Ind.) A form of PITTA, located between the pancreas and the stomach, pachak pitta consists of pancreatic juices, acids and enzymes which aid in digestion of food.

The others of the five forms of pitta are RANJAK PITTA, SADHAK PITTA, ALOCHAK PITTA, and BHARAJAK PITTA. Ayurveda identifies the characteristics of pitta as hot, moving, pungent, sharp, and sour. The aggravation of pitta is normally a consequence of lifestyles and eating habits, including the intake of acidic, hot, oily or spicy food and exposure to the sun. The habitual intake of alcohol, coffee, tea or tobacco also contribute towards creating disorders due to pitta-aggravation.

pada hastasana (Ind.) An ASANA in which one bends forward at the hips while exhaling. Regular practise of this asana is believed to be useful in the prevention of constipation. It also takes care of unnecessary fat accumulation, particularly around

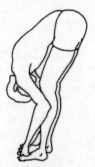

Pada hastasana

the waist. It is also believed to impart flexibility to the spine.

padabhyanga (Ind.) A technique of MASSAGE, restricted to the feet, believed to contain key energy centres of the body. The massage, done with herb-soaked oils, includes a circular massage on the ankle joint, stripping massage to the Achilles, squeezing the heel, pressing and massaging the foot at three planes (i.e., plantar, medial and lateral planes), circular and stripping massage on plantar side, circular massage on each toe and massaging the full legs in two strokes. As circulation improves with this massage, the entire body relaxes. It may also help in the prevention of problems on the legs and feet, including varicose veins, soreness and swellings. The massage usually takes about sixty minutes.

padma mudra (Ind.) A MUDRA formed by gently hollowing the palm, separating and slightly bending the fingers as if holding a round object, 'such as an egg, a bud, a hole of a snake, a fruit or a female breast'. This mudra is said to be helpful in strengthening the nerves.

padmasana (Ind.) Also, lotus asana; from the Sanskrit padma, meaning lotus, and asana, meaning body posture. This ASANA is ideal for undertaking all types of KRIYAS and MEDITATION. This asana, which imparts a pyramidal shape to the body, is considered to help in efficient energy management within the body as a person enters into the stage of SAMADHI. Its most celebrated role is of imparting equilibrium to body, mind and spirit.

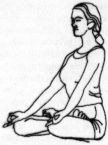

Padmasana

pain (Misc.) A complex experience consisting of a bodily response to a noxious stimulus. This is further followed by an affective or emotional response to that event. Though most pain is associated with tissue damage or hurt and has a physiological origin, some pain experience could emanate from one's mind as well.

> 'Nothing is permanent in this wicked world—not even our troubles.'
> —Charlie Chaplin

pain relief theories (Mod.) There are two important theories which attempt to offer an explanation of analgesic and pain-control action. The first theory, called the gate theory of pain, was postulated by Patrick Wall and Robert Melzack in the second half of the twentieth century. It asserts the existence of gates (filters) in the spinal cord that can either increase or decrease the transmission of pain signals within the nervous system. The second explanation is based on the existence of pain-relieving substances such as endorphins and enkephalins in the central nervous sytem and in other parts of the human body.

pakwashaya gata basti (Ind.) The injection of medicated liquids through the anus and rectum into the colon, as practised in PANCHA KARMA.

palmistry (Occ.) A method of DIVINATION and character-reading by interpreting the lines and bumps on the palm. Palmists are believed to be able to locate the type of illness an individual may be prone to by studying his or her temperament and behaviour characteristics.

palpable Perceptible by touch. In ancient systems, touch was considered an important diagnostic method for examining patients. See also MASSAGE; TOUCH THERAPY.

palpation The act of feeling with one's hands. A common method of diagnosis performed by health professionals, viz., acupuncturists, chiropractors, herbalists, osteopaths and physicians. Palpation is useful in examining oedema, besides abdominal and thoracic conditions.

palpatometry The measurement of the intensity of pressure that does not cause pain.

palpatopercussion (Mod.) A method of diagnosis in which PALPATION is combined with percussion.

Pamula Narasimhiah (Ind.) A popular distant healer who ostensibly helped several snakebite victims through a technique involving CHANTS. Narasimhiah was, in the early-twentieth century, a railway stationmaster at Narasaraopet, a railway station in south India. The victims' families would send telegrams of the incidence of snake bites to the railway station. On receipt of these telegrams, the stationmaster would bathe and chant a set of MANTRAS which was believed to cure the victim from poisoning. A delay in the receipt of telegrams would be attributed to the cause of death.

panchabhuta See FIVE ELEMENTS.

Panchadashanga Yoga (Ind.) Also, fifteen-limbed yoga. An ancient system of YOGA, according to which a serious student of yoga has to take into account the following fifteen aspects to derive maximum benefits: discipline (YAMA), restraint (NIYAMA), sacrifice (tyaga), silence (mauna), right place (desha), right time (kala), posture (ASANA), root-lock (mulabandha), equilibrium (deha samya), stable vision (dhrik sthiti), control of PRANA (prana samrodha), sensory inhibition (PRATYAHARA), concentration (DHARANA), meditation of the self (atma-DHYANA) and ecstasy (SAMADHI).

panchadosha See FIVE BLEMISHES.

panchagavya (Ind.) Five valuable products obtained from the cow, venerated by Hindus, viz., milk, sour milk or yoghurt, ghee or clarified butter, urine (GOMUTRA) and dung. Hindus recognized the anti-microbial properties of its waste products which were employed variously in daily chores.

panchakarma (Ind.) Detoxification procedure. An ancient holistic healing approach in AYURVEDA, aimed at cleansing, detoxifying and rejuvenating one's body, mind and consciousness. The technique involves five interventions, including emesis (VAMANA), purgation (VIRECHANA), enema (BASTI), blood-letting (RAKTAMOKSHANA) and nasal administration of medicines (NASYA).

panchaklesha (Ind.) FIVE PSYCHO-PHYSI-OLOGICAL AFFLICTIONS.

panchamakara (Occ.) FIVE Ms. According to its critics, panchamakara represents a perverted expression of truth and is a travesty of original practises in YOGA. However, its proponents insist on its esoteric meaning, which can be interpreted as the following: destroy the ego, control the flesh, drink the wine of divine-intoxication, unite with the Universal Consciousness or Shiva. According to Shrii Shrii Anandamurti, a spiritual master, the esoteric meaning of panchamakara can be explained as shown in the table:

makara	plain meaning	latent sense
madya	wine	amrita, the divine nectar
mamsa	meat	control of speech
matsya	fish	IDA and PINGALA NADI which are controlled through BREATH
MUDRA	hand gestures	maintaining SATSANG, the spiritual company in life
maithuna	sexual intercourse	union of the individual consiousness with Universal Consciousness (SHIVA); it also refers to the state of SAMADHI

panchakshara (Occ.) FIVE SYLLABLES. The VIBRATIONs emanating from the syllables are used for spiritual elevation in YOGA practices. See also, NADA YOGA. See also FIVE SYL-LABLED INCANTATION.

panchakritya (Occ.) See FIVE FUNCTIONS OF THE DIVINE FORCE.

panchanga (Ind.) From the Sanskrit pancha, meaning five, and anga, meaning limb; an almanac. The five 'limbs' on which the system of casting horoscopes is based are the day of a week (vara), the lunar day (tithi), the lunar mansion (nakshatra), the half-tithi (karana) and time-division (yoga).

panchendriya vardhana (Ind.) A special concoction of oil used in NASYA, meant to stimulate or sharpen the five senses.

paneurhythmy (New Age) Dancing in circles, as in the dances of tribals. A healing process, it is believed to quicken one's attunement with one's nature. Attuning one's subtle energies through rhythmic movements has been practised from ancient times.

pankaj mudra (Occ.) Sanskrit, for lotus gesture. This MUDRA is formed by arranging all ten fingers so that they form the shape of a lotus bud. The thumb and fingers touch each other, and the fingers touch their counterparts on the other hand, tip to tip. This mudra is believed to lead to an interchange of vital energy, resulting in harmony. It is often recommended to be performed in PADMASANA, initially for ten to fifteen minutes with full concentration, in a calm and quiet atmosphere. The practise of this mudra is belived to bring about an enhancement of the beauty of body and mind, gentle behaviour, strong nerves, a healthy spine and blood and the cure of abdominal tumours. The mudra is also said to facilitate detachment, when performed during MEDI-TATION.

papa (Ind.) From the Sanskrit for sin. 1. Wrongful action. 2. Demerit earned through wrong-doing. Papa includes all kinds of wrong-doing, from the simplest infraction to the most heinous crime. Each act of papa is believed to carry its karmic consequence, karmaphala, or fruit of action.

Papa is visualized in the inner conscious aura as a sticky, dark substance and is believed by some to be the reason for the physical and mental suffering of people. However, Hindus believe that through penance (prayaschitta), austerity (tapas) and good deeds (sukritya), disease, depression and loneliness caused by papa can be overcome.

parafango (Spa.) Also, paraffin mud treatment. A volcanic mud, blended with paraffin wax. This mixture is traditionally used in alleviating aches and pains in the body, particularly as caused by arthritis and rheumatism. The combination is believed to make available the benefits of both mud and paraffin treatments.

paraffin bath (Spa.) A healing procedure employing hot paraffin for relief from afflictions including arthritis, rheumatism, sciatica, sprains and stiff joints.

paraffin treatment (Spa.) The application of molten paraffin over the skin to trap heat, absorb toxins and induce relaxation.

paraffin wrap (Spa.) The process of removing dead skin cells with hot oil and Japanese dry brushing techniques. An emollient wax is subsequently applied to the entire body for an intense hydrating treatment.

paraherbalism (Occ.) The administration of herbs based not on the basis of its pharmaceutical content but on other considerations such as ASTROLOGY, AROMATHERAPY, DOCTRINE OF SIGNATURE, superstition and hearsay. Such practices often undermine the credibility of the efficacy of herbs as effective medicine.

paranormal healing (Occ.) The healing concepts and practices, which lie outside the dimensions of normal scientific enquiry. Examples are ABSENT HEALING, BACH FLOWER REMEDIES, CHANNELLING, FAITH HEALING, MAGNET THERAPY, PSYCHIC HEALING, PSYCHIC SURGERY, PSYCHOSYNTHESIS, SPIRIT HEALING, SPIRIT SURGERY and THERAPEUTIC TOUCH.

Paracelsus (1493–1541) (Occ.) A Swiss occultic medical reformer who introduced a new medical philosophy, which combined the esoteric occult teachings of the KABBALAH with science.

parsley (Am.Ind./Chi./Eur./Isl.) *Petroselinum crispum*. baqdounis (Arab.), paseri (Jap.), xiang cai (Chi.) A herb common in Middle Eastern, European, and American cuisines. In Chinese and German traditions, parsley tea is believed to help control high blood pressure. Cherokee Indians use it as a tonic to strengthen the bladder. It is also used as an emmenagogue and a breath-freshener.

'Parsley enhances mental alertness, and affects the immune system.'

—Nutritionist Adam Blackman

parts therapy (Occ.) Also, ego states therapy. A form of HYPNOTHERAPY and a complex hypnotic method in which the therapist talks with various 'parts' of the mind, such as the INNER CHILD and INNER ADULT.

paschat karma (Ind.) A dietetic regimen which is to be followed after a client undergoes the treatment of PANCHAKARMA. Cold food and drink and foods, which may cause indigestion, should generally be avoided after panchakarma treatment.

paschimottasana (Yoga) An ASANA considered conducive for the proper functioning of the heart, reproductive and digestive organs, particularly the bladder, kidneys, liver and the pancreas.

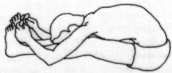

Paschimottasana

past-life regression (Occ.) Also, past-life therapy. 1. A system of PSYCHOTHERAPY involving HYPNOTISM, based on the belief that traumatic experiences that people have could have links with their past births. 2. A regression into a real or imagined past life.

patala (Occ.) From the Sanskrit for fallen or sinful region. 1. A realm referred to as black poison (kakola) in which misguided spirits thrive. 2. One of the seven lower worlds as represented by the LOWER CHAKRAS in the body, corresponding to the state of one's CONSCIOUSNESS. See also NARAKA.

patala yantra (Ind.) An apparatus used in the preparation of medicinal oils in India.

Patanjali (Yoga) A sage who codified the system of YOGA in circa 200 BC with his monumental contribution on ASHTANGA YOGA, RAJA YOGA and SIDDHA YOGA. Considered one of the six classical philosophical systems (darshanas) of the Hinduism, the Yoga Sutras of Patanjali consist of 200 aphorisms which still constitute the foremost text on the esoteric system of Yoga.

patient, the four essential qualities of (Ind.) According to AYURVEDA, recollection, adherence to physician's instructions, courage and the ability to describe his problems constitute the four qualities of an ideal patient.

Pealeism (Occ.) A concept of healing as propounded by Norman Vincent Peale (1898–1993), an American thinker. It is based on the belief that a positive thought properly employed is the most powerful force in the improvement of one's health. Positive thinking, avoidance of negativism, fervent prayer and visualization of goals together, according to him, make the difference.

PEMS (Occ.) An acronym for the four bodies recognized in the system of holistic healing: physical, emotional, mental and spiritual.

pendular diagnosis (Occ.) A diagnostic method, which is common in several systems of VIBRATIONAL MEDICINE. A pendulum suspended from a fixed point is used for DOWSING. See also, IRADIESTHE SIA.

percussion (Mod.) A method of clinical examination; tapping on a body surface to determine if the tissue below is healthy or pathological, and the nature of the underlying structure. While the presence of a solid mass underneath the surface would produce a dull sound, hollow and air-containing structures would produce a sonorous sound. The four types of percussion sounds heard are sonorous, hypersonorous, relatively dull and a completely dull sound.

perfector therapy (Mod.) A method of healing which employs a low current of electricity. As the low current sends tiny electrical impulses to the muscles, they get stimulated. In turn, this leads to toxin removal and lymph drainage which results in a toned and firmer skin and muscles.

performance massage (Mod.) A MASSAGE aimed at improving the athletic performance of sportspersons and those who have active lifestyles and to prevent or reduce injuries. The massage incorporates stretches, which help increase flexibility.

perilla (Am. Ind./Chi./Jap./Kor.) *Perilla frutescens var. japonica*. Also, beefsteak plant, shiso (Japanese), zi su (Chinese). A native of east Asia, it has two distinct varieties: green-leaved and purple-leaved. The essential oil of this plant, which is rich in minerals and vitamins, exhibits anti-inflammatory properties. In Nepal, the seeds of this plant are ground with chillies and tomatoes to make a sauce. In TRADITIONAL CHINESE MEDICINE, the plant is considered useful in stimulating the body's immune mechanism.

person-centered therapy (Mod.) Also, person-centred counselling; an approach to healing in which the patient is encouraged by the therapist to find an answer to his problem himself. The therapist attempts that the client establishes self-acceptance. The approach, developed by Carl Rogers (1902–87), is based on the notion that the relationship between the client and therapist is not a patient–doctor relationship in which the patient submits passively to treatment prescribed by the doctor.

In order to be successful, however, the approach needs a therapist who is a good listener and who really cares about his clients.

personal trainer (Mod.) A health and fitness professional who helps his or her client develop a level of physical condition by designing an exercise regimen and physical training programmes. Personal trainers also help with habitual-behaviour change.

personology (New Age) A recent New Age variant of PHYSIOGNOMY, personology refers to a system of face reading aimed at showing a correlation between a person's appearance and his character. The system was developed in 1930s by Edward Vincent, a Los Angeles judge, who took notes of the behavioural patterns of those who appeared before him in court. He compiled a list of 200 facial features, which were narrowed down to sixty-eight. Some examples of supposed personology correlation are:

Facial features	Probable characteristics
coarse hair	insensitive
fine hair	extremely sensitive
tight skin across the frame of face	meticulously clean and neat
wide jaw	prefers to be in charge of situations
square chin	loves arguments and debates
wide, flared nose	independent

petitionary prayer (Occ.) A type of PRAYER in which a request is repeatedly made to God. Such prayer-songs are common in Indian music.

petrissage A type of MASSAGE which includes kneading, pressing and rolling. Petrissage is considered beneficial especially to muscles.

peya (Ind.) Rice soup, a meal consumed after the treatment of PANCHA KARMA.

Pfrimmer deep muscle therapy (Mod.) Named after Therese Pfrimmer who was affected by partial paralysis and, based on her own experiences, developed this technique in 1940s. The treatment aims at manipulating deep tissues, with a view to stimulate circulation and regenerate lymphatic flow. The deep tissue massage consists of strong strokes which are used across muscle fibres. See also DEEP-TISSUE MASSAGE.

phantom limb The missing limb of an amputee. Most amputees experience warmth, itching, pressure and pain from the missing limb as if it were still part of their body. An explanation for the phantom sensation is that the brain continues to remain connected as if the body were intact.

pharmacopoeia (Mod.) An official publication of drugs in use.

pharmacoproxy (Hom.) A study of the preparation of homoeopathic remedies. The mode of preparation includes the DECIMAL SCALE, CENTESIMAL SCALE, fifty millesimal scale, KORSAKAVIAN METHOD, mixed HAHNEMANIAN and Korsakavian method, Jenichen's potencies, Fincke's method, Skiner's method and Q-potency.

pharmacotherapy The concept and practise of treating diseases with medication.

phase delay Temporal displacement of a rhythm as manifested, usually in teenagers; adolescents often manifest a phase delay in their sleep–wake up cycles, sleeping well after midnight and getting up only ten hours later.

philosophy of biology (Mod.) Also, biophilosophy. A subject which deals with ethical, epistemological and metaphysical issues concerning the biological sciences. Currently, the subject follows an empiristic tradition, advocating naturalistic and physicalistic theories. Contemporary philosophers of biology seem to have largely avoided questions about the distinction between life and nonlife; instead, scientific ideas are handled as philosophical ones and the consequences are explored.

philosophy of mind (Occ.) A study of the nature of the CONSCIOUSNESS, MIND and the nature of their relationship with the physical body. Subjects such as the nature of emotion, memory and perception, questions about free will and the self and its identity, for instance, form its core.

physicalism (Occ.) A hypothesis according to which the mind forms a part of the material (or physical) world. According to some philosophers, physicalism is true and all mental states must be physical states.

phlegm (Ind.) 1. A type of mucous. 2. A sticky water-based gel or fluid secreted in the body by the mucous membranes. While normally clear and white phlegm is considered healthy, yellow, blue or green phlegm may indicate infection, and rusty phlegm, internal bleeding. AYURVEDA counts phlegm (KAPHA) as one of the three bodily humours (DOSHA) and classifies them depending on their location in the human body. The functions of kapha in the body and the ailments caused due to its vitiation are well-known.

phoenix-rising yoga therapy (Occ.) A body-centred PSYCHOTHERAPY which incorporates the techniques of BREATHWORK, ENERGY BALANCING and VISUALIZATION. The therapy is rooted in the concept that unresolved emotional experiences are stored as 'emotional blocks' and that expelling them periodically is necessary for sound health.

phoniatrics (Mod.) Also, speech pathology. A subject of medical research, relating to the treatment of organs involved with speech, viz., the lungs, mouth, throat (larynx) and vocal cords. Phoniatrics deals with areas such as cancer in the vocal cords and their dysfunction and speech disorders. Speech pathologists deal with a wide variety of causes for disorders, from problems in swallowing to laryngeal dysfunction. People with speech disorders, performers with laryngeal problems and those who have undergone laryngectomy are helped by them.

phosphorus (Hom.) A remedy in HOMOEOPATHY, phosphorus is used in the treatment of conditions of excessive thirst, fatigue and nervousness.

photo rejuvenation (Cos.) A cosmetic treatment, aimed at making the skin look healthier and younger. The skin is treated with 'intense pulsed light' technology, to ward off dark spots, freckles, uneven pigmentation and wrinkles with minimal discomfort.

phototherapy (Nat.) The application of regular but moderate sunlight with a view to improve one's health. Exposure to the sun is said to be helpful in overcoming several ailments including depression, eating disorders, insomnia, jet lag, psoriasis and other skin problems.

physiatry (Mod.) Also, physical medicine, rehabilitation. A branch of medicine which specializes in the diagnosis and treatment of chronic disabilities. The physical modes of treatment such as medication, physical exercise and MASSAGE form part of the treatment procedures. Essentially, physiatrists specialize in a wide variety of conservative treatments for the musculoskeletal system and avoid surgical interventions.They also specialize in brain injury (due to stroke), pain management, paediatric medicine, spinal cord injury and SPORTS MEDICINE.

physical education (Mod.) A subject concerned with PHYSICAL EXERCISE and FITNESS.

physical exercise (Mod.) Activating the body with a view to increasing its strength and mobility. Physical exercise, practised regularly and methodically, helps make body movements smooth and easy and muscles firm and joints flexible. Moderately intense physical activity, such as brisk walking, is known to be beneficial when undertaken regularly for at least forty minutes a day. Risk factors for diabetes, high blood pressure, low levels of HDL cholesterols and obesity are effectively overcome with exercise. Active people have also been found to have a lower incidence of strokes.

physical manipulation (Mod.) A healing practice performed by physiotherapists such as chiropractics and osteopaths, the manipulative method is an ancient technique aimed at preventing and treating diseases. Physical manipulation incorporates ACUPRESSURE, MASSAGE, MYOTHERAPY, REIKI, and SHIATSU.

physical therapy (Mod.) Also, physiotherapy. A method aimed at maintaining and restoring maximum movement possibilities in the body so that its functional ability is maximized. The physical functions, when eroded by the process of ageing or due to diseases or injuries sustained can be addressed effectively using the knowledge and skills of a physical therapist. Physical therapy interventions include both manual handling and the use of mechanical and electro-therapeutic agents. Provisions are also made for patient-related aids and appliances. Conditions for physiotherapeutic interventions include conditions such as stroke and multiple sclerosis, pain in the back and neck, spinal and joint conditions such as arthritis, sport-related injuries and stress incontinence.

physician, the four qualities of (Ind.) According to AYURVEDA, an ideal physician is considered to be endowed with the following four qualities: a clear grasp of medical theories, wide clinical experience, personal hygiene and purity of mind.

physiochineitherapy (Mod.) The therapeutic application of heat, light, electrical and mechanical movements. The therapy is aimed at imparting maximum flexibility and strength to the body.

phytoaromatherapy (New Age) A branch of AROMATHERAPY, which exclusively uses essential oils obtained in natural conditions from plants and plant parts. The system avoids synthetic aromatics or those of animal origin.

phytotherapy (New Age) Also, herbalism. The use of plants for their medicinal properties. Phytotherapy is recognized in various systems of medicine such as AYURVEDA, CHEROKEE HERBAL MEDICINE, HOMOEOPATHY, KOREAN MEDICINE, SIDDHA, TRADITIONAL CHINESE MEDICINE and UNANI.

Pilates (Mod.) Also, Pilates method. An approach to physical fitness, developed by Joseph Pilates in the early-twentieth century. Pilates called his method contrology to refer to the way the method would encourage the use of the mind to control the muscles. The programme focusses on the major postural muscles which maintain the balance of the body and serve as the crucial support for the spine. The method teaches awareness of BREATH and alignment of the spine. It is said to help strengthen the deep torso muscles, thereby helping prevent back pain.

pindasweda (Ind.) Also, pindaswedana, NAVARAKIZHI. A procedure of fomentation, performed with a hot bolus of rice, cooked in cow's milk along with medicinal herbs. The bolus is applied or massaged while still hot over affected parts of the body. Performed with two therapists, it is considered cleansing and detoxifying for the body.

pineal gland (Mod.) Also called epiphysis, pineal body. A small endocrine gland situated near the centre of the brain, between the two hemispheres, tucked in a groove. After the 1960s scientists discovered that the pineal gland was responsible for the production of the hormone MELATONIN at night, which is regulated in a CIRCADIAN RHYTHM.

pingala (Yoga) 'reddish conduit'. 1. Psychic nerve-current passing through the right nostril 2. A psychic passageway travelling from the MULADHARA to the AJNA CHAKRA See also, IDA AND PINGALA

pippali (Ind.) Also, Indian long pepper. A pungent shrub, indigenous to north-east and south India. The fruit of the plant is a powerful stimulant for both the digestive and the respiratory systems. It is widely used

in the prevention of recurrent attacks of bronchial asthma in the AYURVEDA, SIDDHA and UNANI systems of medicine.

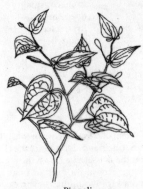

Pippali

pitta (Ind.) One of the three humours (DOSHAS), recognized in AYURVEDA, pitta is considered an outcome of the dynamic interplay between two elements in nature: fire and water. This humour is known for generating body heat and thereby accelerates metabolic processes. See also DOSHA.

pitta churna (Ind.) A dried herbal mixture, containing a number of cooling herbs such as AMLAKI, CARDAMOM, COCONUT, CORIANDER, CUMIN, khas, MUSTARD seeds, NUTMEG, SAFFRON, sesame, star anise and yashtimadhu. The mixture is taken with lukewarm water to counter high acidity in the stomach and to simultaneously ensure digestion. It is believed to be useful in hot weather conditions or when one feels excessive body heat, irritation or impatience.

pitta prakriti (Ind.) The body constitution of a person due to an inherent 'hot quality' of pitta. A tendency to excess consumption of food and drink, having soft hair, being prone to premature greyness, the inability to bear heat, and courageous behaviour are some characteristics of people with pitta prakriti.They are also sharp and quick to grasp knowledge. The categories of pitta are summarized in the table:

pizhichil (Ind.) An ancient MASSAGE technique which comprising the slow, repeated and liberal application of warm medicated oils, layer upon layer, on the body of the cli-

Pitta categories	Location or concentration in the body	Activities affected	Possible ailments due to vitiation
PANCHAKA	stomach, small intenstines	digestion	digestive disorders
RANJAKA	liver, spleen, stomach	blood formation	anaemia, jaundice, etc.
SADHAKA	heart	brain, intelligence, memory	mental disturbances, memory loss
ALOCHAKA	eyes	vision	blindness, cataract
BHARAJAKA	skin	complexion	skin ailments (e.g., leucoderma)

ent by a team of masseurs (two or four). The masseurs, who stand alongside of the client lying on the massage bed, drip the oil in a continuous stream for over an hour as a gentle massage is simultaneously carried out. As the massage progresses, as much as five or six litres of the medicated oil is used. The therapy is indicated in rheumatic problems, as it enhances blood circulation while strengthening the musculo-skeletal system.

placebo (Misc.) An inert or inactive substance used in clinical trials and scientific experiments to study the effect of drugs on animals and humans. A placebo is used to prove whether the experimental substance has a real or imagined effect, hence helping confirm the impartiality of final findings thereof. However, it has also been found that a real physiological effect can be caused even by an inactive placebo, which seems to invalidate the very objectivity attempted to be inbuilt in experiments/trials.

planchette (New Age) From the French word for little plank. Also, ouija; talking board. A triangular or heart-shaped cardboard or wooden 'spirit' board fitted with castors is constructed so that it can move freely around the area where the alphabets are written and can be readily pointed to. The medium and other sitters rest their fingers lightly on the planchette and wait for a contact with the spirit. The board tilts or moves, and knocks on the floor the alphabets, spelling entire messages from spirits. When questions are posed to the invisible medium or spirit, the board, touched by the participants, moves freely and points to the alphabets, spelling out the answers. Designs or symbols expressing emotions such as joy, sadness, anger or love are also used sometimes in place of printed letters, to enable the spirit invited to participate in the session and express itself with regard to questions or incidents pointed out by the participants.

planetary herbalism (New Age) A healing system, which evaluates a herb, not in terms of its chemical or bio-medical profile but by identifying its energy content and intensity. Thus the herbs are described in terms of their 'energetics'. The concept was recently popularized by Michael Tierra, in his book *Planetary Herbology*.

plant alchemy (Occ.) An approach to the therapeutic use of herbs, based on astrological as well as alchemical prínciples, rather than for their bio-chemical or pharmaceutical value. The approach, prevalent since ancent times is now largely forgotten except in some tribal pockets where the use of plants in based on the rich imagery and symbolism of anecdotal and mythological source materials.

plantain (Ind./Chi.) *Plantago major.* A herb known for its role in the health of the urino-genital system of the human body. The seeds are used to promote urination and clear mucus from the body. It is also used in the treatment of cataract and red eyes and to lower blood pressure.

plavini (Ind.) Also, plavini kumbhaka. A BREATHING technique which involves gulping air and swallowing it into the stomach, enabling the body to float on water. It helps belch out toxic gases

play technique (New Age) Also, play therapy. A method of psychoanalysis for children below three years. Developed by

Melanie Klein (1882–1960), a psychoanalyst and author of *The Psychoanalysis of Children* (1932), the technique uses toys which allow children to express their unconscious desires and fantasies, likes and dislikes. The method enables a child to release his or her feelings without the fear of reprisal. The therapist is also able to easily identify the cause of behaviour disorders through this method.

pleasant indifference (New Age) A healthy attitude of being assertively indifferent to unwarranted criticism. In a Jataka fable, a simpleton who abused Gautama Buddha was allowed to have his say by the smiling Buddha. When the man became tired of abusing, Buddha asked him one question: 'My son, tell me, when a man who is offered a gift refuses it, to whom should the gift belong?' The man answered, 'To him who offered it.' Buddha then said gently, 'I decline to accept your abuses. Please keep them with you.'

plunge pool (Spa) Also, mineral pool, Roman pool, sea-water pool; pools or ponds containing cold or hot water, used sometimes alternately in therapeutic or SPA settings. Alternate hot and cold water baths are known in NATUROPATHY for their therapeutic role.

pneumo-acupuncture (Mod.) In ACUPUNCTURE, a technique used to stimulate ACUPOINTS with small doses of medicine-grade carbon-dioxide. The procedure is believed to stimulate acupoints.

point holding (Mod.) An ACUPRESSURE technique that requires multiple practitioners to hold and take charge of acupressure points, designed to achieve emotional release and balance the flow of energy within the meridians. The technique was developed by Karen Peterson and John Walsh.

pointing therapy (Chi.) A classical form of ACUPUNCTURE derived from Chinese martial arts (Chinese Wushu). The therapy involves 'pointing' or poking, pressing, pinching, patting, knocking and pounding ACUPOINTS with the view to stimulate them.

polarity therapy (New Age) From polarity, or the attraction and union of opposites through a balanced middle point; a fundamental law of nature. A healing system based on ancient Eastern concepts relating to energy and developed by Randolph Stone (1890–1982), an Austrian chiropractor, naturopath and osteopath during the first half of the twentieth century. According to Stone, the human body is an energy system like a magnet or battery. It recognizes that energy has to move from a positive to negative pole, through a neutral field. As such, polarity therapy concerns itself with free and easy flow of this energy. To achieve this it uses four different approaches for balancing them including POLARITY BODYWORK, POLARITY DIET AND NUTRITION, COUNSELLING, and POLARITY YOGA EXERCISE. Stone came to hold that health and wellbeing were affected by the balanced distribution of the natural electro-magnetic field existing in living organisms.

polarity bodywork (New Age) A bodywork of POLARITY THERAPY which helps release tension patterns in the body, facilitating the movement of energy. A polarity therapist is said to be attuned to underlying energy patterns and encourages their movement by listening, observing and palpating.

polarity diet and nutrition (New Age) A dietary concept of POLARITY THERAPY, which recognizes that energy cannot flow freely through a congested toxic body. The approach includes a simple, purifying diet, mainly of fruits and vegetables, salads, soups and herbal teas, along with a cleansing regimen for a few days.

polarity yoga exercise (New Age) A part of POLARITY THERAPY, the yoga comprises a group of simple exercises, based on the observation of natural movements people instinctively adopt while wanting to relax in a tense atmosphere. Instead of rigid postures, these exercises use gentle rocking and stretching movements combined with vocal expressions. The movement of the body and use of vocal expressions distinguish polarity yoga from the classical HATHA YOGA.

pomegranate Also, dadima (Ind./Chi.) *Punica granatum*. A popular plant in many parts of the world. Its fruit is rich in antioxidants. Various parts of this plant have been used as medicine from ancient times in Chinese and Indian folk traditions; the fruit rind is used to treat diarrhoea and the juice of the flowers is dripped into the nostrils to control nosebleeds.

positive imagery (Occ.) Training one's mind to think positively about overcoming illness and misfortunes.

positive thinking (Occ.) The practise of thinking positive in real-life situations. Thinking positive is said to help overcome misfortunes, keeping them at least from worsening. AFFIRMATION also equips one to cope with problems and ailments.

posology (Hom.) From the Greek *posos*, meaning how to, and *logos*, meaning study. The study of the dosage of homoeopathic medicine. According to a general law applied to posology, the curative dose, like the remedy, must be similar in quantity and quality to the dose of the causative agent, which caused the disease.

possession (Occ.) A condition in which a person is believed to be under the influence of a spirit.

possibility thinking (Occ.) A derivative of POSITIVE THINKING, propounded by Robert Schuller, an evangelist. According to Schuller, refraining from verbalizing negative emotions could help shape upcoming events so that they are more favourable than the present.

post-hypnotic interview (Occ.) The discussion with the client immediately after the completion of the HYPNOSIS process. This is a review session wherein the hypnotist may suggest to the client the kind of action the client may subsequently undertake.

post-hypnotic suggestion (New Age) A suggestion given to a hypnotized person about the steps to be taken after awakening. 2. A suggestion given during the trance state, which is acted upon after awakening.

post-lunch dip (Misc.) A transitory drop in alertness in the early afternoon. This phenomenon does not necessarily occur after lunch, but a high-carbohydrate lunch could aggravate it.

postural integration (Mod.) A form of DEEP TISSUE MASSAGE, developed by Jack Painter. Directed towards the deeper tissues in the muscle, the technique, which incorporates BREATHWORK, aims at releasing of emotional obstructions in a psychotherapeutic manner.

potencized (Hom.) Diluted to prescription.

potency (Hom.) The dilution of a remedy. The system of homoeopathy assigns higher potencies for greater dilution.

potentization (Hom.) A process of minimizing, rather than negating, the toxic effects of the crude drug substance, while increasing its dynamic and curative properties. This is carried out by SUCCUSSION or TRITURATION.

poultice (Nat.) A long-standing traditional remedy used to relieve swellings and inflammation. Natural ingredients such as mud, herbs and botanicals are heated and applied in a paste-like form, spread between layers of soft, moist cloth. Poultices are known to encourage local circulation, while relieving pain.

portion-controlled meals (Mod.) A weight-loss technique, aimed at limiting the intake of calories to the minimum required by the body. Fatty foods are generally avoided.

power healing (Occ.) An approach to healing in which energy is focused in areas of pain.

power pushing (Occ.) An approach to healing, aimed at expunging stubborn, blocked negative energy out of the system of mind–body complex by simulataneous replacement with healthy and positive energy.

power retrieval (Occ.) An approach to healing, which attempts to retrieve the positive energy for help in healing.

power yoga (Occ.) A system of 'energetic workout' involving a sequence of prescribed postures (asanas) that flow into one another. A Western derivative of ASHTANGA YOGA, the system is said to uncover root-causes of stress through physical practices, attitudes and perspectives.

practitioner A facilitator of healing.

pragbhukta (Ind.) The pre-prandial administration of drugs.

prakopana nidana (Ind.) Exacerbating factors in an infection or disease or infection.

prakriti (Ind.) From the Sanskrit pra, meaning source of origin, and kruti, meaning to perform 1. Natural or original form 2. Original source 3. Body constitution 4. Nature, which is believed to depict its existence in many levels—from subtle (sukshma parvan) to gross realms (sthula parvan).

According to Indian philosophy, all of prakriti is deemed unconscious (achitta) and hence viewed as being in opposition to purusha, the transcendental Self. AYURVEDA insists on examining the prakriti of the patient first, before considering medical intervention. As individuals differ, so would interventions, each one depending on the prakriti.

In terms of the functioning, however, all actions are attributed to the three basic DOSHAs: VATA, PITTA and KAPHA. Most people are influenced by two doshas (dwandvaja prakriti) and they exhibit the characteristics of both. A balanced constitution, in which a balanced state of all the three doshas exist, is considered ideal—though extremely rare, as all ideals are.

The practitioner detetermines prakriti in two ways: QUESTIONING or physical examination.

> 'Prakriti consists of an eternal dimension, called pradhana (foundation).'
>
> —Patanjali

pralepa (Cos.) A plaster with selected herbs in paste form, applied evenly on the face or body and removed before it dries up completely. Such plasters are used to improve the complexion or quell joint-swellings.

prana (Ind.) Sanskrit for LIFE FORCE. The word is used in two wide connotations: physical aspect and abstract sense. In physical aspect, prana, VATA and VAYU are synonyms while in the abstract sense, it means BRAHMAN. According to Jayaratha, the essence of prana is VIBRATION. Prana is also referred to as NADA in the ancient India music treatises. According to AYURVEDA, prana, in combination with the FIVE ELEMENTS, viz., earth, water, wind, fire and ether, facilitates the development of the three humors (DOSHAs), the aggravation of which causes diseases. These humours are also recognized as PRAKRITI (natural characteristics) in terms of the physical, mental and emotional states of a person. Though prana is the recognized one, it assumes five forms each with its own role as given in the following table:

Form	Location in the human body	Role	Colour	Ailments caused by vitiation
Prana	Located in the head region, while moving in the heart and throat regions	Supportive to the functions of the mind, heart, sense organs and intelligence	Coral	Asthma, bronchitis, cold, hiccups, hoarseness of voice
Apana	Located in the colon region, while moving along the waist, thighs and pelvic parts of the body	Excretory functions	Scarlet	Diabetes, anal, bladder, and urinary diseases
Samana	Located in the lungs, while moving in the lungs	Digestive and assimilative functions	Between coral and scarlet	Diarrhoea and Indigestion
Udana	Located in upper chest, while moving in the nose,	Speech initiation, memory, effort undertaken and enthusiasm	Pale white	Diseases of eye, ear, nose and throat

	umbilicus and throat	shown		
Vayna	Located in the heart region, moving all over the body at a very fast speed, attending to the functions related to circulation and movement	Associated with all voluntary and involuntary movements in the body	As in a ray of light	Diarrhoea, fevers, impairment in circulation

'As a mother protects the children, o prana, protect us and give us splendour and wisdom'

—*Prashna Upanishad*

prana ahuti (Occ.) A DHARANA practice, aimed at flooding the body system with the vital force, PRANA.

prana mudra (Occ.) A MUDRA, formed by joining the tips of the thumb, ring finger and little finger. This mudra is said to activate the root-chakra, MULADHARA.

prana pratishtha (Occ.) The ancient act of endowing an image or icon with vital force, PRANA.

prana vata (Ind.) A form of VAYU located in the head, throat, chest and heart. An imbalance of this DOSHA may affect the health of the organs in this region.

prana vidya (Ind.) An ancient healing method which aims at regulating the flow of PRANA. The technique comprises the concentration of prana in the AJNA CHAKRA from where it is directed to move to parts of the body which are diseased from want of prana.While this is a self-healing method, to heal others, the prana is directed towards the healer's right hand, which in turn is placed on the ailing part of the sick person.

'Till you manage your mind, you can not really manage your prana.'

—The Vedas

pranava (Occ.) From the Sanskrit for humming. Also, nadanadi shakti. The primal sound, meditated upon. The mystic syllable AUM. This sound is also transformed into 'inner light', to light thoughts and emotions emanating from inside and to experience the blissful state of AWARENESS. See also AUM.

pranavadin (Occ.) A person who advocates the existence and role of PRANA.

pranayama (Yoga) Sanskrit for 'extending the vital force'. An ancient and essential practice in YOGA and the fourth limb of ASHTANGA YOGA of PATANJALI. It consists of a systematized breathing practice/routine including conscious inhalation (PURAKA), conscious retention (KUMBHAKA) and conscious exhalation (RECHAKA). For trained practitioners who reach advanced states, breath retention occurs automatically and also for a longer durations. The procedure is not just a breath-control exercise, but is aimed at harnessing one's life-energy.

The following aspects of pranayama are also known to the ancient system of HATHA YOGA: SAHITA KUMBHAKA, the practice of retention said to impart agility, flexibility and strength to the body; surya bhedi, the inhalation of breath practised through the right nostril, and exhalation through the left, aimed at detoxifying the body; UJJAYI, the passage of breath between nose and heart, which is said to act as an expectorant, detoxifying nerves; BHRAMARI, a fixed and concentrated breathing practice, believed to help calm the mind; MURCHHA, paving the way towards reaching the near- unconscious stage; vibhaga, a sectional pranayama, concerned with rejuvenating the coarse body; MUDRA, for the rejuvenation of the subtler parts of the body; BHASTRIKA and mahat, cleansing exercises meant for both body and mind; and KEVALA KUMBHAKA, an advanced breath-retention technique, in which the practitioner is able to willfully stop both inhalation and exhalation, which also aids concentration.

'Pranayama is extremely useful in encouraging the appearance of clear mental images.'

—Swami Satyananda Saraswati

pranayama, its ratio (Yoga) The ratio of time-allocation during the practice of PRANAYAMA. The ratio between inhalation of breath (PURAKA), its retention (KUMBHAKA) and its exhalation (RECHAKA) in the practise of PRANAYAMA is usually recommended at 1:4:2. For example, if one inhales for a duration of twelve MATRAS, its retention is prescribed for forty-eight and exhalation twenty-four. This ratio is, however, not fixed and can be varied in accordance with the constitution (PRAKRITI) and experience of a practitioner.

pranayama for the bedridden (Yoga) Also, pranayama on savasana. A method of PRANAYAMA for those who are aged and bedridden: 'With empty stomach, lie down comfortably on the back over a blanket and keep the hands on the ground by the side of the body and legs straight. Keep the heels together, though the toes can be kept apart. Relax all the muscles in the body. Draw in the breath softly and slowly in a happy mood, without making any noise through both nostrils. Retain it as long as possible with ease and comfort and then release it again softly and steadily. Do the exercise ten times and relax in between whenever tired.' Sometimes AUM is chanted mentally during exhalation.

As this exercise combines SAVASANA, PRANAYAMA, meditation and rest, it is considered ideal for bedridden patients.

pranic body (Occ.) The subtle energy body which can be distinguished from the gross, physical body by practitioners of YOGA through their subjective experiences of their own being. The pranic body is said to interrelate with other aspects of the human structure (e.g., mind and body) and is changed by the interactions with them. Death is said to be the disassociation of pranic body from the rest of its associates in the physical and mental realms. See FIVE SHEATHS

pranic crystal healing (New Age) A form of PRANIC HEALING employing CRYSTALS. Crystal is traditionally recognized by psychics for its capacity to absorb negative energies. See also, CRYSTAL, CRYSTAL HEALING, CRYSTAL THERAPEUTICS, CRYSTALOMANCY.

pranic healing (Occ.) An ancient method of healing wherein the energy in PRANA is tapped for curing a variety of psychosomatic diseases and disorders. Healers impart prana to the patients, while recharging themselves from the 'cosmic source' by practising KUMBHAKA or imagining its flow from their hands to the body part of the patient.The patient is believed to feel immediately the warmth of the energy. Pranic energy is used for relief from headaches and colic pain and sometimes in conjuction with MASSAGE, MUSIC THERAPY or TOUCH THERAPY for better results.

pranic psychotherapy (Occ.) A derivative of PRANIC HEALING, this procedure aims at cleansing emotional and psychic energy blocks which cause diseases and discomforts. Negative thought forms and emotional entities, accumulated over a period of time, are believed to get dislodged with this method. In contrast with PSYCHOTHERAPY, no personal information is sought by the healer from his patients in this method .

pranic self-healing (Occ.) A self-healing method in which the energy of PRANA is believed to come as an aid to problems, including pain. The negative energy or pain is visualized to be cleansed at its locus through the practise of PRANAYAMA, while simultaneously infusing positive or healthy energy to replace it. This procedure is sometimes combined with other techniques such as ASANA, MUDRA, THERAPEUTIC TOUCH to enhance its effects.

prasadhana taila (Cos.) Ancient Indian cosmetic and therapeutic unguents applied on the skin to treat cutaneous infections, darkness, eruptions, marks, specks and tans.

prashna (Ind.) Questioning, as a means of diagnosis.

prasvasa (Yoga) Expiratory breath, as opposed to SVASA, the inhaled breath.

prati marsha nasya (Ind.) Also, daily oil nasya. Repeated application of medicated oil to the nostrils. Oil is usually applied by dipping one's cleaned little finger in medicated ghee or oil and inserting it into each nostril, lubricating the nasal passage with a gentle massage. This simple treatment is said to help in opening up clogged channels in the head region, facilitating the movement of the PRANA energy. It is also said to be helpful in relieving mental stress.

pratyahara (Yoga) The withdrawal of senses. The fifth 'limb' of the eight-limbed ASHTANGA YOGA system of PATANJALI, pratyahara is said to pave the way for an effective meditation.

> 'Doing pratyahara successfully depends on one's ability to sit in a comfortable asana.'
>
> —Swami Satyananda Saraswati

pravala bhasma (Ind.) A traditional AYURVEDIC preparation, rich in calcium and prescribed to treat osteoporosis.

prayaschitta (Occ.) Sanskrit for penance. Atonement, aimed at softening or nullifying the anticipated reaction to a past action, particularly a sin (PAPA). Penance is self-inflicted by a person to mitigate his or her karmic burden caused by his or her past wrongful actions. Acts such as prostrating before an image of a deity 108 times, fasting, abstaining comforts or sex, and vow of silence are examples.

prayer (Occ.) People have prayed from times immemorial, even before structured religious concepts and practices developed to institutionalize the faith in human hearts. Verbal and non-verbal communication to the divinity, in the belief that divine logic governs life-processes and that divine assistance can be availed as and when one feels helpless, is attempted through prayer. See also THERAPEUTIC PRAYER.

> 'Prayer can not be verbal; it should be from the heart. To merge into the heart is prayer.'
>
> —Bhagwan Sri Ramana Maharishi

prayer wheels (Tib.) Auspicious devices for spreading spiritual blessings for individual and universal well-being, as used in e.g., Tibetan Buddhism.

precision reflexology (Occ.) A system of FOOT REFLEXOLOGY.

precognition For knowledge of an event, especially of a paranormal kind'.

pre-cognitive re-education (Occ.) A process to release negative thought-forms and re-create within a 'higher self' unconditional love and wisdom.

pre-conscious (Mod.) Unrepressed thoughts which, although unconscious, can eventually become conscious.

pregnancy massage (Mod.) A technique of MASSAGE, to ease common discomforts during pregnancy. The method is aimed at the massage addresses stress during pregnancy, and releases tension in the lower back and other areas of the woman's body promoting maternal and foetal well-being.

pre-hypnosis interview (Occ.) A discussion between a hypnosis client and the hypnotist regarding the nature of the problem, the time when the client became aware of the problem, the remedial action taken by the client in the past to solve the problem, important events in the client's life, and any future events related to the problem. See also, PRE-TALK.

preksha meditation (Occ.) A spiritual-healing method intended to promote pure, simple and genuine emotions based on love and mutual respect.

premonition (Occ.) A warning of an impending event.

press seeds (Occ.) Also, ear seeds, pebbles. Tiny pellet–shaped objects such as black pepper and lentils usually pressed against auricular reflex points with the help of a tape to treat various ailments.

pressotherapy (Mod.) Treatment with pressure cuffs to improve the circulation in the feet.

pressure hosing (Mod.) A form of HYDROTHERAPY which creates the impact of water on the body. Usually sea water is used for pressure hosing in seaside spas.

pre-talk (Occ.) Information provided by the client to the hypnotist before he becomes hypnotized. It also refers to information aimed at overcoming fears and misconceptions about HYPNOSIS in the mind of the client. See also, PRE-HYPNOSIS INTERVIEW.

primal therapy (Mod.) A trauma-based PSYCHOTHERAPY, POPULARIZED BY Arthur Janov. It is based on the notion that therapeutic progress can only be made through direct emotional experience. It holds that simply talking about the problem (referred to as talking therapies) is of limited effectiveness, because the cortex, or higher reasoning area of the brain, has no ability to affect the real source of psychological pain in other areas of the brain. The therapy aims to uncover repressed primal pains (or unpleasant events) experienced by the client in his childhood.

primary emotional energy recovery (Mod.) A method developed by Dan Jones and John Lee, prescribing physical movements and exercises aimed at releasing emotional accumulations locked up inside the body. It is said that this method helps in aligning the body and feelings towards the healing.

pristhabhyanga (Ind.) Back massage, with medicated oil, believed to be helpful to all types of body constitutions (prakriti), but recommended especially for VATA and KAPHA personalities.

prithvi (Ind.) Sanskrit for earth. One of the FIVE ELEMENTS, representing the earth as a constituent of the body. These elements were used to describe interactions and inter-relationships between phenomena in nature. In Japanese philosophy, earth *(tsuchi)* is regarded at the bottom of the asending order of power, followed by the other elements, i.e. water *(sui* or *mizu)*, fire *(ho ka* or *hi)* wind *(fû* or *kaze)* and the void or sky *(kû)*. See also FIVE ELEMENTS IN THE JAPANESE PHILOSOPHY; FIVE ELEMENTS IN THE INDIAN PHILOSOSPHY.

prithvi mudra (Occ.) A MUDRA formed by joining the tips of the thumbs, and the ring fingers. This mudra is said to activate the MULADHARA.

problem-focussed counselling (New Age) Short-term counselling focussed on providing help in overcoming a given problem of the client.

process acupressure (New Age) A healing method which combines the ancient knowledge of ACUPRESSURE with contemporary understanding in psychology, and based on the idea that the body, mind and soul are fundamentally linked, and that the state of one has an effect on the state of the others.

progressive relaxation (Occ.) A simple healing method popularized by Edmund Jacobson (1929) in *Progressive Relaxation*. It involves successive tensing and relaxing of each of the fifteen major muscle groups in the body. Performed lying down, the muscles are tensed, each for a count of five to ten, starting with the head and progressing downwards. Deep breathing may be also combined. This method is said to counter anxiety and stress method. It places emphasis on a slow, disciplined development of muscle tension awareness.

prophecy (Occ.) A divinely inspired vision or revelation of the future. In a broad sense, it refers to the prediction of future events, which includes the spread or alleviation of disease. Prophecies are often based on DIVINATION, or determining the will of gods.

propolis (New Age) Also, bee glue, bee propolis. A dietary supplement made of a resinous compound collected by honey-bees from different flowers. Long known for its antibacterial compounds, propolis is used as a salve for cuts and bruises and is found helpful, particularly in the treatment of swellings in the mucous membrane, sore throats, dry cough, halitosis, tonsilitis and acne.

proto-raga therapy (Occ.) The application of fewer notes (swaras) than the mandatorily required five notes in the Indian raga system. It has been found that mentally challenged children respond more favourably to simple tunes (those with few notes, i.e, four or less in an octave) and active beats than to the elaborate rendering of ragas.

psi Parapsychological or psychic faculties or phenomena.

psyche (Mod.) The spirit or soul.

psychic Occ.) 1. Pertaining to the mind or soul. 2. A person who uses EXTRA-SENSORY PERCEPTION with a view to obtaining information.

> 'To learn the lesson of how to live is more important than any psychic or occult knowledge.'
>
> —Hazrat Inayat Khan

psychic attack (Occ.) 1. Negative intentions of malicious entities attacking the healthy energy pattern in an individual. 2. Energetic pollution from outside, emanating through negative feelings such as anger, jealousy or hatred directed towards the affected person. Negative thought forms are said to adversely affect one's AURA.

psychic diagnosis (Occ.) Holistic or psychic methods and techniques adopted in the field of diagnosis, as in several traditional medicinal practices. Though psychic diagnosis is expected to concur with orthodox methods, occasionally different conclusions are reached. These differences are attributable to the fact that psychic (holistic) diagnosis considers causes other than those considered by orthodox systems.

psychic energy (Mod.) 1. According to a concept developed in the field of psychodynamics by Ernst von Brucke (1874), all living organisms are energy systems, governed by the principle of energy conservation.

2. According to Carl Jung, psychic energy cannot be measured quantitatively as forms of physical energy can. It is considered to express itself in the form of actual or potential forces which induce various psychological activites such as attentiveness, feeling, perceiving, remembering, striving, thinking, wishing or willing. Potential forces of the personality such as inclinations, latent tendencies and predispositions are believed to be induced by psychic energy.

psychic drawings (Occ.) Diagnostic drawings made by psychics, based on the images that emerge from their hands rather than their minds. Depicting possible areas or parts of the body affected by disease, psychic drawings are said to trigger people's insight into their deep-seated problems.

psychic healing (New Age) Also, psychic therapy. An approach to healing with the help of PSYCHIC ENERGY. According to its proponents, a disease is characterized by a deficiency and imbalance of vital energy. Through this method, psychic energy is supposed to get transferred from the healer to the sick, and is believed to help repair and rebalance depleted energy.

psychic medium (Occ.) A person who works as both a PSYCHIC as well as a MEDIUM.

psychic powers (Occ.) 1. SIDDHI 2. The

special ability or skills developed through mental exercises such as MEDITATION, PENANCE, RITUALS and TAPAS.

psychic reading (Occ.) The application of psychic ability to answer a client's question.

psychic self-defence (Occ.) Methods devised to protect oneself from what is referred to as PSYCHIC ATTACKS. Some measures undertaken are closing of the aura to prevent intrusions; utilizing holy and sacred objects, idols, signs and diagrams; special extraction techniques to remove such attacks; the use of charities to pacify the anger of the psychic assailant; and experiencing inner peace and calmness in the middle of chaotic events. See also PSYCHIC HEALING.

psychic sounds (Occ.) Different sound frequencies and timbre, associated with different CHAKRAS. Usually sound is incorporated in the form of chants, or with the help of instruments such as bells, conch-shells, damaru, gongs and drums, to enhance the effect of concentration on specific chakras during MEDITATION. Some sounds used in Hinduism are derived from Sanskrit alphabets. See also, BIJA MANTRA, MANTRA, NADA, NADA YOGA.

psychic surgery (Occ.) A painless, paranormal and non-invasive surgical procedure, practised mainly in Brazil and Philippines. 'Surgery' in this case refers to the removal of diseased etheric tissues in the AURA, either with the bare hands or common instruments like a spoon by a self-appointed psychic surgeon.

'Psychic surgery is pure and unmitigated fakery. The "surgical operations" of psychic surgeons ... with their bare hands are simply phony.'

—Judge Danile H. Hanscom

Psycho-cybernetics (Occ.) A self-help book by Maxwell Maltz, a plastic surgeon. Published in 1960, the book deals with the power and influence of imagination on one's self-image. According to Maltz, patients with poor self-image benefitted little, if at all, from plastic surgery, while patients with a good self-image gained following such surgery.

> 'Your self-image defines and limits your potential.'
>
> —Maxwell Maltz

psychokinesis (Occ.) Also, PK, telekinesis, TK. The paranormal ability of the mind to influence matter or energy. Uri Geller (b.1946) an Israeli psychic, is famous for his spoon-bending demonstrations, allegedly by psychokinesis. See also, GELLER EFFECT.

psychodrama (Occ.) A method of PSYCHO-THERAPY, devised by Jacob L. Moreno (1889–1974), a Romania-born psychiatrist in 1920s. The participants explore their internal conflicts by acting out their emotions and inter-personal interactions. The 'acting' here is a replacement for the 'couch' used by the psychotherapists. This methos is said to enable patients to express their negative emotions and create a scenario that makes them feel better. As the method incorporates strong elements of theatre, the sessions are often conducted on the stage with props.

psychodynamic chirology (Occ.) A comprehensive diagnostic discipline based on the science of dermatoglyphics, it is a method of hand-reading, based on the belief that all events in the human brain are reflected in the hands.

psychoenergetics (Occ.) A healing method formulated by psychiatrist Jordan Weiss, is based on the principle that all matter and creation is 'patterned' energy and that all psychological manifestations, such as thoughts, feelings, and behaviour patterns, are also 'patterned' energy. The method is based on the premise that effective psychological healing, regardless of the method or system, can occur only when there is a change in the basic energies that charge our feelings, thoughts, memories and habits. The practitioner, using a variety of techniques that affect mental and emotional energies at a fundamental level, is believed to develop an access to the source of the individual's discomfort. While going to the core of the matter may be a frightening thought to many, it is considered actually healing, safe and effective. The method is considered useful in anger management and to overcome addiction, depression, low self-esteem and trauma.

psychogenic (Occ.) Symptoms or conditions with a mental origin. The adjective is used for describing disorders that have psychological rather than physiological origins.

psychogenic pain (Occ.) Bodily pain related to mental 'injuries'.

psychology The science that deals with mental states. Empirical methods are generally used to enquire into the mental states like fear, joy or obsessions. See also MIND.

psychomotor (Occ.) Of or relating to movement in the body associated with mental processes.

psychomotor therapy (Occ.) Also, psychomotor activity. A body-centred group therapy involving role-playing as designed by American dancers Albert and Diana Pesso, in 1961. A psychomotor therapist/ movement therapist, like a psychologist, helps people with their psychological problems, but whereas a psychologist only talks with people, a psychomotor therapist actively does things conducive for the patient's relief.

psychoneuroendocrinology (Mod.) A clinical study of hormone fluctuations and their relationship with behaviour and psychiatric illness. A combination of endocrinology and PSYCHIATRY, psychoneuroendocrinology has played an important role in the diagnosis and treatment of mood and anxiety disorders.

psychoneuroimmunology (Mod.) Also, transitional medicine; mind–body–spirit medicine. An inter-disciplinary scientific study of the interaction and inter-connection of psychological, behavioural and neuro-endocrinal factors and the functioning mechanism of the immune system in the body. A humanistic or pluralistic model in medicine, psychoneuroimmunology is a new field of study which considers the interactions and inter-connections between the mind and body. It is based on the inference that the health or well-being of the body has to take into account the mind and emotions. See also, TRANSITIONAL MEDICINE.

psychoneuropharmacology (Mod.) A new branch of study based on the inference that there is a marked impact of psychological processes on physiological functions in an organism. See also TRANSITIONAL MEDICINE.

psychopathology (Mod.) The study of mental and behavioural abnormalities/disorders with reference to their origin, development and manifestations.

psychopath (Mod.) An individual who has problems in coping with his surroundings and situations, with special reference to family and/or social norms. The individual often lacks normal feelings, like empathy and remorse, besides certain unusual physical responses, e.g., showing below average distress when exposed to frightening situations or threats.

> 'A psychopath finds it difficult to process, handle, or use emotional material in the same way the rest of us do.'
>
> —Robert D. Hare

psychosoma (Occ.) A non-physical body whose constituents are energetic, emotional, mental and informational fields.

psychosomatic illness (Mod.) Also, psychophysiologic disorders. An illness whose symptoms are attributed to the mental process of the sufferer rather than any immediate physical (e.g. injury) or physiological (e.g. infection) condition. 2. An illness caused by emotional conditions such as anger, anxiety, depression and guilt.

psychospiritual holistic healing (Occ.) A holistic healing system comprising various methods such as AURA BALANCING, CHAKRA healing, GUIDED IMAGERY, INNER CHILD THERAPY, MEDITATION, POSITIVE THINKING and YOGA.

psychosurgery (Occ.) A modern surgical intervention, performed in the brain, aimed at effecting changes in cognition, with the intent to treat or alleviate severe mental illness. Gamma knife irradiation and deep brain stimulation are some of the minimally invasive techniques which are currently used. Psychosurgery is distinct from PSYCHIC SURGERY, which is a non-invasive method in alternative medicine.

psychosynthesis (Occ.) A system of spiritual therapy, a blend of inner, mystical experience and the new scientific and technological knowledge and skills aimed at achieving health and wellbeing. Developed by Italian psychoanalyst Roberto Assagioli (1888–1974), psychosynthesis refers to the process of one's personal growth, reflecting the natural tendency within everybody to harmonize or synthesize for the same. The guide's role is said to help a client identify his or her inner resources, support the process, and be attentive to what is happening.

psychotherapy (Mod) Also, COUNSELLING. A range of methods aimed at improving the mental health of a client through communication and dialogue. While most forms of psychotherapy use only spoken communication, some use non-verbal forms such as art, music, word and touch. Normally psychotherapy involves discussing the issues in order to arrive at a constructive solution or resolution. See also ART THERAPY, COUNSELLING, MUSIC THERAPY.

pulsatilla (Hom.) A remedy in HOMOEOPATHY, used in the treatment of conditions accompanied by discharges such as bedwetting and sinusitis.

pulse (Mod.) The frequency of the heart beat, measured in beats per minute (bpm). The pulse rate in a healthy adult when resting varies between 60 to 100 bpm. It is as low as 40 bpm during sleep or can rise as high as 200–220 bpm after a strenuous workout. Some common pulse points are:

Pulse points	Location of the pulse point
Radial pulse	On the thumb side of the wrist (radial artery)
Ulnar pulse	On the little finger side of the wrist (ulnar artery)
Carotid pulse	In the neck region (carotid artery)
Brachial pulse	Between the biceps and triceps
Femoral pulse	In the thigh (femoral artery)
Popliteal pulse	Behind the knee in the popliteal fossa, found by holding the bent knee
Dorsalis pedis pulse	On top of the foot (dorsalis pedis artery)
Tibialis posterior pulse	In the back of the ankle (posterior tibial artery)
Temporal pulse	On the temple directly in front of the ear (temporal artery)

pulse diagnosis (Mod.) Also, pulse examination, pulse reading. An important diagnostic tool in several systems of oriental medicine and conventional medicine.

The health of the mind–body constitution, including the vitiation of the DOSHAs, the conditions of various internal organ and problems that may arise in future, can be determined from the pulse.

punnagathi kizhi (Ind.) A form of MASSAGE, in which medicinal herbs are rolled into small cloth bundles, soaked in hot oil, and applied all over the body of the patient. The massage is said to be effective in treating spinal problems and arthritic complaints.

punya (Occ.) Sanskrit for virtuous. A meritorious action, punya includes all forms of doing good. It is seen as light-hued and pastel coloured, in contrast to its counterpart PAPA which is seen as shades of darker colours which are usually static and immovable.

puraka (Yoga) The process of inhalation.

purification rites (Occ.) The ancient practice of cleansing the mind–body–spirit complex. Bronze, circles and wheels, crystals, earth, fire, the fragrance of flowers, ghee, gold, incense, jade, milk, morning, names of gods, perfumes, plants and herbs, sacred objects, sacred personages, silver, sunshine, virgins, the right side and water are believed to represent intrinsic purity.

Purna Yoga (Yoga/New Age) A system of YOGA incorporating the unitive discipline of wholeness or integration as popularized by Sri Aurobindo (1872–1950) of Pondicherry.

purvakarma (Ind.) A set of preliminary procedures in AYURVEDA, undertaken to prepare a patient for PANCHA KARMA. The procedures aim at removing AMA from various parts/organs of the body and restoring vitality, especially in the elderly. The procedures are different for different body constitutions (PRAKRITI) and humour types (DOSHAs)

pustak mudra (Occ.) A MUDRA formed by folding the fingers of the hand into the palm, keeping the thumbs straight. This mudra is believed to help improve the memory.

pyramid (Egy.) A monumental structure incorporating polyhedral geometry, believed to be energy-efficient. As the pyramid energy is spread in all the four directions at its bottom and transcends upwards towards the apex, the sitting posture taken in ASANAs such as PADMASANA is considered highly efficient in uplifting the energy within. It is also believed that water and food kept in a pyramidal structure do not deteriorate as quickly as it would if kept outside.

pyramid therapy (Occ.) Also, pyramidology. The concept and practise of using PYRAMID and pyramidal structures which are believed to accelerate the healing process. According to Dr Sadasiva Rao, an expert on pyramids from Visakhapatnam, Peruvian pyramid structures built by the Aztecs, are preferable to the Egyptian models, as the former show a uniform process of energy distribution.

> 'Pyramids are microprocessors of cosmic energy and wrapped in a hallucinating mystery.'
>
> —Paul Brunton

pyromancy (Occ.) DIVINATION by fire; the shape of the burning flame is usually observed by the diviner. In ancient Greece, virgins at the Temple of Athena are reported to have practised pyromancy. The ancient Chinese are said to have practised pyromancy by burning or heating what was called oracle bones (the shoulder blades of oxen or turtle shells). The cracks developed in them were then interpreted as portents.

Q

qi (Jap.) Also chi, ki. The LIFE FORCE, believed to pervade the human system. Its unimpeded circulation in the body is considered the secret of good health in systems of ORIENTAL MEDICINE. Qi, which signifies both breath and awareness, is said to encompass air and internal qi (referred to as true qi).

The two basic types of qi are congenital or inherited qi, which is gathered and formed at conception and stored in the kidney region, and postnatal or acquired qi, derived from the essence of food (*gu qi*) and air *(kong qi)*. In addition to regulating the diet, training qi is also considered essential in maintaining the condition of HOMEOSTASIS.

> 'That which was from the beginning in heaven is qi; on earth it becomes visible as form; qi and form interact giving birth to the myriad things.'
>
> —Huangdi Neijing

qi in martial arts (Jap.) As a central concept in many martial arts including TAI CHI CHUAN, QI is developed in AIKIDO with a scheme of special exercises. Testing the qi development of a student is done by holding one arm out, as another student attempts to bend it. If the first student tries simply to employ physical prowess, it is believed that he will be quickly exhausted and his arm will bend. On the other hand, relaxing completely and 'extending' the qi is believed to resist the bending more efficiently.

Some QI GONG masters and YOGIS are reported to have demonstrated by tackling or attacking their students from a distance with their vital energy. In a classic story, two opponents meet and hold each other's hands before a fight. While doing so, they feel each other's qi levels, and the one who has the weaker qi simply bows out of the combat without even striking a blow.

qigong (Chi./Jap.) Literally, energy cultivation. From the Chinese *chi*, meaning life energy, and *kung*, meaning achievements. Also, chi gung, chi kung. 1. An approach to healing aimed at releasing blocked-energy 2. A set of popular breathing and movement exercises, an important aspect of Chinese martial arts. The exercises involve contemplation, VISUALIZATION, assumption of postures, and stylized breathing besides body movements. Qigong is also considered useful for therapeutic interventions in some quarters.

Qigong techniques are of two types: DONG GONG, the 'dynamic' qigong, and JING GONG, the 'meditative' qigong.

qi xian (Chi.) QI which is stagnant, due to being blocked in the energy-channels.

qi zhi (Chi.) QI, which is stagnant, due to its sluggishness.

quack (Misc.) An ignorant, illiterate or untrained person, who pretends or imagines that he or she has a skill, particularly in the context of medicine.

> 'The prophet and the quack are alike admired for a generation, and admired for the wrong reasons.'
>
> —G.K. Chesterton

quack medicine (Misc.) A derogatory name for ALTERNATIVE MEDICINE, which is essentially based on one's belief or faith rather than scientific evidence.

> 'And then you have people who know very little about alternative medicine but have a lot of very strong opinions. They are very opinionated about the field, so you have to go up against that.'
>
> —Thomas Leung

quackery (Misc.) The practise of medicine by a QUACK.

quan chi chi gong (Chi./Occ.) A form of QIGONG therapy. Quan chi chi gong is a variant of PSYCHOKINESIS in which the practitioner transfers QI energy, stored in their energy body, into the patient. The method is said to accelerate healing, weight-reduction and drug deaddiction.

quan yin method (Occ.) Also, meditation on inner light and inner sound, quan yin method of meditation. A rediscovery of an ancient, theistic, lacto-vegetarian martial arts method, as popularized by the Vietnam-born Suma Ching Hai (b.1950) in recent times. Quan yin method is said to help conquer negative energies. The five precepts of this system are:

1. Refrain from leading a life of a sentient being
2. Refrain from telling lies
3. Refrain from stealing
4. Refrain from sexual misconduct; and
5. Refrain from using intoxicants

quantum medical consciousness interface system (Mod.) An advanced bio-resonant medical therapy device which gathers bio-energetic data from the body via twenty channels, then sorts and prioritizes the information and automatically begins testing the client's own energetic reactivity. The system also offers many bio-resonant therapies such as COLOUR THERAPY and RIFE THERAPHY.

quantum physics (Mod.) A branch of science which studies the energetic characteristics of matter at the subatomic level.

quantum touch (Occ.) A method of healing which uses simple breathing and body awareness exercises. A quantum-touch practitioner is trained to focus on and amplify LIFE FORCE, by combining various breathing and body awareness exercises.

race walking (Mod.) A method of walking at a fast and energetic pace, aimed at maintaining health. Like walking, it burns calories and tones the leg muscles. It helps in achieving a higher heart rate.

radiance breathwork (Occ.) A body-oriented healing modality aimed at releasing unresolved emotions trapped in the body. In a typical session, a facilitator guides the breather to let go of 'conscious control' and 'take things as they come up'. After a short time, emotional or personality patterns from the unconscious will are said to surface as behavioural patterns. Body-work is also used on occasion to help trigger emotional release. The facilitator encourages the breather to experience feelings fully and move through them. Throughout the session, the material which surfaces gets integrated so that energy blockages are said to get released. Developed and popularized by Gay and Kathlyn Hendricks in the 1970s, the method is also said to facilitate the clearance of the 'effects of birth trauma'.

radiance movement therapy: (Occ.) A form of 'movement work' developed by Gay and Kathlyn Hendricks. The method aims at dialoguing directly with one's 'inner self' and accessing the 'innate intelligence' of the body.

radiance prenatal process (Occ.) A form of BODY-CENTRED PSYCHOTHERAPY, popularized by Gay and Kathlyn Hendricks. The therapeutic session takes place in water, heated to the temperature of the womb. A male and female therapist support the client, ostensibly to induce the client to return to 'the prenatal time', and perform a 'clearing procedure'. The entire procedure is aimed at setting the client free from intense feelings of trauma that he or she might have experienced before his birth.

radiance technique (Occ.) Also, authentic reiki, radiant touch, real reiki, 'The Official Real Reiki'. A form of energy-balancing popularized in 1986 by Barbara Weber Ray, a clairvoyant astrologer.

radiesthesia (New Age) Also, pendulum diagnosis. A paranormal ability to detect radiation in the human body. Such radiations are called AURA. According to its theory, when the pendulum is above a diseased organ, the organ repels it, and the more diseased the organ, the larger the loop the pendulum makes.

> 'Every object in the world has a characteristic 'aura' or electro-magnetic field that can cause a sensitive person to be able to perform dowsing.'
>
> —Solcol W. Tromp

radionics (Occ.) Also, radionic analysis, radionic analysis technique, radionic diagnostic work. A system of DISTANT HEALING, developed by Albert Abrams (1863–1924), radionics consists of a body of concepts and practices concerning medical diagnosis and healing. It is based on the belief that all life and matter contains vibrations and harmonics and that a healthy person exhibits certain 'energy frequencies' different from what a non-healthy person reveals. RADIONIC DEVICES are purported to diagnose and restore persons to health by applying what is called the healing frequencies.

radionic devices (Occ.) Devices which are used for diagnosis of the energy frequencies of a person and to restore health. The two main types of radionic devices include a simple analysis tool for determining what is wrong with the subject being diagnosed and a treatment tool used in healing the subject of whatever is diagnosed. Both these tools may be combined into a single device.

radionic photography (Occ.) An instrument developed in the 1930s by chiropractor Ruth Drown, claimed to be useful for remote diagnosis. Drown was, however, convicted of fraud and medical quackery.

radix (Occ.) Also, radixwork. A form of BODY-CENTRED THERAPY, developed by Erica and Charles Kelly in the 1960s. Based on the Reichian concepts of 'life energy' and 'muscular armour', radix is said to be conceived as a personal psychological growth practice, founded on the principle that each individual is a whole person with a mind, feelings and body. RADIX therefore uses a diversity of mind (verbal), feelings (affective) and body (somatic) counselling techniques to bring lasting change to each level of the whole person. The method is said to reduce the disassociation of body and mind, centering in one's own body experience.

radon therapy (Spa) An inert gas used in many spas, particularly in Europe, as part of a holistic treatment process. It is believed to stimulate organ functions and promote improved secretions of the glands, without the harmful effects of radiation.

raga (Ind.) The unique melodic mode in Indian music, which renders great creative scope for endless improvisation. Ancient music treatises in India referred to the octave divided theoretically into twenty-two microtones (shrutis), but by the sixteenth century, this practice died out. As there is no absolute pitch, each performer treats pitch quite differently, and the precise intonation of a given note depends on melodic context. The performer simply selects a ground note, which serves as the drone.

The raga system is classified into two schools: the Carnatic or south Indian school and the Hindustani or north Indian school. The six fundamental ragas of the Hindustani school are given in the following table:

The Fundamental Raga	Time of the Day with which the raga is associated	The season of the year with which the raga is associated	Mental Attitude or moods with which the raga is associated*
Hindol	Dawn	Spring	To bring in universal love
Bhairava	Mornings	August–September–October	To maintain peace and tranquility
Megha	Mid-day	Rainy season (monsoon)	To summon up courage and to build one's cofidence levels
Deepak	Evening	Summer	To arouse compassion
Sri	Twilight	Autumn	To give and recieve pure love
Malkauns	Midnight	Winter	To develop valour

raga chikitsa (Ind.) Also, raga therapy. 1. An extinct text in Sanskrit by this name. 2. An attempt to revue the ancient system of MUSIC THERAPY, known to AYURVEDA, and prevalent in the Indian subcontinent in ancient times.

The expected therapeutic role of some ragas, both Hindustani and Carnatic, are shown in the following tables. However there is no scientific evidence on the conclusions reached with respect to these ragas. See also, MUSIC THERAPY, RAGA

Some possibly therapeutic ragas of the Hindustani system

Name of the Raga	Expected Therapeutic Role
Ahirbhairav	arthritis, hypertension, indigestion
Basant Bahar	gall stones
Bhairavi	arthritis
Bilaval	tuberculosis
Brindavansarang	leucorrhoea
Chandrakauns	anorexia
Darbari-kanhara	headache, hysteria
Darbari-kalyan	asthma
Des	leucorrhoea
Deepak	acidity, anorexia
Gujari Todi	cough
Gunakali	arthritis, constipation, piles
Hindol	malaria
Jaunpuri	constipation
Jayjaywanti	arthritis, headache
Khamaj	hysteria
Madhuvanti	piles, haemorrhoids
Malkauns	intestinal gas
Marva	malaria
Multani	tuberculosis
Puriya	hypertension, hysteria
Sohani	headache
Tilang	tuberculosis
Todi	hypertension
Yaman	stress

'When I hear music, I fear no danger. I am invulnerable, I see no foe. I am related to the earliest times, and to the latest.'
—Thoreau

Some possibly therapeutic ragas of the Carnatic system

Name of the Raga	Expected Therapeutic Role
Bhupalam	bad mood or depression
Bilahari	bad mood or depression
Dvijaavanti	paralysis
Kedaram	bad mood or depression
Khamaas	marital discord
Nadanamakriya	stress
Nilambari	insomnia
Punnagavarali	violence, anger
Sahana	violence, anger
Sama	stress
Sri	indigestion
Madhuvanti	piles or haemorrhoids
Malkauns	intestinal gas

Marwa	indigestion hyperacidity
Nat Bhairav	indigestion rheumatic arthritis colitis
Puriya	colitis anaemia hypertension
Puriya Dhanashri	anaemia
Ramkali	colitis piles or haemorrhoids
Shree	anorexia common cold cough asthma
Shudh Sarang	anorexia gall Stones (cholecystitis)
Shyam Kalyan	cough asthma
Sohini	headache
Yaman	rheumatic arthritis

rainbow diet (New Age/Occ.) A dietary regimen based on the belief that food articles of a specific colour cleanse and energize CHAKRAs associated with similar colours, and the glands, nerve centres and organs associated with the chakra are favourably affected by the food item.

The food colour	The region of the body affected	General remarks	Sample food items
Violet	Brain	Colour of psychic influence, which is supposed to bring peace and help in solving emotional problems	Violet aubergines, cabbage, jamun, sugarcane and other fruits and vegetables of this colour
Indigo	Forehead	A powerful colour that helps balance the mind by getting rid of obsessions. It is said to be helpful in stimulating intuition and imagination	Aubergine, beet root, blackberry, jamun,
Blue	Throat	Symbolizes peace and tranquility, blue can help one get a good night's sleep	Black cherries, black currants, black dates, black grapes, blue berry, jamun
Green	Heart	Colour of harmony and sympathy and can make one feel more balanced with the surroundings	Artichokes, avocado, basil, bean sprouts, broccoli, cabbage, celery, cluster beans, cucumber, greens, green aubergine, lady's fingers, lettuce, pear, pumpkin, spinach, spring onions, tindas, raw bananas
Yellow	Stomach	Colour of the mind and intellect, it is also considered as the colour of detachment. It is said to be helpful in getting rid of obsessive thoughts and habits, such as over-eating	Banana (yellow-coloured), citrus fruits, cereals, cheese, corn, eggs, grapefruit, melon, muesli, mushroom, pineapple, yoghurt and all yellow fruit and vegetables
Orange	Sex-organs	Colour of joy and happiness, it stimulates the mind, and is a powerful antidepressant	Oranges
Red	Lower regions/limbs	Colour of action, energy and change. Red colour is said to be useful for that initial boost of energy	Apple, cranberry, kidney beans, papayas, pink grapefruits, red pepper, strawberry, tomatoes, water melons

rainbow healing (Occ.) A healing method employing VISUALIZATION. It is based on the belief that visualization, when combined with meditating on the colours of the CHAKRAS ('Cosmic Rainbows Chakra Essences'), can help achieve health and wellbeing.

raindrop therapy (Occ.) Also, raindrop technique. It comprises the application of selected essential oils, dropped on the spine from about six inches above the back. After a massage of the back, a HOT COMPRESS is applied. The method includes AROMATHERAPY and REFLEXOLOGY. The therapy developed by naturopath Gary Young (b.1949), aims at bringing 'structural and electrical alignment' in the body. The 'essential oils' used are valour (a blend of rosewood, blue tansy, frankincense and spruce), thyme, oregano, basil, wintergreen, cypress, marjoram and peppermint.

rajas (Ind.) One of the three GUNAs which represents the movement of energy, vitality and initiative.

rajasic (Ind.) Pertaining to the qualities of RAJAS.

rajasic food (Ind.) Plants and vegetables which enhance RAJASIC qualities by promoting restlessness in the mind. The flesh of animals and 'lower' plants such as mushrooms and tubers are placed under this category. See also GUNA IN FOOD.

raja yoga (Yoga) Also ASHTANGA YOGA; the 'royal path' of yoga. An ancient system focussing on mind and concentration.

rakini (Yoga) The presiding deity of SVADHISHTHANA.

rakta (Ind.) Blood, one of the seven DHATUS in the body.

ranjaka pitta (Ind.) A form of KAPHA, located in the area of the liver and spleen. It aids in the digestion and assimilation of food.

rapid eye technology (Occ.) A self-empowering technique, characterized by the systematic movement of the eyes and eyelids. The technique is said to open up the neuro-pathways where one's personal/inherited traumatic experiences are believed to be trapped. Blinking, breathing and stress-reduction exercises employed are aimed at re-leasing stressful emotions and traumatic memories.

rapport (Occ.) A pleasant, friendly and comfortable interaction between client and hypnotist resulting in a level of trust. A good rapport is found to result in a greater ability to respond to suggestions in HYPNOSIS.

rasa (Ind.) Sanskrit, for essence. The bodily tissue of plasma or nutrient fluid.

Rasa Shastra (Ind.) The medicinal application of mercury as formulated in AYURVEDA and SIDDHA MEDICINE.

rasan kapha (Ind.) A form of KAPHA located inside the mouth, in or near the tongue, taste buds or salivary glands.

rasayana (Ind.) Also, rasayana chikitsa, rasayana therapy, rejuvenation therapy. Sanskrit, for the channel of essence. A medicament or a therapeutic measure aimed at slowing down the process of AGEING, by preventing disease, enhancing youthful looks. Rasayana therapy slows ageing (vayasthapan), enhances life span (ayushkarm), intelligence (medha) and strength (bala) and strengthens immune mechanisms in the body (rogapaharana samartham). See also, KAYA KALPA and REJUVENATION.

rasayana basti (Ind.) A therapeutic form of enema, aimed at REJUVENATION.

rassoul (New Age/Spa.) Also, rasul. A mineral-rich clay, also referred to as Moroccon mud, extracted from the Atlas mountains in north Africa. The clay is widely used in spas as it is found conducive for cleansing the hair and scalp. Some spas even have special 'rassoul chambers' where couples perform what is advertised as an 'oriental ceremony' in which they apply mud on each other and on themselves. The 'ceremony' is followed by a cleansing seaweed soap shower and a hot steam bath.

rational emotive behaviour therapy (Mod.) A cognitive therapy, based on the theory that cognition controls one's emotions and behaviour and therefore, changing the way one thinks about things will help resolve emotional, cognitive and behavioural problems. The method was initially developed in 1953 by American psychotherapist Albert Ellis. The system is based on the assumption that all irrational thought/images block goal achievement, leading to inner conflict, whereas rational thought/images lead to goal attainment and more inner harmony. In other words, rational beliefs are believed to reduce conflicts.

rational fasting (Mod.) A method of fasting as advocated by Arnold EHRET, who also developed the MUCOUSLESS DIET. He discouraged the intake of food, with the exception of water, during a specific period of time. The best time to fast, according to him, was in the spring or summer in winter, the body's resistance to cold weather would be lowered when fasting was undertaken. According to Ehret, drugs cling in the body for fairly long and get released during fasting, causing adverse reactions. He therefore recommended short, periodical fasting in such circumstances. He also suggested that the first meal and the menu for a few days immediately after a fast should be of laxative nature (e.g.

fresh fruits like cherries and grapes, juices, soaked or stewed prunes, munaqqa, raisins and dates, steamed vegetables and honey), rather than nourishing food.

Ravi Shankar, Sri Sri (b. 1956) (New Age) An Indian spiritual leader who popularized SUDARSHAN KRIYA. He established the Art of Living Foundation in 1982 to promote self development and health-related educational programmes.

> 'How far to heaven? Just open your eyes and look. You are in heaven.'
>
> —Sri Sri Ravi Shankar

raw juice therapy (Mod.) The use of freshly extracted juice from fruits and vegetables aimed at cleansing the body and eliminating toxins. Juice therapy also ensures a 'physiological rest' to the digestive and assimilative organs. Some common ailments, responding to raw fruits and their juices are shown in the following table:

Common ailment	Raw juice possibilities
Acidity	Carrot, citrus, grapes, spinach
Arteriosclerosis	Carrot, celery, grapefruit, lemon, lettuce, pineapple, spinach
Anaemia	Apricot, beet, carrot, celery, grapes (red), prune, strawberry, spinach
Arthritis	Beet, carrot, cucumber, grapefruit, lemon, lettuce, pineapple, sour apple, sour cherry, spinach
Asthma	Carrot, celery, lemon, peach, pineapple, radish
Bronchitis	Apricot, carrot, lemon, onion, peach, pineapple, spinach, tomato
Colitis	Apple, apricot, beet, cucumber, papaya, peach, pear, pineapple, spinach
Constipation	Apple, beet, carrot, grapes, pear, spinach
Diabetes	Carrot, celery, citrus, lettuce, spinach
Diarrhoea	Carrot, celery, lemon, papaya, pineapple
Heart disease	Beet, carrot, cucumber, lemon, grapes (red)
High blood pressure	Beet, carrot, cucumber, citrus, grapes
Insomnia	Apple, carrot, celery, lemon, lettuce, grapes
Jaundice	Beet, carrots, grapes, lemon, pear, spinach
Kidney disorders	Apple, beet, carrot, celery, cucumber, lemon, orange, parsley
Obesity	Beet, cabbage, carrot, cherry, grapefruit, lemon, lettuce, orange, papaya, pineapple, spinach, tomato
Piles	Carrot, orange, papaya, pineapple, spinach, turnip
Prostate disorders	All seasonal fruits, asparagus, carrot, lettuce, spinach
Psoriasis	Beet, carrot, cucumbers, grapes
Stomach ulcers	Apricot, cabbage, carrot, grapes
Varicose veins	Beet, carrot, grapes, orange, tomato

rebalancing (Occ.) Also, Osho rebalancing. A combination of therapies which include ENERGY BALANCING, JOINT RELEASE, sensitive DEEP-TISSUE MASSAGE and VERBAL DIALOGUE, aimed at relieving physical pain and tension. The system was founded in 1980 by a group of therapists and practitioners drawn from ROLFING, POSTURAL INTEGRATION, PSYCHOTHERAPY and TRAGER.

rebirthing (Occ.) A BODYWORK method, based on PRANAYAMA, the Indian yoga science of breath which also includes a simple but effective breathing technique. Developed in the 1970s by Leonard Orr and Stanislav Grof, rebirthing uses breathing techniques to alter the normal state of consciousness and pass through emotional blockages. The method also aims at overcoming traumatic experiences of childhood memories.

receptive imagery (Occ.) Also, passive imagery. One of the two forms of IMAGERY (the other is ACTIVE IMAGERY). Receptive imagery aims at getting insight into a particular problem (say, pain or discomfort) by observing the images that come to the mind of the sufferer. It also includes a 'dialogue' with those very images which represent receptive imagery.

Patients can use receptive imagery to help them understand the emotional meaning of their symptoms. On the other hand, active imagery is produced consciously. One can evoke active imagery by making a suggestion, such as the suggestion to make a positive change in a negative receptive image. For example, if the receptive image of a neck pain is solid rocks, one could actively transform this into soft lumps of clay. Thus active imagery aims to relieve distressing symptoms and induce relaxation.

receptive prayer (Occ.) A mental exercise, aimed at drawing spiritual strength from the infinity around. See also, PRAYER.

rechaka (Yoga) Sanskrit for expulsion; exhalation. The system of yoga insists that like inhalation, the exhalation of breath should also be smooth and continuous, though often the tempo of exhaling is somewhat different from that of inhaling.

'One way to break up any kind of tension is good deep breathing.'

— Byron Nelson

red colour therapy (Occ.) Red is considered a powerful colour and is associated with vitality and ambition. In healing, it is said to be useful in curing diseases of the blood and improving circulation. It is also said to help in depression.

red coral (Ind.) A natural substance formed from calcified skeletons of tiny polyps, red coral is traditionally believed to improve the quality of blood and strengthen the male reproductive system.

reductionism (Mod.) A theory in science that the properties of any system made of parts can be understood by knowing its constituents and their interactions with each other. Thus a complex system can be explained by reducing it to its parts. This would imply that the system does not have any characteristics which are beyond the contribution of its constituents. Reductionism is the opposite of HOLISM.

referred pain (Misc.) Pain, which is felt in a part of the body different from the area that is actually affected. Referred pain arises when a nerve is compressed or damaged at or near its origin; the sensation of the pain is felt in the area that the nerve serves, even though the injury originates elsewhere. Relieving the pressure on the nerve root may ameliorate the referred pain.

reflex points (Occ.) Energy centres in the body (on the feet, hands and ears) which act as junctions, relaying and reinforcing energy along the MERIDIANS. It has been found that the representative reflex points can be effectively stimulated in the treatment of pain in a part of the body away from them. Thus the appropriate reflex points situated in the ears, hands, and feet can be stimulated to treat a pain in the neck, shoulders, back, etc., to activate the natural ability of the body to heal.

reflexology (New Age) The art and science of working specific REFLEX POINTS to relax and relieve stress and pain in the body.

reflexology (Occ.) Also, reflex zone therapy, zone therapy. The practice of stimulating REFLEX POINTS on the feet, and less commonly on the hands, in anticipation of it having a healing effect on another part of the body. Reflexology was developed in the 1930s by Eunice Ingham, based on William

Fitzgerald's findings that specific parts of the body could have an anaesthetic effect on another area. Further research by Eunice Ingham led to a map of the body, identifying the reflex areas of the feet. Though reflex points have been identified in the hands, feet, ears and head, the most common form of reflexology is concerned with foot (FOOT REFLEXOLOGY).

reflexology workout (Occ.) A hand and foot MASSAGE, popularized by Stephanie Rick, and consisting of eight workouts which can help in weight-loss, stress control and overall health improvement.

regression (Occ.) Also, regression therapy. A method of healing in which a client is made, during a trance, to slide back in time, to remember past events that may be bothering him or her. The method allows a replaying in the imagination of past events, often with accompanying emotions. It facilitates tracing out the problem areas to their source and releasing the emotion attached to the earlier event or events.

Reich blood test (Occ.) A diagnostic method in ORGONE THERAPY, said to help ascertain the overall energy level in the body. The method is based on the belief that the morphology of erythrocytes indicates the energetic state at the time of their removal.

Reich, Wilhelm (1897–1957) (Occ.) An Austrian-American psychiatrist and psychoanalyst, known for his findings on a physical energy that permeated the atmosphere and all living matter. He called it ORGONE. His views on orgone were never accepted by mainstream science, and his claim on the discovery of 'orgone accumulator' to restore health was found to be bogus. He was imprisoned and died in prison.

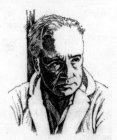

Wilhelm Reich

reiki (New Age) From the Japanese *re*, meaning universal, and *ki*, meaning life-force. An ancient method of healing, employing subtle energy-work with just one's intention, which is believed to help the body to use its 'wisdom' or ability to heal itself through energy flow. In a treatment session, the healing energy is said to be channelled through the hands of a practitioner into the client's body to restore a normal energy balance and health. The most important health benefits from reiki is stress reduction and relaxation.

Reiki was rediscovered by Mikao USUI of Japan in the late-nineteenth century. Reiki healing energy is said to provide means to balance the human energy fields (AURA) and energy centres (CHAKRA) to create conditions needed for the body's healing systems to function by themselves. The training in reiki healing is conducted at three levels, including the following:

Reiki level I The initiate is attuned to the source of healing energy and can heal himself or others, though the sessions are oriented primarily towards self-healing.

Reiki level II The initiate is attuned again to better connect with healing energy and can send energy to others, traversing distance.

Reiki level III The initiate is attuned to unlocked energy and can impart attunements for others to master. See also, ATTUNEMENT.

> 'Reiki is Wisdom and Truth.'
> —Hawayo Takata

rei-so (New Age) A form of spiritual diagnosis based on the belief that dead persons, in the form of 'spirits' (as consciousness, energy or vibration), can influence the living and those who have had intimate relationships with them, when they were alive. It is believed that such spirits create darkness in the 'auras' of people whom they affect negatively.

rejuvenation (Misc.) 1. The act of restoring youth, usually by prescribing various remedies or therapies. 2. A procedure aimed at reversing the ageing process. Historically, all human societies have strived to look for ways to regain qualities of youth. Modern science acknowledges that eight important hormones viz., HGH (human growth hormone), sex hormones, erithropoietin, insulin, DHEA, melatonin, thyroid and pregnenolone are depleted in the human system, and replacing them can bring rejuvenation. See also, KAYA KALPA, RASAYANA.

repaichage (Cos.) A massage and skin treatment for the face and limbs. A combination of herbal, seaweed and clay (mud) masks are used to help deep cleanse and moisturize the face as well as other parts of the body.

relationships, the notion of (Misc.) The idea that a biological system consists not of parts but of relationships.

relaxation methods (New Age) Methods aimed at de-stressing. A simple method of relaxation is to tense the body as much as possible for a few minutes and then release the tension.

> 'The time to relax is when you don't have time for it!'
>
> —*Sydney J. Harris*

remedy picture (Hom.) The collection of symptoms that characterize a homoeopathic remedy. For the dynamic process of cure to begin, the homoeopath matches the remedy with the patient's symptom picture; the two are like two sides of the same coin.

A common symptom (e.g. headache) may be shared by many remedies. It is, however, modified in the characteristic manner of each remedy (e.g. the belladonna kind of headache is sudden, bursting and violent).

remote diagnosis (Occ.) Also, distant diagnosis, telediagnosis. A paranormal method of discovering a particular patient's problems and diseases in his or her absence. The method includes CLAIRVOYANT DIAGNOSIS, PSIONICS, RADIONICS and TELEDIAGNOSIS.

ren (Chi.) A MERIDIAN that runs down the front of the body from the lower lip to behind the genitalia.

repressed memory (Occ.) The memory of a traumatic event unconsciously retained in one's mind, adversely affecting conscious thought, desire, and action. According to some psychologists, the *un*conscious repression of traumatic experiences is a defense mechanism which backfires. The unpleas-

ant experience may be forgotten but never forgiven. It lurks beneath CONSCIOUSNESS, causing psychological and physical problems ranging from bulimia and insomnia to suicide. See also REPRESSION.

repressed memory therapy (Occ.) A form of psychotherapy that encompasses GUIDED IMAGERY, HYPNOTISM and TRANCE WRITING. See also REPRESSION.

repression (Occ.) In psychoanalysis, the term is used to refer to a defense mechanism whereby the most traumatic experiences in life get pulled out of one's consciousness, but are dumped into unconscious. See also, REPRESSED MEMORY.

rescue remedy (Occ.) In BACH FLOWER REMEDIES, an emergency combination of five selected FLOWER REMEDIES: impatiens, star of Bethlehem, cherry plum, rock rose and clematis. It is said that rescue remedy helps cope with everyday situations that may cause tension. It is especially recommended by homoeopaths to counter situations of crisis or trauma, such as bereavement or the breakdown of a relationship.

rescue remedy spray (Occ.) RESCUE REMEDY in the form of a spray is considered handier and faster-acting, especially during emergencies.

resistance In psychoanalysis, the client's refusal or unwillingness to follow the instructions of a therapist.

resonance and entrainment in healing (Occ.) An approach to healing in VIBRATIONAL MEDICINE, based on the notion of ENTRAINMENT. When two entities vibrating at different frequencies come together, there are three possibilities: either the higher frequency matches with the lower one, or vice versa, or they meet somewhere in between. A healer exhibiting an extraordinarily high vibration, is said to match his vibration with the patient without any exhaustion.

resort spa (Spa) A SPA facility, which offers professionally administered services and a variety of health treatments (QI GONG, MASSAGE, VIBRATIONAL MEDICINE, YOGA) at a vacation spot within a resort or hotel with various leisure activities including golf, tennis, horse-riding, skiing, water sports and children's programmes.

response prevention (Mod.) A therapeutic method wherein the client is advised not to respond to the stimuli administered by the practitioner. This technique is prescribed in the treatment of anxiety disorders and phobias.

resveratrol (Mod.) A phyto-medicine, found in the skin of red grapes and sold as a nutritional supplement. The supplement is said to have anti-tumour, anti-ageing and anti-inflammatory properties. Resveratrol seems to explain the so-called 'French paradox' of why the incidence of coronary heart disease is relatively low in southern France despite the high consumption of foods rich in saturated fats.

revivification (New Age) 1. Reliving an event in a session of HYPNOSIS. During revivification, the hypnotized client is said to be able to hallucinate, re-experiencing a past event which has remained dumped in his or her unconscious for a long time. 2. Renewal or restoration of life; the act or state of being recalled to life.

rhabdomancy (Occ.) A type of DIVINATION in which the diviner uses a hazel rod to trace the presence of minerals or metals below the ground. See also, DOWSING.

rhus toxicodendron (Hom.) Also, poison ivy, rhus tox. Used in the treatment of conditions with symptoms of fever, restlessness and swollen glands.

rhythm healing (Occ.) The therapeutic application of complex rhythmic patterns in music, believed to affect the internal rhythms in the body, such as heart beat, respiration and brain-wave patterns.

'Rhythm is the essence of music, as it finds its counterpart in man's innermost self.'

—Georg Wilhelm Friedrich Hegel

rhythmic entrainment intervention (Occ.) Also, RET. A rhythm-based programme in MUSIC THERAPY, using auditory rhythmic stimulation (usually the rhythm from percussion instruments), aimed at stimulating and improving brain function. See also RIFE THERAPY.

rhythmical breathing (Occ.) A form of PRANAYAMA in which the ratio of time taken for exhalation and inhalation is 1:1. Rhythmical breathing is said to generate energy in the body.

rhythmical massage (Occ.) A form of MASSAGE, which is characterized by an EFFLEURAGE in the form of the figure '8'. Developed by Ita Wegman (1876–1943) a physician, the massage through its gentle rhythmic quality of touch is said to penetrate deep and help harmonize the imbalances in the system.

rhythms, biological (Misc.) Also, body rhythms. The rhythms found inside (endogenous) and outside (exogenous) the body, which determine the health and quality of human life. For example, the pulsation to secrete growth hormone is reported to occur a few hours after one goes to sleep; thus, it depends upon the sleep–wake cycle. This rhythm is found inverted in night workers who go to bed during the day. (Reilly et. al. 1997). However, most biological rhythms have both exogenous and endogenous influences. It is difficult to determine the endogenous nature of a rhythm unless the exogenous influences are first removed.

rib breathing (Occ.) A form of CHEST BREATHING, wherein the abdomen is drawn in as the diaphragm is pushed upwards, while the chest is somewhat expanded. This form of breathing ensures a better supply of oxygen to the lungs, compared to COLLARBONE BREATHING. It is also considered beneficial for trimming excess fat deposits in the stomach region, particularly in men.

Rife therapy (Occ.) Devised by Royal Raymond Rife, an American microbiologist, in 1930, as a method to cure cancer. The therapeutic intervention, with what is called Rife instruments, is based on the concept that every specific disease has a unique, modifiable electromagnetic signature. Due to technical difficulties and stringent laws in the US, Rife abandoned research in this area. However, in 1986, Barry Lynes, a medical journalist, researching information on cancer cures, stumbled on Rife's discovery and found that his research was very well documented in the scientific and medical journals of the thirties. Lynes subsequently authored a book *The Cancer Cure that Worked* (1987) and brought Rife into focus again.

The therapy makes use of the Rife resonators which generates resonance waves in the required frequencies so that they destroy harmful bacteria without doing any harm to the user. Rife therapy is claimed to be fast and painless, and has proven to be entirely free of side effects. See also, MUSIC THERAPY, RHYTHMIC ENTRAINMENT INTERVENTION.

ritual (Misc.) 1. A set of actions, performed mainly for their symbolic value as mandated by religion or tradition. 2. The performance of acts or ceremonies as prescribed by tradition. The objectives of rituals are many; while they comprise compliance with religious obligations or ideals, they also achieve a sense of satisfaction of spiritual or emotional needs for those who perform them. They also strengthen social bonds; even actions like hand-shaking and sending greetings to others can be considered common rituals.

ritucharya (Ind.) A seasonal regime, prescribed in AYURVEDA for the maintenance of health and well-being.

RL-test (Mod.) A modern diagnostic method in ACUPUNCTURE. Which aims at diagnosing the conditions of MERIDIAN.

ro-hun therapy (New Age) A healing method which aims at exploring how 'energies' accompanying birth, childhood, adulthood, and 'past lives' affect the client's life, and how such 'energies' can be transformed for the overall benefit of the client's health and wellbeing. It helps in identifying and releasing 'faulty thought patterns which block us from attracting our highest good.' It aims at clearing the seven major CHAKRAS, creating an even flow of energy.

rock salt (Ind.) Traditionally considered the healthiest form of salt in AYURVEDA, rock salt is used to pacify all the three DOSHAs. It is also used as an appetizer, a laxative and digestive.

rock water (Hom.) Pure, clean water filtered through layers of rocks, often originating from an underground spring and believed to be health-enhancing. Though not a flower essence, rock water is included among the original BACH FLOWER REMEDIES. According to Bach, rock water softens the hardened 'personlity' in people imparting them a spontaneous, flexible and fluid approach in their lives.

roga pariksha (Ind.) 1. The examination of disease. 2. Diagnosis

rogi pariksha (Ind.) 1. The examination of a client or a patient.

> 'The art of medicine consists of amusing the patient while nature cures the disease.'
>
> —Voltaire

role-playing (New Age) A widely popular method in the sessions of BEHAVIOUR THERAPY, wherein the therapist demonstrates effective behaviour, taking into consideration real-life situations encountered by the client. 2. Enacting the role of a character as in theatre. Role-playing also includes computer-role playing games, play-by-mail games, etc. Simulations and role-playing exercises which have been among the oldest educational methods, have also seeped into healing. See also PSYCHODRAMA.

Rolfing (Mod.) Also, structural integration. A codified series of soft-tissue manipulations, referred to as DEEP-TISSUE MASSAGE or deep-tissue therapy, Rolfing aims at enhancing vitality and wellbeing by realigning the body structurally, thereby harmonizing its fundamental movement patterns. It was developed in the 1950s by physiotherapist Ida Pauline Rolf (1896–1979). The method is oriented towards developing a method of organizing human structure in relationship with gravity, which Rolf referred to as structural integration. According to her, bound-up fascia (or connective tissue) often restricted opposing muscles from functioning independently from each other. The technique aims at separating the bound-up fascia by deeply separating the fibres manually so as to loosen them to ensure smooth

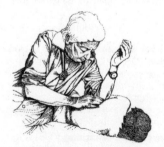

Rolfing; Ida Rolf at work

movement patterns. The process of breaking down old muscle patterns by massage contemplated here is somewhat akin to Wilhelm Reich's technique in which massage was used to break down what he referred to as armour. According to sceptics, however, there is no scientific evidence connecting muscle movements with trapped emotional experiences. See also, ORGONOMY; REICH, WILHELM.

Roman bath (Rom.) A local bath complex in ancient Rome. Traditionally, the term referred to a series of pools: hot (caldarium), warm (tepidarium) and cold (frigidarium) pools. A public bath at Pompeii contained two tepidariums and caldariums, along with a PLUNGE POOL and a large exercise area. In contemporary SPAS, however, the term Roman bath refers to a hot whirlpool or JACUZZI.

root chakra (Yoga) See MULADHARA CHAKRA.

rosary 1. A set of prayer beads and a system of prayer, which combines PRAYER and MEDITATION. Roman Catholics and Hindus wear rosaries as an outward symbol of their faith.

Rosen method (Occ.) Also, Rosen technique. A non-invasive approach, named after Marion Rosen, a Germany-born physiotherapist, who discovered that in physiotherapy settings, verbalization of sensations and emotion play an active role in helping clients recover faster than in sessions without them. The system also uses gentle touch to detect areas of muscular contraction, referred to by Rosen as holding breath. By enhancing the client's self-awareness, the method is said to be of use in cases of chronic health conditions.

rosemary (Eur.) *Rosmarinus officinalis.* From the Latin *rosmarinus*, meaning dew of the sea. A woody herb with fragrant evergreen needle-like leaves, native to the Mediterranean region. Rosemary has been long-known for its role in memory-enhancement. It is also useful in the treatment of fever, halitosis, headaches and rheumatism and is also reported to control dandruff. Hungary water, prepared by seeping fresh rosemary tops in wine for a few days and then distilling it, is rubbed vigorously on hands and feet for relief from gout.

royal jelly (Nat.) A milky white substance formed in the salivary glands of worker bees, meant for feeding the queen bee. It has traditionally been used as medicine to treat loss of appetite, fatigue, infertility and asthma. It is also said to help prevent the development of leucoderma. Though there is no scientific evidence to support the claim that it plays an important role in retarding AGEING, royal jelly commonly finds use in anti-wrinkle creams.

ruah (Heb.) The soul, represented by emotion and corresponding to the *heseddindtiferet* triad.

Rubenfeld synergy (Mod.) A blend of BODYWORK and psychotherapy developed in the 1960s by Ilana Rubenfeld, an orchestra conductor. As therapies were divided into physical or psychological approaches, she found that no clinician was able to cut across disciplines to directly address the mind–body interaction on both fronts. Based on her experience with ALEXANDER TECHNIQUE, FELDENKRAIS METHOD, GESTALT THERAPY and HYPNOTHERAPY, this method was created so as to allow the address of interplay between physical and psychological factors. This method is said to be useful in the treatment of headaches, lower-back pain, stress, anxiety disorders and depression.

ruby (Gem.) Wearing this red-coloured gem-stone is believed to strengthen the heart, stimulate circulation and improve digestion.

Rudra (Ind.) The destroying force of the Universe; the presiding deity of MANIPURA CHAKRA.

Rudra granthi (Yoga) A GRANTHI or a psychic knot situated between the throat and the eyebrow. When 'pierced', through KRIYA practices, a yogi is said to overcome illusion (maya), experiencing a constant sensation of bliss.

Rudraksha (Ind.) From the Sanskrit, for the eye of Rudra. The seeds of the blue marble tree (*Elaeocarpus* spp.), described in Indian legends as 'the tears of Shiva', are widely used in making ROSARY. A garland of rudraksha seeds from one face to twenty-one faces is called Inderakshi mala and is believed to bring great luck to its wearer; otherwise, the bigger the seeds the better.

The therapeutic benefits from the various varieties of Rudraksha are indicated in the table below:

Type of Rudraksha	Probable therapeutic impact
1-faced	To cure chronic diseases like asthma and tuberculosis
2-faced	For mental peace
3-faced	Fights jaundice
4-faced	For curing diseases of the brain
5-faced	For general wellbeing
6-faced	To cure epilepsy and gynaecological problems
7-faced	For a long, healthy life
8-faced	For mental concentration
9-faced	For spiritual progress
10-faced	For whooping cough
11-faced	For issueless women
12-faced	For vitality and personality
13-faced	For virility
14-faced	Cures several diseases
15-faced	Cures skin ailments
16-faced	For general wellbeing
17-faced	For physical assets
18-faced	For pregnant women
19-faced	For good health
20-faced	For improving eyesight
21-faced	For general wellbeing

'Rudrakshas and Shivalingas—the bigger they are, the more powerful.'

—Meru Tantra

Rudraksha dowsing (Occ.) Also, Rudraksha lolaka. A method of DOWSING, employing RUDRAKSHA, aimed at detecting any inner growth such as cancer, pregnancy or cardiac disorders. The dowser's concentration, experience and extra sensory perception are pivotal for the accuracy of this method.

rue (Am./Ind./ Chi.) Also, Chou cao (Chi.) *Ruta graveolens.* Also, garden rue, herb of grace. TRADITIONAL CHINESE MEDICINE uses this herb for cooling and relieving swellings, boils and eczema. It is also used in the treatment of difficulties in urination, epilepsy, fever, hernia, influenza, physical injuries, rheumatoid arthritis etc. Rue is also a remedy in HOMOEOPATHY.

rutucharya (Ind.) The adaptation of diet and lifestyle, based on seasons, in AYURVEDA. Adapting food regimen in accordance with the season was considered a means to prevent various ailments, as each season had its own impact on the balance of the DOSHAs.

sabhukta (Ind.). The administration of medicine along with food.

sacred psychology (New Age) A form of 'experiential psychology', as developed by American philosopher, Jean Houston. According to this theory, three realms of experience exist: ordinary reality, the collective unconscious, and 'the realm of God'. CONSCIOUSNESS has been the original focus of psychological research in the past and has in recent years been revised as a central topic of enquiry.

> 'We all home the extraordinary coded within us, waiting to be released.'
>
> —Jean Homston

sadhak pitta (Ind.) A form of PITTA, located at the area of the heart. It is associated with the perception and intelligence of an individual. In derangement, this DOSHA is said to create anger, anxiety, fear and mania.

saffron (Misc.) *Crocus sativus*. Saffron, the most expensive spice in the world, is extracted from the flowers of this plant; the style of the flower is collected and dried before being used as a seasoning or colouring agent.

An Assyrian dictionary of botany, written in 668–633 BCE, refers to the medicinal use of saffron: dyspnoea (breathing difficulty), painful urination, menstrual disorders, and 'diseases of the head'.

sagarbha pranayama (Yoga) A form of PRANAYAMA in which a MANTRA is chanted repeatedly as breathing exercises are undertaken.

sahaja samadhi (Occ.) ENLIGHTENMENT. The final attainment of a spiritual path, considered the most healthy condition in humans, embodying the transcendence from selfishness and yielding to the condition of natural and spontaneous ecstasy.

Sahaja Yoga (Occ.) Sanskrit, meaning the easy path. A natural and spontaneous approach to self-healing, based on the notion of thoughtless state of mind (nirvichara). A simplified version of RAJA YOGA, Sahaja Yoga is based on the notion that God is simple and hence the way to reach him is also simple. It believes that like power, thought and speech, spirituality can also be transmitted without much effort. In this practice, negative thoughts, which are believed to act as poison in the system, are purged through MEDITATION.

sahasra lekhana sadhana (Occ.) Sanskrit, for 'thousand-times writing discipline'. A spiritual practice, of repeatedly writing a selected MANTRA, for, say, 108 or 1,008 times. The practice is believed to focus one's concentration, bringing relief from mental tension or stress. Phrases or passages from sacred texts from religions can be used for meting technique.

sahasrara (Occ.) Sanskrit, for the lotus of a thousand petals. 1. 'The crown chakra'. The seventh chakra representing SUPERCONSCIOUSNESS. 2. A meeting point of KUNDALINI with SHIVA, pure consciousness. 3. The cranial psychic force centre considered as midway between psychic and spiritual realms in human existence. There is some disagreement about the location of sahasrara in the body. According to Sir John Woodroffe and C.W. Leadbeater, it is located at the crown point at the very top of the head, while others (e.g. Sri Aurobindo) held that it is situated at a distance above the head. However, there is unanimity about the higher chakras representing varying degrees of transpersonal or intuitive divine consciousness.

> 'It's hard to think at the top.'
>
> —Stringfellow Barr

sahita kumbhaka (Yoga) From the Sanskrit sahita, meaning accompanied by. A form of PRANAYAMA emphasizing the retention of breath (KUMBHAKA). The method is said to keep the body agile, strong and flexibile, calm the mind, and control hunger and thirst during long sessions of meditation.

Saiva Yoga (Yoga) A form of YOGA based on the belief that the mind cannot be effectively controlled through compulsion and repression. Gradual taming of the mind 'as that of a young steed', instead, is advocated.

shakti (Yoga) 1. Primal energy 2. Manifested consciousness 3. Energy, personified as female and distinguishable from its male or passive aspect, SHIVA, representing pure consciousness.

shaktichalini (Yoga) Sanskrit, meaning conducting the thought-force. A DHARANA practice involving regulation of breathing and focussing AWARENESS on CHAKRAS.

shaktipat (Yoga) The transmission of spiritual energy. It can be accomplished in four ways: through touch, word, look or thought. It is essential that the receiver remains in a state of readiness to receive such transmission.

> 'You can pour tea only into an empty cup.'
>
> —A Zen saying

salakya tantra (Ind.). A branch of AYURVEDA dealing with the organs above the head, viz., ear, nose, throat and eyes.

salamba sarvangasana (Yoga) Shoulder-stand. An ASANA aimed at integrating the body, it is also referred to as the mother of asanas. The shoulder-stand is suggested as an integral part of physical exercises for its health benefits.

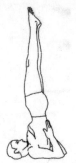

Salamba sarvangasana

> 'People with high blood pressure should only attempt this asana immediately after holding the final pose of halasana for at least three minutes.'
>
> —B.K.S. Iyengar

salt glow (Spa) Also, salt-rub therapy. A SPA treatment in which the client's skin is rubbed with a coarse salt, sometimes in combination with fragrant oils. This exfoliating treatment helps remove the top layer of dead skin, stimulating circulation. The treatment is, however, not recommended for the face or damaged skin.

salya tantra (Ind.) Also, salya chikitsa. From the Sanskrit salya, meaning broken parts of an arrow or other sharp-edged and pointed weapons. Surgery, a branch of AYURVEDA. This ancient method was used to remove, by surgery, broken parts of arrows and other sharp-edged and pointed weapons from the bodies of soldiers.

samadhi (Yoga) 1. A state of mind in which the seer and the seen unite through the very act of seeing. 2. A blissful and illumined state of CONSCIOUSNESS, devoid of any thinking process.3. The state of meditative union with God.

Of the many types of samadhi, the most significant distinction is between conscious (samprajnata) and supraconscious (asamprajnata) ecstasy; the latter is expected to pave the way towards the dissolution of the karmic factors deep within one's mind. Beyond both these types of ecstasy lies enlightenment, which is also sometimes referred to as the condition of natural or spontaneous ecstasy (sahaja-samadhi). PATANJALI dealt with the following categories of samadhi: distinguished contemplation (samprajnata samadhi), non-distinguished contemplation (asamprajnata samadhi), deliberated absorption (savitarka samadhi), non-deliberated absorption (nirvitarka samadhi), reflective meditation (savichara samadhi), non-reflective meditation (nirvichara samadhi), meditation in which the mind continues to carry the seeds of earthly impressions (sabija samadhi), and where each seed of such earthly impressions are erased (nirbija samadhi).

> 'A man who has experienced samadhi even once is a completely changed man. He has raised himself above the average and he sees everything in a totally new light.'
>
> —Swami Satyananda Saraswati

> 'By not thinking of external things and simultaneously by keeping away from inner thoughts, one experiences samadhi.'
>
> —Hathayoga Pradipika

Samadhi Yoga (Yoga) A system of yoga, which is said to lead one to ecstasy.

> 'Death or fear, have I none,
> Nor any distinction of race;
> No father, no mother,
> Not even a birth I own.
> No friend, no foe
> Neither disciple, nor guru.
> For, I am eternal–bliss–awareness
> I am Shiva! I am Shiva!'
>
> —Adi Shankara

samagni (Ind.) A balanced state of digestive fire, which ensures good health. According to SUSHRUTA, JATHARAGNI (digestive fire) is of four types. These are samagni (normal), visamagni (abnormal), teekshagni (above normal) and mandagni (below normal). Samagni is considered balanced when all three doshas, VATA, PITTA and KAPHA are in a balanced state. When agni is disturbed by the vata, the resulting condition is known as vishamagni. When pitta affects agni, teekshagni results and when kapha affects agni, mandagni results.

samana (Ind.) A form of PRANA associated with the gastro-intestinal tract and lungs and which aids the absorption of nutrients and oxygen. It is also said to homogenize sensory, mental and emotional experiences. Its movement is said be a churning action from the periphery towards the centre.

samanu (Occ.) A method of cleansing energy channels with the help of BIJA MANTRA (seed-syllable). Eastern systems of medicine rely heavily on the clearance of the energy channels to facilitate healing.

saman vata (Ind.) A form of VATA, existing at the area of stomach and duodenum, saman vata is said to help in the digestion of food and in isolating its essence from the wastes for supply to blood stream.

samanvay mudra (Occ.) A MUDRA formed by joining all the fingers, symbolizing the coordination between the Five Elements that constitute the universe. Practising this mudra is said to help in developing strength.

samatva (Occ.) Evenness. The mental condition of harmony and balance, considered essential for good health.

sambhavi mudra (Occ.). A DHARANA practice of gazing forward and then upwards, as high as possible, without tilting one's head, while focussing on the centre of the eyebrows, i.e. the THIRD EYE. The practice also involves breath-control, focussing awareness on the CHAKRAs and VISUALIZATION. Its practise is said to help awaken the eyebrow chakra (AJNA), considered the seat of union of the lower and the higher forms of CONSCIOUSNESS.

samayama (Ind.) The integration of the body, breath, mind, intellect and self. PATANJALI grouped DHARANA, DHYANA and SAMADHI under this broad category.

samayik (Occ.) A spiritual practice aimed at SELF-REALIZATION, and one of the most important ritual practices of Jainism.

Samkhya Yoga (Yoga) A system of YOGA, aimed at the development of insight.

samprapti (Ind.) Also, agati, jati. 1. The process of development of diseases, which starts from a disturbance of the DOSHA equilibrium. 2. Pathogenesis.

Samputa Yoga (Yoga) A practice in TANTRISM, which involves sexual intercourse (maithuna).

samskara (Ind.) 1. The 'root' impressions derived from past experiences. In the Hindu tradition, it represents subconscious impressions, not only of the present life, but also of the past (or prenatal tendency), left behind by each act of volition. The countless impressions, encrusted in the mind, are believed to get eliminated through YOGA. 2. Sacraments or rites, performed to mark a significant transition in one's life.

samyama (Yoga) The simultaneous, spontaneous and effortless flowing of attention, awareness and energy in MEDITATION. In RAJA YOGA, the process of samyama consists of three stages: focussing attention on the object meditated upon (DHARANA) and contemplation (DHYANA) and absorption of the object meditated upon (SAMADHI). Each of these stages can help in altering one's awareness from the normal waking state to a healthy state of profound depths of absorptions in the continuum of CONSCIOUSNESS.

samudrika lakshana (Ind.) The ancient science of understanding the state of the body, mind and spirit from the physical features of a person. See also, PHRENOLOGY.

santhara (Ind.) An age-old Jain ritual, in which aged devotees volunteer to give up food and water. It is practised by the faithful to purify the body and sublimate desire.

sangoma (Afr.) A traditional herbalist of South Africa.

sankhaprakshalana (Ind.) Also, sankhaprakshalana kriya. In AYURVEDA, an approach to COLON-CLEANSING. It comprises the rapid gulping of large volumes of saline water and doing twenty-five ASANAs.

sankirtana yoga (Ind.) A system of YOGA which seeks to find union with the Divine through songs and chants. Emotion-rich melodies are said to facilitate focussing one's awareness on the object of MEDITATION. It is an effective way of practicing MANTRA YOGA and japa yoga.

> 'Singing is the best way to get rid of the blemish of one's ego.'
>
> —Sai Baba

shanti (Yoga) Sanskrit, for peace. A religious rite or ceremony to remove evil influences. Several BIJA MANTRAS referring to various parts of the body are recited to bring peace.

> 'We do not need guns and bombs to bring peace, we need love and compassion.'
>
> —Mother Teresa

> 'When the power of love overcomes the love of power, the world will know peace.'
>
> —Jimi Hendrix

santosha (Occ.) 1. Contentment.

> 'Not external contentment to impress other people, but inner contentment (requires cultivation).'
>
> —Swami Satyananda Saraswati

Sanyasa Yoga (Yoga) A system of YOGA, with its emphasis on renouncing the world as an illusion (maya).

> 'So long as one has a longing to obtain any particular object, one cannot go further than the object.'
>
> —Hazrat Inayat Khan

sapta dhatu (Ind.) The seven DHATUs in the human body, viz., fluid (ras), blood (rakta), muscles (maans), fat (meda), bones (asthi), bone-marrow (majja) and semen (shukra). Anomalies in these tissues are believed to cause various diseases.

Saptanga Yoga (Yoga) From the Sanskrit saptanga, meaning seven limbs. A system of YOGA which emphasizes the following seven 'limbs' as essential for this yoga practice: good deeds, consisting of six purificatory methods (SHAT KARMA); posture (ASANA); seal (MUDRA); sensory inhibition (PRATYAHARA); breath-control (PRANAYAMA); MEDITATION (DHYANA); and ecstasy (SAMADHI).

sarasvatarishta (Ind.) A formulation in AYURVEDA containing 4–6 per cent alcohol from natural fermentation. It also contains BRAHMI, SHATAVARI, PIPPLI, vidari, usira, honey and gold ash (svarna bhasma), all considered to help in developing one's mental faculties and treating nervous anxiety, diminished libido, mental confusion, tremors, and memory loss.

sardius (Gem) A gemstone believed to prevent nightmares.

sarpagandha *Rauwolfia serpentine*. Also, Indian snakeroot. The trade name *rauwolfia* relates to the sixteenth-century German botanist Leonard Rauwolf who introduced this indigenous herb to the West. The plant is believed to have been in use in the Indian system of medicine for about 4,000 years. In ancient times, Indian physicians used its roots as an antidote for the bites of poisonous reptiles and snakes. In Indian folklore, the herb is used to reduce fever during delivery and to stimulate uterine contractions and promote the expulsion of the foetus. It is also said to lower blood pressure and treat insanity.

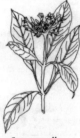

Sarpagandha

sarira durgandha haranam (Ind.) Body deodorants, commonly used in ancient India.

sarsaparilla (Am.Ind./Ind.) *Smilax regelii*. Also, nannari (Tam.) A vine whose roots are considered highly medicinal. Sarsaparilla is grown in parts of south India, and also in Central and South America and Mexico. In American folk medicine, it has been used as a general tonic for physical and sexual weakness. In Tamil Nadu, it is mainly used in flavouring summer beverages. It is also used in HOMOEOPATHY as a remedy.

sarvangasana (Yoga) An ASANA recommended for the maintenance of the thyroid and as a cure for hernia, menstrual disorders, piles, reproductive malfunctions and varicose veins.

Sarvatobhadra Yantra (Num./Occ.) An auspicious YANTRA believed to bring good luck to its wearer. In the yantra shown below, the total of the numbers, counted from any side, of all sides and angles is 36.

10	17	2	7
6	3	14	13
16	11	8	1
4	5	12	15

satavari (Ind.) *Asparagus racemosus* Also, sparrow grass, wild asparagus. Considered a powerful RASAYANA drug which can improve physical as well as mental performance by slowing down the ageing process. It is also a galactogogue and is widely used in the treatment of amoebiasis, diabetes, diarrhoea, dyspepsia and tumours.

satmya (Ind.) Homologation or suitability as an indicator of health or morbidity.

satori (Jap.) Japanese, meaning to understand. Also, *kensho*. A Zen Buddhist term for ENLIGHTENMENT. It is also taken as a transitory state of epiphanic enlightenment.See also, SELF-REALIZATION.

> 'Satori is the raison d'être of Zen, without which Zen is no Zen.'
>
> —D.T. Suzuki

sattva (Ind.) A GUNA representing purity and 'uplifting' tendencies, towards clarity, light or awakening, and conducive to the overall health of an individual and society. It is also believed to awaken one's CONSCIOUSNESS.

sattvavajaya (Ind.) Psychotherapy in the system of AYURVEDA. According to AYURVEDIC texts, sattvavajaya is based on three principles: a) replacing undesirable emotions by other incompatible emotion; b) repetitive assurances and c) psychological shock.

sattvic (Ind.) 1. Of SATTVA 2. Pure 3. Genuine

sattvic food (Ind.) Foods which are digested easily and promote mental clarity, calmness and harmony. Sattvic foods are closest to their natural forms and include honey, milk, milk products, fruits, dry fruits, nuts, grains, sprouts, most fresh vegetable except garlic, onion, scallions, and chives. Sattvic food is moderately cooked with few spices and little fat. See GUNA IN FOOD.

satya (Yoga) Truthfulness. Freedom from falsehood is an attitude to be developed by those who wish to advance in the practise of YOGA; one of the FIVE MORAL RESTRAINTS, spelt out by PATANJALI in his ASHTANGA YOGA.

sauna (Spa) A SPA treatment in which dry heat, intense, but tolerable, is used to induce perspiration in the body. In combination with refreshing cold showers, sauna is said to enhance circulation and activate the body's immune system. It also helps relieve stress.

savasana (Yoga) An ASANA wherein the body is kept motionless so as to imitate a corpse. It is aimed at relaxing the body to make the breathing process soft and easy.

> 'Relaxation begins from the outer layer of the body and penetrates into the deep layers of our existence.'
>
> —B.K.S. Iyengar

saw palmetto (Am. Ind.) *Serenoa repens* A fan palm whose fruits were used as food by native Amerians. It is also reported to be used in the treatment of urino-genital problem including prostate enlargement.

scalp acupuncture (New Age) A healing system developed by Toshikatsu Yamamoto of Japan in 1973, aimed at relieving neurological diseases and dysfunctions.

scarring moxibustion (Chi.) A form of MOXIBUSTION, which is used along with Chinese medical astrology for longevity.

Schroth cure (Nat.) Also Schroth fast. A method of FASTING, developed in 1830 by Johann Schroth (1798–1856), a Silesian naturopath. The fasts, undertaken as a treatment for rheumatism, is observed on alternate days over a period of two to three weeks.

Scotch hose (Spa) Also, Scotch hose massage. A HYDROTHERAPY treatment in which an alternate hot- and cold-, and fresh- and saltwater jet at high velocity is directed on a standing client through a high-pressure hose. This invigorating treatment method is said to help relieve sore muscles and stimulate circulation.

Schuessler Biochemic system of Medicine (New Age) An alternative healing system, using twelve cell-salts, also known as BIOCHEMICS developed in 1873 by Wilhelm Heinrich Schuessler, a German physician.

scientology (Occ.) A philosophy and quasi-religious movement and a system of psychotherapy. The Church of Scientology was founded in 1953 by Lafayette Ron Hubbard (1911–86), a science-fiction writer. The theory which posits reincarnation aims at the liberation of one's 'essential' or 'true, spiritual' self.

sclerology (Occ.) Also, sclera diagnosis. A diagnostic method in which the location and shape of blood vessels visible in the sclera are said to broadly indicate the health condition of an individual.

Scottish douche (Spa) A DOUCHE in which water jets are directed up and down against the spine to stimulate the nervous system. In modern SPAs, SAUNAs are constructed with Scottish douches.

scrying (Misc.) Also, crystal ball, crystal gazing, CRYSTALOMANCY. The ancient 'art' of seeking information on occult matters or the future by looking at a candle flame, a transparent object, or an object with a reflective surface (e.g. a globe of quartz glass, mirror, etc). Scrying also includes HYDROMANCY, in which the practitioner looks for water.

séance (New Age) French, for seat. 1. A get-together for the purpose of experiencing psychic or supernormal phenomena. 2. An assembly to communicate with the dead. The séance or sitting is led by a MEDIUM who is believed to be under the control of a spirit during the séance, usually conducted in a dark or semi-dark room. See also OUIJA, PLANCHETTE.

seasonal ailments (Ind.) In ancient systems of medicine like AYURVEDA, diseases associated typically with specific seasons were said to flare up when the characteristics of a particular season manifested themselves in excess or were marked by deficiency.

seaweed wrap (New Age) Also, seaweed therapy. The application of concentrated seawater and seaweed (e.g., iodine-rich algae) containing nutrients including minerals, rare trace elements, vitamins, and proteins. Aimed at DETOXIFICATION and increased circulation, the wraps are said to counter CELLULITE. See also ALGOTHERAPY, BODYWRAP.

see-and-be technique (New Age) A method of direct image substitution, which involves repeatedly picturing one's body as perfectly healed (or healthy). A three-dimensional image of one's body, or a part thereof, may also be mentally constructed over which an image of whatever is needed for healing is superimposed. See POSITIVE IMAGERY.

seed-pressure method (Chi./New Age) A form of AURICULAR THERAPY in which the practitioner tapes a bean or seed to ACUPOINTS so as to keep them pressed. See also PRESS SEEDS.

seichim (Egy./New Age) Pronounced say-keem. The healing art of the ancient Egypt, said to be rediscovered in 1992 in New York. The method includes visualizing what is referred to as the goddess energy for health and wellbeing. See also, VISUALIZATION.

seicho-no-ie (New Age) Japanese for house of growth. A movement founded in Japan in 1930 by writer Masaharu Taniguchi (1893–1985). Its 'divine message of great harmony' insists upon the development of an attitude of gratitude, and reconciling with one's surroundings. Spiritual healing forms a major component of seicho-no-ie, which combines elements of Christianity with those of Buddhism, and considers that no illness exists in reality and whatever appears as illness is a false experience.

seiki (Jap.) Universal healing energy. See also PRANIC ENERGY.

seiki-jutso (Jap.) A method of healing in which SEIKI, universal energy, is said to get transferred to a patient through the whorl of hair at the crown.

seitai (Jap.) 1. A natural movement-based therapy that works with the body's natural ability to correct and align postural faults and injury sites. 2. Body alignment adjustments.

seitai control technique (Jap.) Also seitai technique. A healing method which aims at restoring SEITAI, the 'true' and 'perfect' state of physical and mental health, to those who suffer from ailments and diseases.

self (Occ.) 1. The complete individual distinguishable from another being. 2. Ego. 3. Consciousness of one's identity. 4. One's own interest or benefit.

'The perfect man has no self; the spiritual man has no achievement; the sage has no name.'

—Chauang Tzu

self-applied health enhancement methods (Occ.) Also, SAHEM. An approach to health which applies time-tested and cost-effective knowledge and procedures. Developed by Roger Jahnke, the methods include gentle movements and postures (e.g.TAI-CHI), self-massage (e.g. AURICULAR THERAPY), and other exercises of BREATHING and RELAXATION.

self-care modalities (Occ.) Self-treatment methods which can be learnt with the aid of instructional books or videos or by attending training programs.

self-expansion therapy (Occ.) A form of PSYCHOTHERAPY as developed in New York by Ralph Gray. It is based on the concept that one can attain growth and transformation by listening carefully to one's inner self—reconnecting one's thoughts and feelings, recovering one's authenticity and releasing physical and emotional blockages.

self-healing (Occ.) Also, self-help treatments. An independent approach to health, without the involvement of a therapist. The method, which aims at tapping one's innate healing potential, commonly employs several traditional time-tested measures such as the use of affirmation, QIGONG, PRAYER, SELF MUSIC THERAPY, VISUALIZATION, YOGA and PRAYER.

'The aim of medicine is to prevent disease and prolong life, the ideal of medicine is to eliminate the need of a physician.'

—William J. Mayo

self-help for stress and pain (Occ.) A system of APPLIED KINESIOLOGY, as developed by Elizabeth and Hamilton Barhydt to combat stress and pain. The method is also said to be helpful in the treatment of back pain, carpal tunnel pain, foot-ache, headache, knee pain, neck and shoulder pain, tendonitis etc.

self-hypnosis (Occ.) 1. A self-induced TRANCE state. 2. A self-healing practice, through AUTO-SUGGESTION. This method is used as a cure for several psychosomatic disorders, including addiction, depression and insomnia.

self-intercourse (Chi.) A Taoist technique of MEDITATION and VISUALIZATION, in which the practitioner visualizes the co-mingling of energies of fire ('universal energy from the heart') and water ('sexual energy from the kidney') inside a person's body. The result is said to be the formation of an imagined vapour spreading through the length and breadth of the body, cleansing the MERIDIANS, cells, tissues, organs and glands.

> 'To love oneself is the beginning of a lifelong romance.'
>
> —Oscar Wilde

self-music therapy (Occ.) A concept and practice of MUSIC THERAPY, developed in its current form by T.V. Sairam (b. 1946), an Indian writer on alternative medicine. The selection of appropriate melodies and rhythms is emphasized in his works for self-healing.

self-realization (Ind.) Also, nirvikalpa samadhi. Considered the ultimate spiritual attainment, self-realization refers to a state of CONSCIOUSNESS which is said to occur when the KUNDALINI energy, located in the root-chakra (MULADHARA), rises and pierces through the crown chakra (SAHASRARA). It refers to the realization of that which exists beyond the mind, time, form and space.

self-reflection (Occ.) 1. observing oneself—one's mind, emotion and thinking 2. Introspection. 3. Playback of impressions and memories stored in the SUBCONSCIOUS. Self-reflection is said to lead towards relaxation.

self-suggestion (Occ.) A method of healing through imagining that one is getting healed through repeated self-suggestion. See AUTO-SUGGESTION THERAPY.

self-talk (Occ.) A method of healing, by adopting what is referred to as 'positive self-talk', carried out as a soliloquy to overcome adverse situations and trauma in one's life. According to some psychologists, many gains in life can be attributed to the quality of one's 'inner conversations'; negative self-talk could lead to negative feelings about oneself, resulting in low self-esteem, affecting one's performance. A technique for arresting negative self-talk is referred to as 'thought stoppage' which is said to help student athletes identify and eliminate negative thought-patterns so as to achieve mental strength and increased ability.

semi-vegetarianism (New Age) Also, demi-vegetarianism, fishetarianism, pescetarianism, pesco-vegetarianism, pollo-vegetarianism, vegequarianism. A lifestyle which eliminates specific foods from the diet. A semi-vegetarian may eat sea-food but avoids red meat, beef, pork and lamb. A pollo-vegetarian eats chicken, while a fishetarian allows fish in his diet.

sensate focus (Mod.) Also, sensate focussing. An expression associated with a set of specific sexual exercises for couples or for individuals. First introduced by Masters and Johnson, the exercises are aimed at increasing personal and interpersonal awareness. The participants are advised to focus on his or her own varied sense-experience for mutual sexual enjoyment, rather than see orgasm as the only goal.

sepia (Hom.) Also, ink of cuttlefish. The discharge used by a cuttlefish to change their skin-colour and pattern and slip away from the predator. Homoeopaths use sepia in the treatment of apathy, a weak mind or memory.

seven malas (Ind.) The seven waste-products excreted by the human body. The quality, quantity and frequency of discharge of malas are said to determine the health or lack of it in an individual. The AYURVEDIC system pays special attention to malas such as faeces, urine, and sweat. In the TIBETAN SYSTEM OF MEDICINE, urine evaluation is a central tool diagnostic.

The overall quality of a person's health depends on the condition of OJAS which comes from the refinement of sukra or semen. Both AYURVEDA and TRADITIONAL CHINESE MEDICINE (notably the Daoists) advocate the retention of semen as far as possible or practicable and specific restraint techniques with regard to sexual activity are recommended.

AYURVEDA postulates that every refinement process undertaken in the body results in a pure substance and a waste (mala) as indicated in the following table:

Process	Pure substance generated due to the process	Toxins or wastes generated due to the process
Refinement of food in the body (ahara	Rasa dhatu (an activated nutritive essence)	Faeces and urine

rasa)	corresponding to the Chinese concept of YINGQI	
The refinement of rasa dhatu	Rakta or blood	MUCUS
The refinement of rakta	Mamsa or flesh	Bile
The refinement of mamsa	Meda or fat	Excretions from the eyes, nose and ears
The refinement of meda or fat	Asthi or Bones	Sweat
The refinement of asthi or bones	Majja or Marrow	Hair and nails
The refinement of majja or marrow	Sukra or bindu or semen (corresponding to the Chinese concept of JING, it is also found in women.)	Oil of the skin
The refinement of sukra or bindu or semen	OJAS	Nil

> 'Semen is under the control of the mind; life is dependent on semen. Mind and semen, therefore, need to be protected by all means.'
>
> —*Hatha Yoga Pradipika*

seven keys meditation programme (Occ.) A system based on seven spiritual tools, called keys, said to unlock one's inherent healing potential. Popularized by David Wheele, the method is based on the belief that the universal energy, present in all human beings, can be transmitted for healing purposes.

seven tissues (Ind.) SAPTA DHATU, the seven body tissues including plasma (rasa), blood (rakta), muscle (mamsa), fat (meda), bone (asthi), marrow (majja) and semen (shukra). These dhatus are said to support and derive energy from each other and are affected by each other both in health as well as in diseased conditions.

sex surrogate (Mod.) A member of a SEX THERAPY team, who may engage in physical relations with a client. This practice was conceived by the American authors, William Masters and Virginia Johnson (1970) in their work *Human Sexual Inadequacy*. It has been reported that since the 1980s female clients have also opted for male surrogates with whom they try and sort out their sexual dysfunctions.

sex therapy (Mod.) A form of PSYCHO-THERAPY dealing with problems faced by couples in sexual encounters. The procedure, which takes place in an intensive marital workshop, includes talking about one's sexual history, physical check-ups and specific physical movements or exercises. Sexual dysfunctions, such as impotence, low desire, premature ejaculation, erectile dysfunction, sexual fetishes, painful sex and lack of sexual confidence are treated in strict confidence. In what is referred to as comarital therapy, both members of a couple are treated by a team comprising one male and one female therapist as it is recognized that sexual dysfunction takes place in the context of the interaction between the two partners and is not a consequence of the problem of one partner alone. In individual therapy, however, for only one of the partners, the services of a SEX SURROGATE, considered unethical in many parts of the world is used. Group therapy programmes are also conducted—for both single-sex or male–female groups—in which individuals discuss their feelings with fellow participants.

> 'Sex is one of the nine reasons for reincarnation... The other eight are unimportant.'
>
> —Henry Miller

sexual energy massage (Occ.) A MASSAGE on the genitals, along with BREATHING exercises. The MASSAGE aims at releasing the energy blocked in the genitals (*ching chi*) for dissemination in the body and absorption by the bones. *Ching chi* is believed to be a combination of sex hormones and sex energy that can regenerate bone marrow.

shabda Brahman (Occ.) The healing rhythms or vibrations, considered divine and protective. The ancient system of NADA YOGA had acknowledged the healing effects of intonation.

shabda Yoga (Occ.) An approach to ENERGY HEALING which employs intonations (NADA); sound vibrations in chanting are employed for dissolving energy blockages.

Shadanga Yoga (Yoga) A system of YOGA which emphasizes on the following six 'limbs' as essential for this yoga practice: breath-control (PRANAYAMA); sensory inhibition (PRATYAHARA); MEDITATION (DHYANA); concentration (DHARANA); examination (TARKA); and ecstasy (SAMADHI).

shadow sound therapy (Occ.) Also shadow therapy. A combination of MUSIC THERAPY and GUIDED IMAGERY, as developed by a Jungian psychotherapist Elidé M. Solomon. The therapy is based on the belief that interpreting images of the UNCONSCIOUS could quicken the process of healing.

shakti (Ind.) 1. Energy or power. 2. The ultimate Reality in its feminine aspect.

shalakya tantra (Ind.) A branch of AYURVEDA akin to ophthamology and otorhinolaryngology, essentially eye, ear, nose and throat medicine. Surgical techniques as well as herbal treatments for conditions such as cataracts are included in this branch.

shalya (Ind.) Also, shalya tantra. The ancient method of surgical practice in AYURVEDA which uses 101 types of blunt and twenty-one types of sharp surgical instruments. Shalya covers topics such as anatomy, physiology and the surgical treatment of conditions such as bowel obstructions.

'The hand of the surgeon is the best, the most useful and the most important of all surgical instruments.'

—Sushruta

shaman (Occ.) A man or woman capable of entering into a TRANCE or dream state or an altered state of CONSCIOUSNESS. Techniques employed by shamans to achieve such states include chanting, dancing, drumming, rattling or the consumption of hallucinogenic drugs.

shamanic extraction healing (Occ.) Also, shamanic healing. An ancient practice of accessing the realms of spirits for guidance and healing. The procedure includes sensing and removing illness or pain localized in one's body. A SHAMAN professes to 'extract' the misplaced energy from a person's body by pulling it out and putting it inside the saline water.

shamanic psychotherapy (Occ.) A form of SPIRITUAL HEALING, based on SHAMANISM and the concept of REINCARNATION, shamanic psychotherapy combines traditional shamanic methods with modern psychotherapeutic knowledge and is found to be effective particularly in the treatment of trauma.

shamanism (Occ.) A traditional religious and healing concept and practices rooted to the belief that the spirits (both good and evil) can be influenced by SHAMANs who serve as intermediaries between man and such spirits.

shankh mudra (Occ.) Also, shell-posture. A MUDRA, formed by placing firmly the left-hand thumb on the right palm and wrapping the fingers of the right hand around it. The right-hand thumb is made to touch the fingers of the left hand. The mudra is said to remove speech disorders, impart sweetness to the voice and aid digestion.

sharira (Ind.) AYURVEDA believes that the human body comprises three bodies: sthula sharira or annamaya kosha, the gross, physical body; SUKSHMA SHARIRA or linga sharira , the SUBTLE BODY (which in turn includes pranamaya, manomaya and vijnanamaya Koshas) and karana sharira or ANANDMAYA KOSHA, the causal body.

shashankasana (Yoga) The rabbit-in-the-moon posture. Considered a cure for impotency and sexual debility, this ASANA is believed to influence the flow of adrenaline, be responsible for the fight-or-flight response mechanism and tone up the lumbo-sacral nerves.

shat karma (Ind.) Also, shat kriyas. The six purificatory processes recommended to be undertaken before PRANAYAMA, are indicated in the following table:

Name of the process	Description
Neti	Nasal cleansing
Dhouti	Cleansing the alimentary canal
Nouli	Abdominal massage
Basti	Enema
Kapalabhati	Purification of the frontal portions of the brain
Trataka	Developing the power of concentration

shaucha (Yoga) Purity, one of the five methods of self-regulation in the yoga system of PATANJALI. It refers not only to regular baths for cleansing the body, but also to the cleansing of emotional or mental dirt.

> 'In deep meditation the flow of concetration is continuous like the flow of oil.'
>
> —Patanjali

shavasana (Yoga) Sanskrit, for a corpse-like posture. An ASANA recommended for relaxation.

sheaths See KOSHAs.

shell scrying (New Age) A method of SCRYING, using shells which sound like the ocean.

shen (Chi.) The mind or spirit, designed to unlock blocked energy.

shen tao (Chi.) A system of healing, combining ACUPRESSURE and TAOISM.

shiatsu (Jap.) From the Japanese *shi*, meaning finger, and *atsu*, meaning pressure. An ancient and commonly practised Japanese version of ACUPRESSURE in which rhythmic pressure is applied on specific points by the practitioner for three to ten seconds along the MERIDIANs (energy channels), using the fingers, hands, elbows, knees and feet. The shiatsu technique also involves patting, rotating, sweeping and vibrating affected areas. For the purposes of treatment, the human body is divided into three centres:

Centre	Activities	Chakra(s)
Head	Imagination and intellectual pursuits (mental activities)	Eyebrow (AJNA) chakra
Heart	Social interaction (emotional activities)	Throat (VISHUDDHI) and heart (ANAHATA) chakra
Abdomen	Survival and practical concerns in life (physical activities)	Base (MULADHARA), sacral (SVADISHTHANA) and solar plexus (MANIPURA) chakra

While dividing the energy equally between all three centres is considered an ideal health situation, because of various factors such as education, culture, diet, lifestyle, or habits, energy is not equally divided, with an adverse impact on the chakras/organs where there is reduced energy. To overcome this, shiatsu has formulated a variety of exercises.

shilajit (Ind.) A bituminous substance obtained from rocks, as a black, sticky mineral that leaks out of them. Shilajit is used in AYURVEDA to cure diabetes.

shinkiko (Jap.) From the Japanese *shin-ki*, meaning healing energy). Also, energy flow, true ki, true-ki energy flow. A system of healing, based on the relationship between the material (e.g., illness) and non-physical world (e.g., energy), shinkiko, devised by Japanese healer Masato Nakagawa, aims at synchronizing one's vibration with the healing vibration of QI. Healing is believed to take place as one learns to keep the healing vibration within oneself and heighten it continuously in one's body. Apart from increasing the levels of energy in the body, shinkiko is also said to impart an intuitive sense.

shiroabhyanga (Ind.) Head massage in AYURVEDA.

shirodhara (Ind.) Dripping of warm medicated oil in a steady flow over the forehead of a patient. The treatment lasts for seven to ten minutes or more. One of the adjunct procedures of PURVAKARMA designed to calm the mind and pacify VATA in the central nervous system, it is believed to help one focus, concentrate and relax the mind. The treatment is also recommended for insomnia, memory loss, mental disorders, neurological disorders, senile dementia, and paralysis. Medicated oil may be, at times, replaced with milk or sour milk.

shirovirechana (Ind.) Medicated powder or oils administered through one's nasal passage. One of the five methods of SHODHANA, shirovirechana is said to eliminate the excessive DOSHAs in the head region and enhances the functional capacity of eyes, ears, nose, throat and tongue. It also helps the breathing process, making it smooth and steady. During nasya, a patient is advised to avoid speech, laughing and swallowing. See, NASYA.

Shivambu (Ind.) Also, water of life, water of Shiva. The age-old practice of using one's own urine as a remedy, especially in treating serious or terminal illnesses. According to ancient texts such as *Shivambu Kalpa Vidhi*, urine is the most potent and readily accessible cure, and is referred to as 'holy water'. See also AUTO-URINE THERAPY.

'Shivambu is a divine nectar.'

—*Shivambu Kalpa Vidhi*

Shivambu kalpa (Ind.) The ancient technique of using one's own urine (SHIVAMBU) as medicine. See also AUTO-URINE THERAPY.

shleshman kapha (Ind.) A form of KAPHA, located between two joints or layers, providing lubrication to save the vital parts and organs from friction.

shodhana (Ind.) 1. The procedure of PANCHAKARMA 2. Cleansing of the body, by eliminating deposits of toxins (AMA). AYURVEDA prescribes five effective methods for cleansing the whole body: blood-letting (RAKTAMOKSHANA), emesis (VAMANA), enema (BASTI), nasal cleansing (NASYA) and controlled purgation (VIRECHANA).

shodhana nasya (Ind.) The administration of medicated oil into the nostrils for eliminating toxins accumulated in the paranasal sinus zone. See also, NASYA.

shoshuten (Chi.) A Taoist method of purifying SUSHUMNA, by the circulation of energy in the upper part of the body.

showers, cold (Nat.) Recommended for bringing down the temperature and to overcome fatigue.

showers, hot (Nat.) Recommended for reducing the pain and to soothe irritation.

showers, localized (Nat.) The beneficial effects of showers on localized areas are indicated in the following table:

Areas	Therapeutic benefit	Remarks
Soles of feet	Cold feet, weakness, bladder incontinence, impotency	Strong cold jet from ½ to 2 minutes
Entire feet	Headache, congestion in head	Strong cold jet for ½ to 2 minutes
Abdomen	Constipation	Cold jet for a few seconds
Abdomen	Pain in bladder, uterus, ovaries and in pelvic areas	Hot jet for 3 to 5 minutes
Abdomen	Chronic ailments, irritation in lower back, weak abdominal organs.	Alternate jets (3 minutes hot and 3 minutes cold repeated for a number of times)
Chest	Deficiency in circulation particularly in pelvic regions	Cold jet for a few seconds
Shoulder	Bladder malfunction, constipation, incontinence	Cold jet for a few seconds
Face and scalp	Fatigue and brain disorders	Very cold jet for a few minutes
Face and scalp	Tension, trauma	Neutral jet for a few minutes
Anus	Haemorrhoids, constipation	Cold jet for a few minutes
Anus	Fissures, rectal ulcers	Hot jet for a few minutes

showers, lukewarm (Nat.) Recommended for bed-wetting, nervousness and pelvic problems.

shuddhi (Yoga) Sanskrit, meaning purification. A state of purity, a synonym of SHODHANA.

shukari mudra (Occ.) A MUDRA that resembles the pig's snout; See SAMANVAY MUDRA.

shukra (Ind.) The male and female reproductive tissues in the human body, often translated as semen.

sialogogue (Mod.) An agent that stimulates salivation.

siddha medicine (Ind.) From the Sanskrit siddha, meaning perfect. Also, Shaiva school of medicine, Siddha system of medicine. An ancient Indian system of medicine, based on humoural pathology (i.e., bile, phlegm and wind) like AYURVEDA and UNANI. It is, however, distinguished by the herbs and medicines it uses in its treatment procedures.

The popularity of Siddha medicine is somewhat confined to south India, particularly Tamil-speaking areas. According to Siddha philosophy, the human body (microcosm) represents the universe (macrocosm) as both are made of two essential entities: matter and energy. Both the body and the universe are made of five primordial elements: munn (earth), neer (water), thee (fire), vayu (wind) and aakasam (ether).

siddha meditation (Yoga) An ancient method of MEDITATION, which combines BREATH CONTROL and MANTRA.

siddha pulse diagnosis (Ind.) An ancient method of pulse-reading in SIDDHA MEDICINE. In this system, pulse is considered the manifestation of PRANA. Traditionally, reading the pulse was taught by gurus to their disciples.

siddhasana (Yoga) An ASANA, believed to facilitate the maintenance of both spinal and mental steadiness, essential for prolonged MEDITATION.

Siddha Yoga (Yoga) A system of YOGA which emphasizes on the role of a guru (sidddha guru or the perfect master) in the disciple's achieving the higher levels of CONSCIOUSNESS. According to siddha traditions, knowledge and wisdom can be transmitted to disciples more easily by a guru than by scriptures or manuals. Gurus of this lineage include Guru Dattatreya, Sai Baba of Shirdi, Nityananda and Swami Muktananda.

siddhayoni asana (Yoga). A variation of SIDDHASANA, recommended for women.

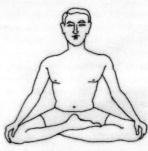

Siddhayoni asana

siddhi (Yoga) 1. Psychic achievements 2. A supernormal perceptual state 3. Powers achieved through occult practices.

> 'Destiny is not a matter of chance, it is a matter of choice; it is not a thing to be waited for, it is a thing to be achieved.'
>
> —William Jennings Bryan

silent hikes (Occ.) A leisurely long walk in natural settings in which the walker is supposed to connect with the natural surroundings. See also, WALKING MEDITATION.

silica (Hom.) Also, flint. In HOMOEOPATHY, silica is used in the treatment of conditions that cause sweating, weakness and sensitivity to cold.

silk reeling (New Age) Also, winding-silk power, foundational training. The name is used allegorically for a set of exercises in which movements are smooth and consistent, just like the action of reeling out silk successfully; reeling too fast would make the silk break as reeling too slow would make it tangled. These exercises are choreographed to be continuous, with cyclic patterns performed at constant speed. The patterns are performed in a concentrated, meditative state with an emphasis on relaxation.

similia principle (Hom.) A homoeopathic tenet according to which to cure a sick person with a remedy, one should look at the remedy that provokes similar symptoms in a healthy person. The similia principle was postulated by HAHNEMANN.

simonton method (Occ.) A form of GUIDED IMAGERY as developed by Oscar Carl Simonton, a radiation oncologist, and Stephanie Mathhews-Simonton, a psychologist. The method is based on the ground philosophy that cancer is a message of love and an invitation to become 'who you truly are'.

sirobasti (Ind.) Also, sirovasthi. Pouring down of warm, medicated oil on the head, through a special hollow cap kept on the head of the patient. The oil is allowed to remain there for about forty-five minutes. The procedure is intended to stimulate brain function. The treatment is also recommended for chronic colds, facial paralysis, headaches, insomnia, sinus and several diseases of ears, eyes, nose and throat.

sirolepana (Ind.) The application of a paste of herbs on the scalp. This treatment is recommended to treat mental and neurological disorders.

sirsasana (Yoga). Headstand. Known as the king of ASANAS, this posture is believed to strengthen the musculoskeletal system, and improve respiration and digestion.

sitali (Yoga) Also sitali pranayama. A form of PRANAYAMA in which one's tongue is stretched a little away from the lips and folded like a tube through which air is sucked, with a hissing sound. After retaining the breath so inhaled for as long as easily possible, the air is exhaled slowly through the nostrils. Sitali can be practised seated (in PADMASANA, SIDDHASANA or VAJRASANA), standing or while walking. It is said to help purify blood and to be of use in 'disaster management', when there is a shortage of drinking water as by practising it one is said to be able to overcome thirst.

sithikarana vyayama (Yoga) Loosening exercises such as jogging, running, rotation and stretches.

sitkari (Yoga). Also, hissing breath, sitkari pranayama, teeth hissing. A form of PRANAYAMA characterized by a hissing sound, produced by the tongue touching the upper palate, when the breath is drawn in through the mouth. After the breath is held (KUMBHAKA) for as long as one comfortably can, it is released through both the nostrils. While assuaging thirst, hunger, indolence and sleep, sitkari pranayama is believed to make the practitioner both vigorous and beautiful.

sitz bath (Nat.) Also, hip bath. A type of bath in which only hips and buttocks are soaked in water or saline solution. The name is derived from *citizen*, German for 'to sit'. It is needed to ease the pain of hemorrhoids, uterine cramps, painful ovaries and testicles. Inflammatory bowel diseases are also treated with sitz baths.

Sitz bath (cold water)	Sitz bath (tepid)	Sitz bath (hot)
Circulation in abdominal organs is improved, relieving from problems relating to constipation, delayed menstruation, impotence, vaginal discharge	Works as a sedative, tepid sitz bath can be helpful in the treatment of colic, fevers and uterine spasms	Hot sitz bath is said to be useful in the treatment of cystitis, haemorrhoids, respiratory difficulties, sciatica, spastic constipation, vaginal spasms

Sivananda, Swami (1887–1963) (Yoga) An Indian allopathic doctor who alleviated human suffering through YOGA and Himalayan herbs. He established the Divine Life Society at Rishikesh.

Sivananda Yoga (New Age) A school of YOGA which includes the application of ASANAS, breathing exercises, MEDITATION, deep relaxation, vegetarianism and study of scriptures. This variety of yoga was founded by Swami Vishnu-Devananda, author of the contemporary Yoga classic, *The Complete Illustrated Book of Yoga*. (1960), and named after his teacher, Swami Sivananda.

six healing sounds (Chi.) Also, six-syllable secret, six basic soundless sounds for health. A series of arm movements and vocalizations accompanied by VISUALIZATION, aimed at releasing negative energies. Inhalation of the breath is done through the nose and a much slower exhalation is through the mouth.

The practice is said to help develop concentration and strengthen the body through the synchronization of sound vibrations with that of the internal organs. There is one way of inhaling and six of expelling the breath, sounded by using six different syllables whose significance is shown in the table:

Syllable	Healing significance
Hsü	To display malaise
Her	To release anger
Hoo	To expel cold
Sss	To regain equilibrium
Chway	To expel heat
Shee	To relieve tension

'Each of the six vibrations has a psychic influence on its corresponding organ sphere which prompts the expulsion of impurities from the sphere and its manifestations, and the gathering of fresh energy into each system.'

—Ni Hua-Ching

sixty-one point relaxation exercise (Occ.) Also, sixty-one-point shavayatra, sixty-one-point exercise. A method of relaxation aimed at REJUVENATION. The sixty-one points refer to the specific parts of the body taken up for relaxation. The exercise is believed to affect one's energy field, eliminating muscular tension.

The following sixty-one points are travelled through slowly by being aware of each one of them as blue-coloured marbles located at their respective areas in the body, while remaining motionless in SHAVASANA, the corpse pose:

1. Point between the eyebrows
2. Hollow of the throat
3. Right shoulder joint
4. Right elbow joint
5. The bend of the right wrist
6. Tip of the right thumb
7. Tip of the right index finger
8. Tip of the right middle finger
9. Tip of the right fourth finger (ring finger)
10. Tip of the right small finger
11. The bend of the right wrist joint
12. Right elbow joint
13. Right shoulder joint
14. Hollow of the throat
15. Left shoulder joint
16. Left elbow joint
17. The bend of the left wrist joint
18. Tip of the left thumb
19. Tip of the left index finger
20. Tip of the left middle finger
21. Tip of the left fourth finger (ring finger)
22. Tip of the left small finger
23. The bend of the left wrist joint
24. Left elbow joint
25. Left shoulder joint
26. Hollow of the throat
27. Heart centre
28. Right nipple
29. Heart centre
30. Left nipple
31. Heart centre
32. Solar plexus (just below the bottom of the breast bone)
33. Navel center (two inches below the physical navel)
34. Right hip joint
35. Right knee joint
36. Right ankle joint
37. Tip of the right big toe
38. Tip of the right second toe
39. Tip of the right third toe
40. Tip of the right fourth toe
41. Tip of the right small toe
42. Right ankle joint
43. Right knee joint
44. Right hip joint
45. Navel center (two inches below the physical navel)
46. Left hip joint
47. Left knee joint
48. Left ankle joint
49. Tip of the left big toe
50. Tip of the left second toe
51. Tip of the left third toe
52. Tip of the left fourth toe
53. Tip of the left small toe
54. Left ankle joint
55. Left knee joint
56. Left hip joint
57. Navel center (two inches below the physical navel)

58. Solar plexus
59. Heart centre
60. Hollow of the throat
61. Centre between the eyebrows

smoke scrying (Occ.) A method of scrying using smoke. See also SCRYING.

smokey quartz (Gem.) Also stabilizing stone. A protective stone said to impart stability and protection and believed to bring good luck to its wearer.

smudging (Am. Ind./Occ.) The use of a smoking stick made from dried herbs including cedar, juniper, lavender, sage and sweet grass, intended to cleanse the human AURA. It is believed that by burning herbs the surroundings are cleansed and purified; the smoke is said to banish negative energies from the atmosphere. The term smudging is Native American.

snehana (Ind.) Also, oleation therapy. The administration of fatty substances such as ghee, marrow or vegetable oils through ingestion, enema or the skin (ABHYANGA). Snehana is performed on weak people and the elderly. It rejuvenates the skin and restores the appetite.

snehan kapha (Ind.) A form of KAPHA, located in the head region. Besides nourishing the brain, this DOSHA is said to support vital sensory functions (smell, sight, taste, etc) which results in overall efficiency of the human organism in terms of knowledge, intelligence, behaviour and memory.

snehapanam (Ind.) A diet regime comprising the ingestion of medicated oils on an empty stomach, aimed at curing afflictions including constipation, hyperacidity, osteo-arthritis and ulcers.

snow quartz (Gem.) A stone that is believed to bring good fortune. It is also considered helpful in meditation.

soaring crane qigong (Occ.) A 'fast acting' form of QIGONG, developed in the 1970s by Zhao Jin-Xiang. It is said to clear MERIDIANS.

so-hum meditation (Occ.) An approach to healing through meditation. Deeply inhaled breath (sounding like 'so') and slowly exhaled breath (sounding like 'hum') form the main focus of concentration.

solution-focussed brief therapy (Occ.) An approach to psychotherapy which focusses on building a 'solution', rather than solving a 'problem'. Attention is given to developing a picture of the 'solution' and discovering the resources to find it; current resources and future hopes are relied on, with present problems and the past causes overlooked. The method encourages the formulation of future goals as it is believed that clarity of one's goals makes them all the more achievable. The method is said to be useful as an adjunct to other treatments.

somato emotional release (New Age) A system of BODY-ORIENTED PSYCHOTHERAPY which aims at helping the mind to get rid of the adverse effects of past trauma and associated events. John E. Upledger and Zvi Karni who developed this system were of the view that the body often retained, rather than dissipated, physical forces as the result of accident, injury or emotional trauma. The procedure of somato emotional release is said to help the client physically identify and expel the 'energy cyst' by re-experiencing and resolving the unpleasant incidents.

'The shock of any trauma, I think, changes your life. It's more acute in the beginning and after a little time you settle back to what you were. However it leaves an indelible mark on your psyche.'

—Alex Lifeson

sonopuncture (Occ.) An approach to healing in which an ultrasound device transmits sound waves directly to the body's ACUPOINTs. Apart from sound waves, ACUPUNCTURE also uses heat, friction, laser beam, magnets and suction.

soul retrieval (Occ.) A form of spiritual healing addressed to trauma patients, soul retrieval is based on the belief that when faced with trauma, either physical or emotional, one's soul may lose a part of itself for the benefit of the whole. In a soul retrieval session, a shamanic healer supposedly traces out the lost part and returns it to the client.

soul energetics (Occ.) An approach to healing, in which one's voice is analyzed to identify and apply its sound frequencies, capable of releasing psychological and emotional energies. The system, developed by Helena Reilly, is based on the belief that one's voice is a reflection of one's overall energetic vibrations in the body.

> 'The body is a truly sensitive and receptive instrument and its vibrations, like sound, express the harmony or dissonance within it.'
>
> —B.K.S. Iyengar

sound probe (Mod./New Age) A device which is said to emit a pulsed tone of three alternating frequencies that can destroy the microbes not in resonance with the body in the atmosphere.

sound therapy (New Age/Occ.) An approach to healing in which sound vibrations, are believed to play a therapeutic role in the prevention and treatment of several mental problems. By directing selected sound waves to areas of the body where the body's resonant frequency is out of balance, it is believed that balance can be restored.

This therapy is based on the premise that every individual emits non-verbal sounds or frequencies called 'essential silent perceptors', which characterize his or her psychological and physical status. A cymatic computerized system devised by Peter Manners has some 800 sound frequencies, identified for treating specific health complaints. See also CYMATICS, MUSIC THERAPY, NADA YOGA, RAGA CHIKITSA, SELF-MUSIC THERAPY.

> 'First of all, you must use your ears to take some of the burden from your eyes. We have been using our eyes to judge the world since the time we were born. We talk to others and to ourselves mainly about what we see. A warrior always listens to the sounds of the world.'
>
> —Carlos Castaneda

sound touch therapy (Occ.) A form of TONING, developed by Wayne Perry, aimed at the identification of 'personal missing notes' and making an attempt to facilitate their return. Using a chromatic tuner, the client's voice is assessed for pitch, octave and notes that are either missing and/or in stress. Energy blockages in the body, causing disease or pain, are also attempted to be eliminated with appropriate sound waves. See also, SOUND THERAPY

South Beach diet (Mod./New Age) A modern approach to DIET which advocates eating high-fibre carbohydrates which offer nutritional benefits, such as brown bread instead of bread made of refined flour.

spa (New Age) Originally, the name of a small town near Liege in Belgium, the term has come to refer to all leisure resorts with thermal or mineral water, used for drinking and bathing, offering solace to the diseased and the convalescent. Currently, the term refers to a place devoted to enhancing one's overall wellbeing through a variety of professional services that encourage REJUVENATION.

spanda (Ind.) 1. Vibration, creative spark, movement or motion associated with waves of activity emanating from an unseen source of spontaneous outcome. 2. The subtle creative pulse of the universe found in the dynamism of all living forms. Spanda also refers to CONSCIOUSNESS, and is an essential feature of KUNDALINI YOGA. Oriental healing techniques encourage the development of an intuitive consciousness of spanda for overall health and wellbeing.

Sparsha Yoga (Ind.) An ancient system of YOGA, which stresses on contact or touch exercised with MANTRA recitation and breath-control (PRANAYAMA).

> 'Touch is as essential as sunlight.'
>
> —Diane Ackerman

specific human energy nexus therapy (New Age) A form of TOUCH THERAPY, based on the belief that an emotional energy field (chi field) permeates and surrounds one's physical body.

> 'We must fully embrace each level and then move higher—as if ascending the rungs of a ladder.'
>
> —Ken Wilber

speech therapy (Mod.) Also, speech and language therapy, speech-language pathology. A rehabilitative or corrective treatment of disorders resulting in difficulty with communication, both verbal and non-verbal. Depending on the severity, disorders can be treated in a variety of ways, including instructive and repetitive practice sessions and the introduction of strategies to improve the client's functional communication level. Speech therapists also advise for swallowing difficulties.

> 'While uttering a word, the speaking desire inspires our mind to speak, after referring to the intellect.'
>
> —Panini

spinal balancing (New Age) An approach to healing through the manipulation of the spine, referred to as the 'tree of life'. The spine is first evaluated structurally and energetically through visual observation and palpation. Then specific manipulations are carried out so as to align the sacrum or 'sacred bone' with the spine and cranium so as to facilitate the flow of energy to all parts of the body. Techniques include muscle release, vertebra release, stretch release, pelvis adjustment and sacral balancing.

spinal touch (New Age) A method of holistic healing aimed at postural correction, developed by John Hurley, a mechanical and structural engineer. Spinal touch is said to be useful in the correction of chronic and acute pain conditions. This simple technique is used by many professionals including chiropractors, masseurs and physical therapists.

spirit guide (Occ.) A term used in the Western traditions to describe an entity that remains a disincarnate spirit in order to act as a spiritual counsellor or protector to a living incarnated human being.

spirit healing (Occ.) An ancient system of healing in which healing is ascribed to disincarnate spirits. Unlike in hand-healing and SPIRITUAL HEALING, spirit healing comes directly, not through healers.

spirit releasement (Occ.) Also, depossession. An ancient form of EXORCISM said to remove 'negative' energy from persons and property. In ancient traditions, diseases were believed to be caused by the presence of attached spirit entities in one's AURA. It was believed that the spirit entities could be removed by dealing directly with the victim, using various techniques. The principal requirement seems to have been a degree of assertiveness on the part of the facilitator.

spirit surgery (Occ.) A form of surgery performed by other-worldly healing entities at the behest of a spiritual leader.

spiritual beauty care (Occ.) A part of alternative beauty care, aimed at restoring the balance of bodily energies, as developed by writer Jacqueline Sinnige.

spiritual counselling (Occ.) An approach to healing, including CHAKRA HEALING, INNER CHILDWORK and TOTEM PSYCHOLOGY.

spiritual hypnosis (Occ.) The use of HYPNOSIS to achieve insight, enlightenment or other experiences, aimed at having a healthy disposition.

spiritual integration therapy (Occ.) A form of VIBRATIONAL MEDICINE, developed by Lynda Darbes which includes concepts and practices from BODYWORK, DREAMWORK, IMAGERY and MEDITATION.

spiritual medicine path (Am.Ind./Occ.) A form of CHEROKEE medicine, which includes giving thanks to God. See also PRAYER.

> 'Only faith in God and His remembrance is demanded for speedy recovery in addition to perseverance.'
>
> —Bhag Singh Lamba

spiritual psychology (Occ.) A healing modality that springs from concepts and practices from ANTHROPOSOPHY, ARCHETYPAL PSYCHOLOGY and JUNGIAN PSYCHOLOGY.

> 'Both modern psychology and yoga stress the importance of evolution of continual growth of each individual from "less wholeness" to "more wholeness".'
>
> —Swami Satyananda Saraswati

spiritual psychotherapy (Occ.) An approach to healing, as developed by Carol Weidberg which includes DREAMWORK. The approach is based on the Jungian theory of synchronicity.

spiritual practices (Occ.) An approach to good health and wellbeing with activities which are believed to purify and strengthen one's mind and body, paving way towards a spiritual path. Such activities include CHANTS, CONTEMPLATION, JAPA, MEDITATION and seva or selfless service.

> 'Science is not only compatible with spirituality, it is a profound source of spirituality.'
>
> —Carl Sagan

> 'The spiritual is the parent of the practical.'
>
> —Thomas Carlyle

spiritual surgery (Occ.) A form of SPIRIT SURGERY, as popularized by Lorna Green.

spirulina (New Age) Blue-green alga, rich in gammalinoleic acid (GLA) and other nutrients, used as a high-protein food supplement.

sponge bath (Nat.) Also, sponging. Sponge baths are recommended particularly for bedridden patients. While cold sponge baths are recommended for bringing down fevers, hot sponge baths have a sedative effect.

sports massage (Mod.) A MASSAGE used before, during or after athletic events to prevent injuries and to promote circulation.

sports psychology (Mod.) A specialization in psychology, aimed at understanding the mental factors that affect a sportsman's performance and the application of this knowledge for the improvement of individual as well as team performance. It includes minimizing the psychological pressures of injury and poor performance and managing emotions in sportsperson.

> 'If you can't accept losing, you can never win.'
>
> —Vince Lombardi

sports spa (New Age) Also, adventure spa. A SPA resort providing specialized services for sportspersons and adventure enthusiasts. Facilities include therapeutic baths and body treatments, suitable for such sports/adventure.

spring dragon qigong (Chi.) A traditional Taoist approach to healing through a series of eight movements, aimed at increasing the flow of QI energy through meridians and strengthening the immune mechanism.

srota (Ind.) Energy channels in the body, in which blockages usually take place. The flow through srota may be affected variously: through deficient or excess flow of energy or by forming blockages or overflows (bypass). In addition to the body, the mind is also considered to have a srota, the mandvaha srota, that can affect the flow of emotions, sensory impressions, and thoughts in the same way as physical srotas affect energy flow. In many ways, srotas are akin to the Chinese MERIDIANS, in as much as the types of disorders perceived (deficiency, excess, blockage, overflow) are similar in both.

sroto-shuddhikara chikitsa (Ind.) A procedure to regulate the energy flow in SROTA for health and wellbeing.

St John's Wort (Chi.) *Hypericum perforatum*. Also, goat weed, klamath weed, Quan ye lian qiao (Chi.) TRADITIONAL CHINESE MEDICINE uses the plant in the treatment of anxiety, nervousness, sleep disorders and depression.

standing meditation (Chi.) A system of QIGONG, consisting of simple postures which can be done in unusual places, such as the grocery store or in waiting halls. See also TADASANA, ZHAN ZHUANG.

steam room (Spa) In a SPA, a special room which is kept at 110 to 130° F and in which humidity is generated. A steam room is used for maintaining clean and soft skin and calming down nervous tensions.

steam therapy (Spa) The therapeutic use of steam, particularly in pulmonary and respiratory problems. It is also widely used to open up the pores of the skin and increase circulation to eliminate toxins. See also, BASHPA SWEDANA.

step aerobics (Spa) Stepping up and off a platform during an aerobic-exercise session. The workout is aimed at toning the hips, legs and buttocks.

sthala basti (Yoga) Also, dry basti, sushka basti. Sucking of air through the anus, while remaining in an inverted ASANA like VIPAREETAKARANI. According to *Hatha Yoga Pradipika*, the enlargement of the glands and spleen and all diseases arising from excess wind, bile and mucus can be eliminated from the body by this method. Basti cures digestive disorders and is said to help relieve constipation.

sthula sharira (Ind.) The gross physical body. See also, KOSHA.

stichomancy A 3000-year-old practice of seeking metaphysical insight by opening a book at random and reading a passage.

Stone, Randolph (1890–1983) The founder of POLARITY THERAPY. Interested in both medicine and mysticism, he roamed far and wide in search of medical insights to alleviate human sufferings. His conclusion in this regard: 'Whatever works, works!'

stress management (Mod.) A combination of physical exercise, deep relaxation and VISUALIZATION techniques to counter the ill effects of stress on the body.

'The first step towards conquering stress is to accept that it is not created by external events so much as by how we deal with them.'

—Dadi Janki

structured spa (Spa) A SPA meant exclusively for goals such as weight loss, de-addiction, fitness and sports (e.g., golf).

structural integration (New Age) See ROLFING.

sub-atomic healing (Occ.) An approach to PSYCHIC HEALING, consisting of several methods, including AURA BRUSHING, the laying of hands, photographic and telepathic healing as developed by Heshheru Amenrahetep, a hypno therapist. The approach is said to be of use in the treatment of AIDS and cancer, besides psychological problems.

subconscious (Occ.) Also, samskara chitta; subconscious mind. 2. A part of one's personality, which exists below the surface of waking state or CONSCIOUSNESS. The unconscious mind is said to be affected by the sensory inputs and can be conditioned and programmed by punishments or rewards. Positive and negative affirmations are also said to affect this part subtly.

subh mudra (Occ.) A MUDRA formed by joining the fingers and thumbs of both the hands with each other and putting the thumbs over the index fingers. This mudra is said to bring peace, prosperity and happiness and help concentration and memory.

subliminal (New Age/Occ.) Below the threshold of CONSCIOUSNESS or apprehension. For example, an attitude of which one is never aware.

subsequent sensitizing event (Occ.) Also SSE. In HYPNOSIS, events that occur after the INITIAL SENSITIZING EVENT.

submodalities (Misc.) The components that comprise a sensory modality. For example, in the visual modality, the submodalities would include colour, brightness, focus and dimensionality.

subtle aroma therapy (Occ.) An approach to healing and wellbeing, in which one combines AROMATHERAPY with CHAKRA THERAPY. The approach, developed by Patricia Davis, is claimed to affect the subtle ('energetic') body.

subtle body (Occ.) Also, sukshma sharira. A term referring to any of the subtle-energy bodies which exist in the higher frequency octaves, beyond the physical body. The subtle body includes the PRANAMAYA, manomaya and vijnanamaya KOSHAS.

subtle energy (New Age) A general term that denotes energy that exists outside our physical reality (sometimes referred to as electromagnetic energy). The energy is therefore not bound by the physical laws. This energy is supposed to move at a speed greater than that of light energy.

succussion (Hom.) The shaking method used in preparing soluble, homoeopathic remedies.

Sudarshan kriya (Occ.) An approach to healing comprising the practise of a set of breathing exercises. Based on the assumptions that keeping biological rhythms with nature's rhythm produces a sense of harmony and wellbeing, this rhythmic breathing pattern is said to harmonize the rhythms of the body and emotions and, as a consequence, lower levels of stress experienced by its practitioners.

'The words that enlighten the soul are more precious than jewels'

—Hazrat Inayat Khan

Sufi healing (Per.) A tradition of faith healing, which has its roots in the teachings of the Chishti order of SUFISM, and which includes a number of methods such as ABJAD, BREATHWORK, FASTING and PRAYER. The system, developed mainly in Persia (Iran), views disbelief in God as the severest 'imbalance' in an individual.

Sufism (Per.) A Persian mystical religion, based on the tenets of Islam.

suggestibility (New Age/Occ.) The ability of being influenced by suggestion, an essential factor in generating the effects of HYPNOSIS. The greater the suggestibility, the greater the effect that suggestions offered will affect a person's perceptions of reality. In high levels of suggestibility, suggestions can cause amnesia, anaesthesia and both positive and negative hallucinations.

suggestion therapy (Occ.) Also, suggestive therapy. A healing method in which positive suggestions are made in the hypnotized state which are believed to replace negative thought patterns and quicken the healing process.

> 'Stand up, be bold, and strong. Know that you are the creator of your destiny. All the strength and succour you need are within you!'
>
> —Swami Vivekananda

su jok acupuncture (Occ.) A form of ACU-PUNCTURE, as developed by Korean practitioner Sir Park Jae Woo. The hands and feet are used to achieve the same results as body acupuncture does. In this method, laser, moxa, needles, seeds, stimulators, etc., are employed to treat various problems, more particularly, addiction, cardio-vascular diseases, constipation, cramps, epilepsy, eye diseases, fibrositis, headache, lumbago, nausea, rheumatism, sexual and urino-genital disorders. See also MOXIBUSTION.

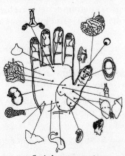

Su jok acupuncture

sukha puraka (Yoga) A form of PRANAYAMA in which inhalation of air, its retention and exhalation are done without any prescribed duration; its practise is left entirely to one's comfort and free will.

sukhasana (Yoga) A meditative asana in which one sits cross-legged, with spine erect and abdomen drawn in, on a mat placed on the floor. The hands are on the knees, palms downwards, shoulders and elbows relaxed. With the eyes closed, concentrate on the breath. This asana is said to help in stress relief, mental stability and peace.

sukla (Ind.) The male and female reproductive tissues in the body; semen. AYURVEDA considers semen as one of the seven DHATUS in the body.

sulphur (Hom.) A remedy useful in the treatment of conditions connected with symptoms of allergy, itching, odour and pain.

sumirani japa (Occ.). The repetition of a MANTRA, as a healing ritual.

sun-bath (Nat.) The application of the sun's rays and heat for health purposes. Sunlight is found to be beneficial especially in the treatment of skin infections.

sunfood diet (Mod.) A dietary regimen, based on the notion that raw plant food is the key to unlocking the dormant or latent powers.

sun mudra See SURYA MUDRA.

sun-sign lucky trees (Num./Occ.) An ancient practice of identifying trees which are compatible with one's sun-sign and planting and growing them for his or her health, luck and prosperity. The sun-sings and the corresponding lucky trees are shown in the following table:

Sun sign	Lucky trees
Aries	Amal, garmado, sadar
Taurus	Borsali, gulmohar, siras
Gemini	Champa, neem, papal
Cancer	Ashoka, kher, neem
Leo	Asopalav, papal
Virgo	Ardusi, bili, papal
Libra	Borsali, gulmohar
Scorpio	Gugar, khakro, nagor
Sagittarius	Banyan, mango, shimdo
Capricorn	Banyan, khijdo, rukhdo

| Aquarius | Garmado, kadamb, khijdo |
| Pisces | Bili, bahedo, mahudo |

sunyamudra (Occ.) A MUDRA formed by conjoining the thumb and the middle finger so that the nail touches the soft part of the thumb, keeping the other fingers straight. The mudra is believed to benefit ear diseases and congenital deafness. It is often suggested that one practises a MUDRA for as long as ailments stay.

superconscious (Occ.) 1. A part of MIND, wherein higher wisdom is supposed to lie. Though one may not be usually conscious of this, it is said to contribute towards one's personality. 2. A state during meditation (SAMADHI), wherein there is only consciousness of the object and no concurrent consciousness (or self-consciousness) of the mind. The duality of object and the perceiving subject is supposed to be non-existent in this state.

superior fast (Occ.) Also, superior fasting. An ascetic mode of fasting, aimed at reaching a higher mental state.

superior herbalism (Chi.) A form of Chinese herbalism which prescribes the so-called 'superior' herbs also referred to as 'tonic' herbs. These herbs are considered efficient in balancing body energies.

super-shape permanent weight-control system (Occ.) An audio-course programme aimed at weight loss, body shaping and the maintenance of ideal body size.

superesonant wavenergy programmme (Mod.) An approach to healing with exercises, as prescribed by ex-surgeon Irving I. Dardik. This method refers to wavenergy, i.e. waves of energy, a language understood by cells, hormones, genes, and molecules in the human body, which are believed to speak to one another.

superior fasting (Occ.) An ascetic mode of fasting, intended to achieve higher realms of consciousness.

superior herbs (Chi.) Also, tonic herbs. Special herbs, fewer than a hundred, recognized in Chinese herbal medicine, for their immense potential in balancing psychic and emotional energies.

superior herbalism (Chi.) A form of Chinese herbal medicine, in which SUPERIOR HERBS are included.

surabhi mudra (Occ.) A MUDRA formed by touching the tip of the index finger of one hand to that of the middle finger of the other hand and vice versa with the other hand. This mudra is said to aid in digestion.

surya mudra (Occ.) Also sun mudra. A MUDRA formed by conjoining thumb and ring finger while keeping the other fingers straight. It is said to activate the thyroid glands, reduce fat in the body and remove mental tension. As this mudra is said to produce heat in the body, water intake before commencement is often advised.

surya namaskara (Occ.) Salutation to the sun. A set of exercises which blend ASANA and PRANAYAMA. The set of exercises consists of the following twelve movements:

Step 1. Stand erect, legs together and palms together. Raise the hands above the head, palms together and bend the body backwards. Inhale fully as you bend backwards.

Step 2. Bend the body forwards and touch the knees with the head. Keep the palms on the floor on either side of the legs. Exhale fully while doing so.

Step 3. Kick the right leg back, take the left knee forward, look up straight and inhale.

Step 4. Take the left leg back, resting only on palms and toes. Exhale completely.

Step 5. Bend at the knee and rest the knees on the floor. Rest the forehead on the ground. In this position, inhale while moving backwards and then exhale completely.

Step 6. Come forward on the chest and rest the forehead on the ground. Eight organs, viz., forehead, chest, palms, knees and legs should touch the ground. Here, the breath-out condition (baahyakumbhaka) is reached.

Step 7. Raise the head and trunk making the spine concave upwards without changing the position of the palms and feet, keeping the knees off the ground. Inhale.

Step 8. Raise the buttocks, push the head down with heels touching the ground and palms the floor.

Step 9. Same as Step 5. Inhale and exhale.

Step 10. Bring the right leg between the two

palms and in line with them, as in step 3. Inhale.

Step 11. Bring the left foot forward next to the right foot and touch the knees with forehead as in step 2. Exhale.

Step 12. Stand erect with hands along the body and relax. Inhale while coming up.

(Note: Sometimes, Step Nos. 5 and 9 are omitted).

> 'The movement of the body and the intelligence of the brain should synchronize and keep pace with each other.'
>
> —B.K.S. Iyengar

> 'Sun salutations can energize and warm you, even on the darkest, coldest writer day.'
>
> —Canol Krucoff

Sushruta (Ind.) A surgeon who lived in ancient India, known for his seminal contributions to the science of surgery. Referred to as the 'father of surgery', Sushruta describes in his *Sushruta Samhita* over 120 surgical instruments and 300 surgical procedures. The *Samhita* contains some writings that date as late as the first century. Cosmetic surgery was also his forte, as his technique of forehead flap rhinoplasty (repairing a disfigured nose with a flap of skin from the forehead) is still practised. Sushruta reconstructed noses that were amputated as a punishment for crimes.

Sushruta Samhita (Ind.) An ancient commentary on AYURVEDA, authored by SUSHRUTA. *Susruta Samhita* contains the earliest written descriptions of several surgical interventions, which include the joining of the intestines, removal of the cataract and prostate gland and draining of abscesses.

sushumna (Occ.) Considered as the most important of all NADIs, sushumna is the central channel which extends from the base of the spine to the crown of the head. It is said to be the pathway for the awakened serpent-power (KUNDALINI), facilitating its ascendance towards the crown of the head.

sushumna darshana (Occ.) Visualization of SUSHUMNA. A DHARANA practice involving breathing with awareness, IMAGERY and VISUALIZATION of CHAKRAS.

sutala (Occ.) Sanskrit for great depth. One of the lower CHAKRAS (the third chakra from MULADHARA), centred in the knees, representing feelings of obsessive jealousy and retaliation. Sutala is considered to correspond to the third astral netherworld beneath the earth's surface called samhata (abandoned).

sutra neti (Ind.) A form of NETI, nasal irrigation in which a rubber catheter is used to facilitate the flow of saline.

svadhyaya (Yoga) Self-study or self-enquiry. One of the five forms of observances (NIYAMA) in the yoga system of PATANJALI. It implies continuously watching and analyzing one's actions and reactions to different situations with more awareness, including, for instance, why one becomes happy, sad or angry.

> 'Self-study should also extend to your meditations, however deep, so that you progressively understand more about yourself.'
>
> —Swami Satyananda Saraswati

svadishthana (Occ.) Also spleen chakra, swadishthana. One of the CHAKRAS, located in the spleen region, representing the higher realms of CONSCIOUSNESS, a rational approach.

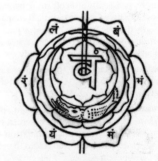

Svadishthana

svana (Occ.) Also swana. Breathing like a dog. An ancient yogic breathing exercise, consisting of the following steps:

Step 1. Stand and bend forward a little.

Step 2. Open the mouth widely fully stretching out the mouth. Step 3. Inhale and exhale rapidly through the mouth. Repeat several times. The exercise is said to aid detoxification of the body.

svarasa (Ind.) Extract of herbs and other plant parts prepared by pounding the plant parts in a mortar, expressing the juice and straining it through a cloth filter.

Svara Yoga (Occ.) A yoga system, based on the science of BREATHING.

svarupadarshana (Yoga) Sankrit for 'the vision of the Self'. A DHARANA practice, during which the body is kept motionless and often visualized as an immovable solid mass, as full focus of awareness is kept over the process of BREATHING.

svasa (Occ.) The inhaling breath, as distinguishable from the expiratory breath (PRASVASA).

svastikasana (Yoga) A basic form of ASANA, considered the easiest to perform. It is said to enhance blood-circulation in the legs and is therefore recommended for those who remain on their feet for long hours, such as security personnel.

svedana (Ind.) Also, sudation. A herbal steam bath with AYURVEDIC medicinal plants, aimed at inducing perspiration in the body, so as to eliminate body toxins through the pores of the skin. Svedana liquefies vitiated DOSHAs and removes stiffness in the body. Usually after oleation, patients are administered fomentation. Svedana is prescribed in the treatment of facial paralysis, headache, hemiplegia, oedema, sciatica and feeling of heaviness in the body.

svastha vrutta (Ind.) the maintenance of positive health, which is considered a distinguishing feature of AYURVEDA.

sweat diagnosis (Ind.) A diagnostic measure in SIDDHA MEDICINE. When in excess, sweat indicates an aggravation of VATA. Sweat on the forehead is said to indicate constipation.

sweat lodge (Am. Ind.) A traditional Native American place for ceremonial purification and meditation using intense heat in a sauna-like environment.

Swedish massage (Eur./New Age) A classical European MASSAGE technique with special oils. It includes therapeutic stroking and kneading of muscle tissues mainly aimed at

promoting stress relief, with long relaxing strokes on the body. The technique was popularized in 1812 by Per Henrik Ling, a Swedish physiologist. While Swedish massage was developed as part of gymnastics, seeking to affect specific muscles, joints and organs so as to relieve pain and increase mobility, the Esalen Institute, located in California, subsequently extended some basic Swedish massage techniques and worked to bring this massage into the human development/awareness movement. See also ESALEN MASSAGE.

sweetgrass (Am.Ind.) *Hierochloë odorata*. A popular grass in CHEROKEE rituals, sweet grass used to be burnt after smudging with sage. The grass is burnt to welcome good influences after driving out the bad.

Swiss shower (Spa) A hydropathic treatment that involves powerful shower jets directed at the body from various heights, creating the effect of an invigorating massage.

sympathetic vibratory physics (Mod.) Based on the ancient idea that everything in the universe vibrates, and that the vibration forms the connecting link to everything in the universe, it has been postulated that by studying the physics of vibration, one can see 'beyond material matter' and into the nature of the causative forces of nature operated by immutable universal laws.

symptom-producing event (Occ.) In HYPNOSIS, the event that either causes the problem or reinforces the cause in such a way that it assumes an active role in the client's life. (see also, INITIAL SENSITIZING EVENT, SUBSEQUENT SENSITIZING EVENT).

synchronization (Misc.) An adjustment that causes something to occur or recur in unison.

synchronized massage (Spa.) A form of MASSAGE in which more than one masseur participates to massage in a rhythmically synchronized manner.

systematic desensitization (Mod.) The use of programmed IMAGERY in a systematic way so as to help desensitize someone from an anxiety or phobia.

tadasana (Yoga) Also, mountain pose. An ASANA wherein the practitioner stands still, firm and motionless like a mountain. This asana is said to be helpful in correcting faulty posture, acquired over years, by straightening the spine and improving body alignment.

> 'Mountain pose teaches us, literally, how to stand on our own feet ... teaching us to root ourselves into the earth ... our bodies become a connection between heaven and earth.'
>
> —Carol Krucoff

TaeUIJu healing meditation (Occ.) Also TaeUIJu, TaeUIJu healing, TaeUIJu meditation. A form of MEDITATION, described as a process of returning to the 'magnanimous bosom of the original mother' and as the 'first step to eternal life'. In the practice of TaeUIJu, one sits comfortably and patiently repeats the 'mantra' aimed at returning to one's own original place. By going back to one's own roots through this meditation, it is believed that illnesses—mental and physical—can be cured.

tagara (Ind.) *Valeriana xallichii*. Also, all-heal, amantilla, balaka, great wild, Indian valerian, sugandhbala. A medicinal herb, found in Afghanistan, Bhutan and India, used in a variety of pharmaceutical preparations. An oil obtained from the plant is used to massage the spine as a pain-reliever. It is also used in relieving migraines.

t'ai chi chih (Chi.) A system of physical exercises, comprising twenty prescribed movements, aimed at harmonizing and balancing the body and mind.

tai chi-chi kung (Chi.) Also, taiJi-qigong. A simple combination of TAI CHI CHU'AN and CHI KUNG exercises. Eighteen specific exercises are designed to re-train the breath and develop energy within MERIDIANS and inner organs. The chi kung exercises are believed to release the powerful healing energy inside the body, assuring health benefits to its practitioners.

tai chi ch'uan (Chi.) Also, meditation-in-motion, tai chi, tai ji, tai ji ch'uan, tai ji juan, tai ji quan, tranquility-in-motion. A Chinese martial art, tai chi uses gentle, dance-like, stylized gestures with synchronized breathing. Traditional tai chi prescribes about 108 to 128 postures, including repetitions. Each movement is conceived in harmony with the direction of the energy in and around the body, leading to the next, without any pause. CHI energy, developed through smooth movements, is believed to be helpful in achieving a state of harmony and relaxation, besides spiritual development.

tai chi, five essential features of (Chi.) Five essential features in the practice of TAI CHI CH'UAN, and their significance are indicated in the following table:

Features	Significance
slowness	conducive for developing one's awareness
lightness	conducive for creating a flow in movements
balance	conducive for preventing strain

calmness	conducive for maintaining continuity
clarity	conducive for focussing the mind

taido (Occ.) A healing technique, developed in the 1980s by Toshihisa Hiraki, in which hands 'empowered by universal energy' are used. Taido, which resembles reiki, is a form of energy-field work that does not encourage physical contact.

t'ai hsuan ching (Chi.) An ancient Chinese text, consisting of eighty-one four-line graphs, called tetragrams. These lines, when unbroken, represent heaven, when broken, the earth and when twice-broken, the human.

taiji wuxigong (Chi.) A form of QIGONG, which when practised regularly is said to guarantee fitness, mental stability and restoration of vitality. It is also believed to 'open up' the body's 'middle energy channel' (SUSHUMNA). Regular practise is believed to improve one's health and increase mental stability.

takionic (Chi.) A technology for CHI enhancement and optimal health as promoted by Yung Chia.

tala (Occ./Yoga) Also, chakras of darkness, LOWER CHAKRAS. The name of the seven realms of lower consciousness, centred in the seven chakras located in the lower part of the human body, below the MULADHARA. See also, NARAKA.

> 'Never in the world can hatred be stilled by hatred; it will be stilled only by non-hatred—this is the Law Eternal.'
>
> —Gautama Buddha

talatala chakra (Yoga/Occ.) 'Lower region'. The fourth CHAKRA below MULADHARA, located in the calves. This is said to be the region of prolonged chaos and unreasonable stubbornness. This state of consciousness is born of the sole motivation of self-preservation.

talisman (Occ.) From the Arab *tilasm*, meaning to initiate into the mysteries. An object of stone, metal, wood or paper inscribed with magical signs, symbols, alphabets, numbers, characters or drawings, believed to bring luck and good health to the person who owns it. See also, AMULET.

Tamang shamanism (Tib.) A form of SHAMANISM as practiced by the Tamangs, a group of Tibetan Buddhists settled in Nepal. The rituals here are borrowed from both Hindu and Buddhist practices. In this healing system, all diseases and disorders are assumed to be acts of evil spirits. The Tamang shamans of Nepal also function as community psychotherapists, treating a wide range of symptoms by redressing family or social conflicts.

tamarind (Ind.) *Tamarindus indica*. A large, evergreen tropical tree. The fruit pulp, rich in sugar, vitamin C, and tartaric and citric acids, is used in syrup, juice concentrates and condiments like chutney and pickles, as well as curries and meat sauces. It is also an ingredient in cardiac- and blood-sugar reducing medicine. The bark is traditionally used in the treatment of diarrhoea. Bathing with an infusion of its leaves helps against skin ailments such as scabies.

tamas (Ind.) From the Sanskrit, for darkness. One of the three GUNAs, traits or tendencies. Tamas is characterized by lethargy, heaviness, inertia, ignorance, delusion, indecision, obstructiveness, stubbornness, stillness and stability. It is represented by the Vedic deity Rudra, the god of dissolution.

tamasic (Ind.) Of or pertaining to tamas.

tamasic food (Ind.) Acidic, frozen, processed, preserved, stale, overcooked and over-ripe foods, and bottled drinks and alcohol are tamasic foods, considered to promote negative characteristics and tendencies (such as anger, envy, selfishness) and induce heaviness of the body and dullness of the mind. Overeating also has a tamasic effect. According to traditional advice, the stomach should be half-filled with food, one-quarter with water, leaving the last quarter empty for air.

> 'Fast food is equivalent to pornography, nutritionally speaking.'
>
> —Stere Elbert

tanden (Jap.) Japanese for red field. Also, hara. 1. The centre of gravity in the human body, located in the abdomen, three fingers-width below and two-fingers width behind the navel. 2. The alleged seat of 'spiritual power', it is an important focal point in QIGONG and in other breathing techniques. 3. The psychic centre of the human body. See also DANTIEN.

tanden breathing (Chi.) In ZEN YOGA, an approach to healing, aimed at tapping TANDEN. The procedure involves slow ABDOMINAL BREATHING, directing the breath energy into the lower abdomen. By making the breath deep and slow, one can make his or her mind steady and relaxed.

tangerine peel (Chi.) Also, Mandarin-orange peel. *Citrus reticulate*. A remedy for stomach-upset, nausea and vomiting.

tanmatra (Yoga) The five rudimentary principals of the elements which are unmanifested, including sound (shabda), touch (sparsha), form (rupa), taste (rasa) and smell (gandha). Tanmatras are considered the special modifications of one's CONSCIOUSNESS.

tan tien See DAN TIEN

tan tien breathing (Chi.) From the Chinese *tan tien*, DAN TIEN, meaning area beneath the navel. A natural and powerful BREATHING exercise, said to stimulate the VITAL ENERGY in the body, particularly in the lower abdominal area. The method involves natural diaphragmatic breathing, wherein one inhales through the nasal passage while directing the breath energy down into the area below the navel (tan tien). While exhaling slowly through the nose or mouth, the practitioner simultaneously condenses the breath energy into the cells of tan tien by intentionally prolonging the exhalation. The method is said to help in achieving deep relaxation and self-healing.

tan tien chi kung (Chi.) An approach to healing which consists of BREATHING exercises. Aimed at developing the power of DAN TIEN, (the lower abdominal area) by increasing the VITAL ENERGY stored therein, in this method one learns to develop the CHI pressure, which results in increasing one's vitality and strengthening the organs, thus promoting self-healing .

tantra (Occ.) Also, tantrism. An esoteric system of spiritual practice and healing, a precursor of the world's existing religions Most yogic practices, such as ASANA, KRIYA YOGA, PRANAYAMA, TRATAKA and YOGA NIDRA owe their origin to tantras. There are two paths of tantra: the 'right-handed' (dakshinachara), a marga considered sattvic or rajasic, and the 'left-handed' (vamanachara), considered to be rajasic or tamasic. They relate to the two main tantric lineages: 'rule-based' (samaya) and 'heritage-based' (kaula). While the 'rule-based' lineage follows strict spiritual practices, the 'heritage' aims at achieving expansion of consciousness and liberating the mind through sensuality, through the FIVE Ms (makaras)

'This embedded openness to the world is metamorphic, deepening vision, strengthening the heart. As such, systems of control based on fear and obedience have always viewed tantra as suspicious, if not seditious.'

—Phil Hine

tantra toning (Occ) An approach to healing, by raising and releasing energy in the body. The exercise makes use of the power of sound vibrations emanated while engaged in breathing.

Tantra Yoga (Occ.) An ancient system of YOGA, which seeks to raise sex-energy with the help of a partner but makes use of it up in the CHAKRAS. TANTRISM believes that sex energy, viewed as sacred energy, can be tamed and mastered for SELF-REALIZATION.

tantric sex (Occ.) A holistic view of the sex-act, as a forerunner for the spiritual growth of an individual. In this system, sex is considered as an act of MEDITATION and YOGA. By denying the normal, natural outlet for the reproductive juices (SHUKRA), it is believed that they get transmuted into a powerful sex-energy capable of activating the crown-chakra (SAHASRARA), thus facilitating spiritual attainments (SIDDHIs). See also, OJAS.

tantsu (Occ.) An acronym of tanric shiatsu, a form of BODYWORK in which the practitioner holds a partner continuously and touches various parts of his or her body.

Tao (Chi.) Also, dao, from the Chinese for the way. The central concept of Chinese religion, translated as 'way' or 'path', it also refers to a flow in the universe. Tao is never stagnant, is very powerful and keeps things in the universe balanced and in order. It also refers to the law of nature. Though TAOISM is traditionally considered impossible to translate, Tao is often understood as cosmic order.

> 'The Tao has its reality and its signs but is without action or form. You can hand it down, but you cannot receive it; you can get it but you cannot see it. It is its own source, its own root. Before heaven and earth existed it was there, firm from ancient times. It gave spirituality to the spirits and to God; it gave birth to heaven and to earth. It exists beyond the highest point, and yet you cannot call it lofty; it exists beneath the limit of the six directions and yet you cannot call it deep.'
>
> —Chuang Tzu

Taoism (Chi.) Also, Daoism. From the Chinese word, meaning the way. 1. A philosophical school, based on the teachings of the Tao Te Ching, ascribed to Laozi, and Zhuangzi and believed to have been written around 600 BC. 2. A family of organized Chinese religious movements, Zhengyi and Quanzhen, tracing back to Han dynasty. 3. Folk religion of China. Several ancient healing practices such as FENG SHUI, Chinese martial and healing arts including many styles of QIGONG and the TRADITIONAL CHINESE MEDICINE trace their roots to Taoism.

Tao of Health (Occ.) Also, Tao of Healing, Tao of Healing method. An approach to health as promoted by the School of Classical Taoist Herbology, in Manhattan (New York City). Based on the notion of original and 'rightful' state of health, practices relating to ENERGY BALANCING, ENERGY DIAGNOSIS, SELF-HEALING, SEX THERAPY, TAOIST DIET and TUINA are included.

Tao rejuvenation (Occ.) A simple, easy-to-learn, self-massage technique which is said to increase healing energy flow in the body. Chi self-massage, a hands-on self-healing method using one's internal energy to strengthen and rejuvenate the sense organs, is taught. Using internal power (CHI) and gentle external stimulation, this simple technique is said to help in dissolving energy blocks and stress points, which are otherwise responsible for diseases or triggering the process of AGEING.

> 'Energy is equal to desire and purpose'.
>
> —Sheryl Adams

Taoist diet (Occ.) A system of healthy food combinations, based on the notion of balancing the YIN AND YANG nature of food. There are many different historical and modern schools of TAOISM with different ideas on diet. While contemporary diets advocate the consumption of whole grains, planned on the premise that the rotting of the grains in the intestines would attract demonic creatures known as the 'three worms'. An early text, the *Taipingjing*, suggests that people 'live on air', and that it is best to be satiated without eating solid food. In effect, it suggests that people eat non-corporeal food such as QI. A Taoist diet could however be frugal, focussing on whole grains, vegetables, fruits, nuts seeds and tofu, while discouraging red meat, refined flour, dairy products and soft drinks.

Taoist numerology (Occ.) The science of numbers according to Taoist traditions; numbers are used to facilitate an understanding of life-events. Taoist numerology, in which a person's name is converted to numbers, is used to forecast destiny, past life, compatibility with others and suitability of one's profession. Taoist numerology is different from western numerology in that a number in Taoist numerology has both positive and negative meanings, YIN AND YANG. See also, NUMEROLOGY.

Taoist personology (Chi.) A method of face-reading, based on the belief that the conditions of the body can be gauged by facial features. The method was originally used for diagnostic purposes. The colour, shape and any disfigurations on as many as 108 areas in a face are studied individually; each of these areas is believed to represent an aspect, e.g., spouse, children and property, in an individual's life. It also represents how an individual fares in his life at a particular age.

Taoist qigong (Chi.) A form of QIGONG, focussed on slowing down the process of ageing.

Taoist sexology (Chi.) Sex taught and practised in accordance with the principles of Taoism which holds that while correct sex spreads happiness among individuals, their progeny, and society, incorrect sex causes pain. *Su Nu Ching* (Classic of the White Madam) is the basic book of Taoist sexology.

tapa svedana (Ind.) The application of dry heat to the body, aimed at reducing swellings in the joints. See also SAUNA.

tapotement (New Age) A specific stroke used in SWEDISH MASSAGE which refers to a rhythmic percussion most frequently administered with the heel of the palm. Tapotement is said to help soothe nerves and strengthen muscles.

Taraka Yoga (Yoga) From the Sanskrit word, meaning that which delivers. A system of YOGA, based on the non-dualistic philosophy of Shankaracharya which aims at delivering the practitioner with the unconditioned reality of the Absolute. The system is based on the belief that the infinite universe (BRAHMAN) and the self (ATMAN) form one entity; that there is no division between them. The goal of Taraka Yoga is to lift one's ordinary, unhealthy consciousness to a healthy level of continuous awareness of this Absolute Reality. To achieve this, the practitioner is trained to see and experience a light phenomenon of the inner dimensions of reality by focussing his or her attention on the THIRD EYE.

tarot (Occ.) A deck of seventy-eight cards, used for fortune-telling and predictions relating to health. The tarot deck comprises cards which represent archetypal images, rooted in EUROPEAN MYSTICISM. The images on the cards are believed to usually correspond with 'unconscious intent, potential and destiny' of the guidance-seeker and can be considered as representations of his or her archetypal qualities.

taste (Ind.) The detection and identification of dissolved chemicals associated with taste buds by the sensory system. In AYURVEDA, the six qualities of sensory reception, viz., astringent, bitter, pungent, salt, sour and sweet, are often associated with diagnosis and treatment.

taste blindness (Chi./Ind.) The inability to detect the taste of a substance. In feverish conditions, patients become taste blind. To activate the taste-buds, a dose of tangerine peels is usually administered.

teekshnagni (Ind.) A very quick digestion of whatever a person eats.

telediagnosis (Occ.) Also, distant biological detection. A paranormal method of distant diagnosis wherein the practitioner holds a pendulum over a photo of the patient for examination. See also DISTANT TELEDIAGNOSIS.

teletherapy (Occ.) A paranormal method of diagnosing and treating ailments without the physical presence of the patient. See also, DISTANT HEALING, TELEDIAGNOSIS.

telepathy The psychic communication of thoughts or ideas by means other than the known senses.

temazcal (New Age) A SWEAT LODGE. A traditional gathering of participants around a pit where water is poured over heated stones. The steam arising is meant to relax and create a balanced state of mind.

ten jin do (Jap.) From the Japanese, for the way of angels. An approach to healing, which includes a meditative form of ABSENT HEALING, as developed by Japanese nun Anju Tenbu Myodo.

ten mudras (Yoga) The ten MUDRAS in YOGA, which are considered essential are PRANA MUDRA, JNANA MUDRA, BAYAU MUDRA, PRITHVI MUDRA, SURYA MUDRA, VARUNA MUDRA, LINGA MUDRA, SHUNYA MUDRA, VAYU MUDRA and APANA MUDRA.

Tenrikyo (Jap.) A sect founded by a Japanese housewife, Miki Nakagama (1798–1887), in which faith healing is the major component.

Tensegrity (Occ.) A series of twelve movements popularized by Carlos Castaneda (1925–98), who learned them from his teacher, Juan Matus (Don Juan), a sorcerer, in Peru. The exercises aim at gathering energy to promote health and wellbeing.

tepidarium (New Age) A heated open space which in ancient Roman baths was used as a room where visitors would prepare for a bath. Contemporary tepidaria often feature lounges and comfortable furniture.

> 'There must be quite a few things a hot bath won't cure, but I don't know many of them.'
>
> —Sylvia Plath

Thailand medical massage (New Age) A Thai traditional massage administered without oils, on a floor mat as the recipient is advised to wear comfortable clothing. The massage is performed slowly with gentle and rhythmic movements, with appropriate pressure applied on points and muscles by using hands, thumbs, fingers, elbows, knees and feet. The massage is practised in the university-affiliated hospitals in Thailand as a treatment for certain ailments. A prayer is said at the beginning of each massage session. The massage is said to provide stimulation to the MERIDIAN.

thakradhara (Ind.) A technique in AYURVEDA in which medicated and diluted yogurt is poured on to the forehead continuously for 40-60 minutes. The treatment is said to cure depression, insomnia, psoriasis, stress and stress-related disorders and cool the eyes.

thalassotherapy (New Age) SPA treatments in which sea and seawater products such as seaweed and seaweed wraps are used. The treatment normally includes daily bathing in a heated sea-water pool with jets, mud bath, seaweed bath (ALGOTHERAPY), hydro-massage and AROMATHERAPY. Thalassotherapy is found useful for relaxation, stress management, muscle and skin restoration and weight-control. Mineral-rich Dead Sea water and Dead Sea weeds are used for better results.

tharpanam (Ind.) Also, netra tharpanam. A popular treatment in AYURVEDA in which medicated ghee is applied gently for twenty or thirty minutes. The treatment is said to have a cooling effect on the eyes, prevent eye diseases and relieve eye strain.

theocentric therapy (New Age) Also, Christian psychological counselling; theocentric counselling, theocentric psychological Counselling, theocentric psychological and educational therapies, theocentric psychology. A Christian healing system as propagated by LaSalle University in Mandeville, Louisiana.

theotherapy (Occ.) A form of self-healing as developed by Peter Lemesurier, based on the notion that every divine characteristic is positive and sustainable and works as a therapy. Theotherapy involves determining, more or less unconsciously, which Greek god or goddess best symbolizes one's disease, and treating the disease by trying to adopt those godly characteristics one considers positive and sustainable. According to its theory, every divine characteristic is a therapy and every symptom is a healing tool.

therapeutic kinesiology (New Age) A form of KINESIOLOGY as developed by Tom Little, based on the concept that releasable energy is often attached to one's negative emotions.

therapeutic massage (New Age) A relaxing form of massage consisting usually of soothing strokes and rubbing.

therapeutic prayer (Occ.) A powerful form of expression of one's gratitude to nature and god, and the energy obtained in the process is utilized for the welfare of others, through mind, words and actions.

therapeutic shiatsu (Occ.) A form of SHIATSU in which gentle massage is used to remove energy blocks in the meridians, along with trapped emotion.

therapeutic touch (Occ.) A form of laying on of hands, based on the premise of the transmittable nature of energies as developed by Dolores Krieger, an American nursing professor in 1972.

therapeutic touch inner work (Occ.) An expansion of THERAPEUTIC WORK, based on the notion that the most profound healing originates in a transpersonal realm.

therapy A treatment or process, done with the intent to move someone into a state of health and wholeness, or to remove blockages which inhibit health or wholeness, or inhibit one's reaching one's full potential.

third eye (Yoga) Also, AJNA CHAKRA, sixth chakra, third eye chakra. The psychic centre of MEDITATION located in the centre of the brain, between the eyebrows and believed to be the centre of psychic vision. The pineal gland, the last endocrine gland to have its function discovered by science, is associated with this sixth chakra.

third position (Yoga) A mental attitude, developed to observe events in one's life with detachment, as if observed by an observer from the outside. Such an attitude could work one to cope with any stress and trauma. See also ATTITUDINAL HEALING.

thirty-day body purification programme (New Age) An approach to healing, consisting of a variety of purification techniques: 'cleansing the body's internal ecosystem with herbs' and 'pure nutrients', AROMATHERAPY, MACROBIOTICS, TISSUE SALTS. The 'purification' is also based upon VISUALIZATION, wherein one visualizes dust, toxins and the colour gray leaving one's body.

thirty-day energetic workout (New Age) An approach to healing consisting of a series of exercises designed by Richard M. Chin (1992), aimed at removing energy blocks in the body, thus balancing the body, mind and spirit. While removing energy blocks, it is also believed that the flow of CHI is infused automatically.

> 'Flow with whatever may happen and let your mind be free. Stay centred by accepting whatever you are doing. This is the ultimate.'
>
> —Chuang Tzu

Thomsonianism (Am. Ind./New Age) A form of HERBALISM, popularized in the US in the nineteenth century by Samuel Thomson (1769–1843) who studied both native and settler folklores and evolved this system. According to him, the selection of a medicine should be based exclusively on observation; theories obscured the simplicity and created a needless mystery about medicine. He considered that disease was caused by the decrease or derangement of vital fluids, brought about by a loss of animal heat. He believed that by restoring the heat by means of steam baths and cayenne (capsicum annum), toxins which obstructed health would be thrown into the stomach from where they would be eliminated.

thought (Occ.) A private conversation with oneself, thought has become synonymous with one's MIND. 'Making up one's mind', 'changing one's mind' and 'remaining in two minds' all indicate the thought-process which may or may not be explicit to others unless one communicates verbally or non-verbally. According to Indian philosophy, there should be harmony between thought, speech and action, without which one's health could be severely affected.

> 'Thought makes the whole dignity of man; therefore endeavour to think well, that is the only morality.'
>
> —Blaise Pascal

thought energy (Occ.) The energetic expression of human consciousness, revealing the power of THOUGHT and emotion whose hidden potential in making or marring one's life were recognized in early human societies; suitable measures were worked out to regulate the thought process by inculcating love for fellow-beings and eliminating negative thoughts and emotions from the mental realms. Ancient religions, rituals and rites have all played an effective role in binding communities together, especially at the time of crisis, natural or manmade. The essence of all religions, too, is love for fellow-beings. See also THOUGHT ENERGY FIELD.

> 'Change your thoughts – and you change your world.'
>
> —Norman Vincent Peale

thought energy field (Occ.) A collection of thoughts, interrelated by their common theme and bound together as a functional unit. The disruption of the free flow of energy within the thought field is seen as the fundamental cause of all negative emotions, which cause an imbalanced (diseased) mind, body or both. Several psychotherapeutic measures make an attempt to balance or synchronize through their interventions.

> 'Breath is thought. If you stop breathing, thoughts immediately stop. Try it for a second. Stop breathing. Immediately there is a break in your thinking process; it is broken. Thinking is the invisible part of the visible breathing.'
>
> —Swami Chaitanya

thought field therapy (Occ.) Also, TFT. A form of meridian therapy, addressed to psychological and emotional disturbances as developed by Roger Callahan, a Californian clinical psychologist in the 1980s. The theory is based on the idea that there exist invisible energy fields called thought fields whose occasional blockages cause psychological problems. The therapy endorses overcoming one's self-sabotaging behaviour with optimism. The procedure includes the manual tapping of ACUPOINTS to add energy to the system and help rebalance energy flow.

> 'Remember happiness doesn't depend upon who you are or what you have; it depends solely upon what you think.'
>
> —Dale Carnegie

thought-forms (Occ.) An energy structure, induced by strong thoughts or emotions, which are said to be clairvoyantly seen in AURA.

thought therapy (Occ.) A healing system, aimed at relieving depression and pain and improving the quality of sleep. It comprises ways to distract one from brooding over the past loss, betrayal, humiliation or other disquieting memories. Simple acts, such as walking to a pharmacist, meeting a friend over breakfast or starting a challenging project could ease the dread of failure or disappointments, by diverting one's thought habits.

> 'When thought becomes excessively painful, action is the finest remedy.'
>
> —Salman Rushdie

three bodies of human beings (Yoga) Also tri sharira. The system of YOGA recognizes three bodies in the human beings:

The Body	Meaning	Remarks
Coarse, physical body (sthula sharira)	Gross and mortal physical frame, made of food. The outermost and visible of all the three bodies.	A seat of sensory equipment; fully dependent on sensory stimulation for action or reaction.
Subtle or Pranic body (sukshma sharira)	The psycho-mental complex. Though not seen by the naked eye, it is identifiable through a higher level of intuition.	Subtle body is known to influence the coarse physical body.
Causal Body (karana sharira)	The infinite potential that permeates time and space.	The 'essence' of one's existence.

Since the system is intertwined, all bodies remain connected to each other. Physical acts are influenced by the SUBTLE BODY as well as the quality of the passages to the CAUSAL BODY and vice versa; there exists a two-way traffic functioning of the energy body between all these three bodies.

They are therefore supposed to act in harmony for the very survival of the system. Once the connections get disturbed, stress and confusion occur, paving the way for discomfort, ill-health or even death.

three-phase workout (Occ.) A routine workout, designed by chiropractor John Douillard, aimed at reaching the 'zone', described as a 'quasi-mystical state of consciousness'. The routine consists of (a) the 'salute for the sun', consisting of a series of ASANAS aimed at integrating the mind and body; (b) performance, in three phases, of the exercise of one's choice, with what is referred to as mind–body breathing and (c) a cool down.

throat chakra See VISHUDDHI CHAKRA.

Tibetan eye chart (Tib.) A mandala-like chart created by Tibetan monks, aimed at training the optic nerves and muscles for correcting eye problems.

Tibetan medicine (Tib.) An ancient system of medicine, bearing some similarities with other traditional systems of the Asian region: AYURVEDA, SIDDHA, TRADITIONAL CHINESE MEDICINE and UNANI. The system is based on intricate theories of disease causation, diagnosis and therapeutics. It works on the principle that humans and the surrounding environment in which they live are interconnected, as both are made of the same basic FIVE ELEMENTS (earth, fire, water, wind and space). The interaction between a person and the world at large—through diet, human relationships and climate—is believed to trigger disease. An individual's own mind and feelings can also contribute towards inducing a disease in as much as its curing. Traditional Tibetan Medicine makes use of animal, vegetable and mineral components of the universe to restore health and balance. The treatment is offered in five main areas: general advice on behaviour to be adopted or avoided, dietary counseling, the prescription of herbs, external treatments such as MOXI-BUSTION, and mind exercises to be practiced.

Tibetan pulse-reading (Tib.) The most essential diagnostic method in TIBETAN MEDICINE, pulse reading helps the Tibetan physician diagnose the nature of disease. The physician takes not only the pulse but also gauges the degree of tautness and warmth in the vein to determine the thickness of blood, its rapidity and other subtle vibrations transmitted by the pulse from the interior organs, visualized by the pulse reader. A special feature in pulse reading is that six points on both wrists of a patient are palpated simultaneously, as each point is believed to carry information about one of the six organ systems in the body. A physician thus has access to the whole body of the patient. See also, PULSE READING.

Tibetan pulse healing (Tib.) Also, Tibetan pulsing. An ancient form of healing, based on the belief that working through the body, it is possible to reach areas of emotional and mental tension. Tibetan pulse healing uses gentle pulsations in rhythm with the heart beat to bring loving energy into the areas needing healing. Tibetan pulsing is reported to be useful in a wide variety of conditions such as addictive behaviour, eating disorders, emotional trauma, low immune system and stress.

Tibetan reiki (Occ.) A form of REIKI, which traces its origin to Tibet, although it was rediscovered in the twentieth century. The healing system has eighteen symbols and practitioners channel VITAL ENERGY to places where it is needed most within the body. It is believed to help people overcome their pain, stress and emotional problems.

tikta ghrita (Ind.). Medicated ghee with a predominantly bitter taste, used internally and externally. According to AYURVEDA, it has a purifying and strengthening effect on the liver and deep tissues. It is also said to protect OJAS. It is recommended for PITTA or KAPHA imbalances.

Tila (Ind.) *Sesamum indicum*. Also, sesame. A flowering plant, whose oil-rich seeds are used in cookery and in medicine. Sesame oil is used for massage and health treatments of the body in the ancient Indian AYURVEDIC system with ABHYANGA and SHIRODHARA MASSAGE. The unhulled seeds of sesame are reported to be rich in manganese, copper and calcium (90 mg per tablespoon in unhulled seeds). The oil is used in ayurvedic massage.

tisane (Chi./Ind.) Also, herbal 'tea', ptisan. An infusion made of fresh or dried herbs, flowers, leaves, seeds or roots, generally by pouring boiling water over them and letting them stand for a few minutes. The tisane is then strained, and sweetened, if necessary, before serving. Tisanes are often consumed for their medicinal effects, especially for their stimulant, relaxant or sedative properties. Some common tisanes are made from anise, roasted barley, bissap, catnip (relaxant and sedative), chamomile (sedative), chrysanthemum, citrus, lemon and orange peel, roasted corn, echinacea (to prevent cold or flu), FENNEL, GINGER, GINSENG, hibiscus, LEMON GRASS, LIQUORICE, lotus flowers (stamens), mint, NEEM, rosehip, ROSEMARY, sage, thyme, TULSI and VETIVER.

tissue salts (Hom./Mod.) Also, SCHUSSLER BIOCHEMIC SYSTEM OF MEDICINE. An inorganic compound essential to growth and functions of the body's cells. They are prepared in very low homoeopathic potency (6X usually) and pass rapidly into the body through the bloodstream.

tolle causam (Nat.) Also, find-and-treat-the-cause. The foremost principle of NATUROPATHY, which stresses on identification of the cause of a disease and treatment of the cause, rather than the symptoms. According to this theory, symptoms are expressions of the body's attempt to heal and naturopathy therefore advocates that they should not be suppressed with medicine.

Tomatis, Alfred A. (1920–2001) (New Age) A French ear, nose, and throat doctor who made medical and psychological discoveries that led to audio–psycho–phonology, or the TOMATIS METHOD.

> 'We sing with our ears.'
> —Alfred A. Tomatis

Tomatis method (New Age) Also, auditory training, auditory stimulation, listening therapy. A system of auditory stimulation, designed by Alfred A. Tomatis, a French otolaryngologist. It is based on the theory that high-frequency sounds (charging sounds) such as those found in Gregorian and Tibetan chants, energize the brain and awaken the higher consciousness, and low-frequency sounds, predominant in certain drumming have hypnotic effect on the body and make the body move.

tone acupuncture (New Age) Also, sonopuncture. The application of sound frequencies on ACUPOINTS instead of needles. Sound frequencies are used to activate the acupuncture point in a similar but more subtle way. Sonopuncture is painless, and can be used alone or in combination with other therapies.

tongue acupuncture (Chi.) A form of ACUPUNCTURE, based on the ancient Chinese medical book, *Wang Di's Internal Medicine*. This method focusses on the tongue which is considered to be the intersection site of all fourteen meridians in the human body. Specific ACUPOINTS on the tongue are identified and linked with various functional aspects of the body.

tongue diagnosis (Chi.) A distinguishing feature of clinical diagnostic examination in TRADITIONAL CHINESE MEDICINE. The tongue, the only body organ exposed and seen externally, has rich nerve and blood supplies. By observing its colour, thickness, dryness, superficial growth and smell, practitioners can learn patients' health conditions and check whether their qi (energy) and blood have a smooth flow. As different areas of the tongue correspond to different organs of the body, by correlating the location of the blemishes on the tongue, one can determine which organ of the body is afflicted. Some diagnostic indicators in the tongue are:

Indicator	Inference
A pale tongue	Anaemic condition
Yellowish tongue	Excess bile in the gall bladder
Blue tongue	Heart ailments
Whitish tongue	KAPHA imbalance
Red or yellowish green tongue	PITTA imbalance
Black or brown colouration of the tongue	VATA imbalance
Coating on the tongue	Presence of toxins in the stomach and/or intestines

tonification (Chi.) Also, stimulation. An acupuncture technique devised to stimulate the QI energy levels in the body. It consists of a straight insertion of a needle, without manipulation to ensure that the point receives a boost of energy at once. All tonification measures are closely related to parallel concepts of regeneration, rejuvenation, and longevity.

> 'Happiness is the absence of the striving for happiness.'
> —Chuang Tzu

toning (New Age). A healing procedure developed by Laurel Elizabeth Keyes, an American healer. It aims at bringing 'new life energy' to 'inhibited' or 'unbalanced' parts of the body. The method involves standing with eyes closed, relaxing the jaws, and expressing feelings with vocal sounds. See also SOUND THERAPY.

touch and breathe (Occ.) A natural healing method in which the patient fingers the areas selected for treatment and lightly keeps the fingers there as he or she respires once.

touch therapy (Occ.) A basic human need, touch is also considered therapeutic. Touch therapy refers to a variety of treatments in which the hands are used for healing, including OMEGA, RADIANCE TECHNIQUE and REIKI. The physical and psychological role of touch is long recognized and has been part of all traditional systems of medicine.

tourmaline (Gem) A black-coloured stone, recommended for guarding against negative energies, evil eye and situations that cause emotional distress and trauma.

tracing (Occ.) A healing technique akin to TOUCH THERAPY, involving the use of hands or fingers along the meridians.

traditional acupuncture (Chi.) A classical form of ACUPUNCTURE based on the meridian theory of Traditional Chinese Medicine.

Traditional Chinese medicine (Chi.) An ancient system of health care, based on the Chinese concept of balance in the body as well as harmony between the body and its outside environment. Techniques used in TCM include ACUPRESSURE, ACUPUNCTURE, CHINESE MARTIAL ARTS, CHINESE PULSE DIAGNOSIS, CUPPING, FOOD THERAPY, HERBOLOGY, MOXIBUSTION, QIGONG and SHEN.

The history of Chinese Medicine dates back to the 3000-year-old seminal medical text of ancient of China, *Huang Di Nei Jing* (Yellow Emperor's Inner Cannon). Traditional Chinese Medicine is largely based on the philosophy that the human body is a mini-universe with a set of complete and elaborate interconnected systems which usually work in balance to maintain the healthy function of the human body

traditional chiropractic (New Age) A form of CHIROPRACTIC as popularized by Daniel David Palmer (1845–1913).

'We chiropractors work with the subtle substance of the soul. We release the imprisoned impulses, a tiny rivulet of force, that emanates from the mind and flows over the nerves to the cells and stirs them to life. We deal with the magic power that transforms common food into living, loving, thinking clay....'

—Daniel David Palmer

Trager (New Age) Also, psychophysical integration, Trager approach, Trager bodywork, Tragering, trager psychophysical Integration®, Tragerwork. Also referred to as a 'Movement education approach', this method was developed in the US in 1958 by Milton Trager (1909–97), a former boxer and acrobat. Practitioners are said to work in a meditative state called 'hook-up'. The system is designed to help polio victims and those with other neuro-muscular disorders.

trance (Occ.) A mental state of inwardly directed attention and oblivion to the external environment. It is a state of awareness marked by a relaxed body and focussed mind. It is, in general, a condition of altered consciousness, a state of intense concentration, introspection and MEDITATION.

'The timeless in you is aware of life's timelessness.'

—Kahlil Gibran

transcendental meditation (New Age) A simple means of meditation that allows one to quieten the mind through repetition of a personal MANTRA.

transitional medicine (New Age) An approach to healing , based on concepts of psycho–neuro–immunology. The approach recognizes that the mind can and does play a significant role in diseases and the healing processes. Many different areas, including medicine, psychiatry, counselling, spirituality, art, colour, poetry, and bibliotherapy, are used in combination to enhance the mind–body–spirit connections and create the healing experience.

transliminal hypnotherapy (THT) (New Age) A form of HYPNOTHERAPY in which no verbal suggestion is used to reach the subconscious mind; instead, sounds having specific frequency is used through audio-cassettes. The efficacy of transliminal suggestions are attributed to the fact that they bypass the conscious mind and are picked up by the subconscious only. As the sub-conscious mind does not know the difference between a real and an imagined experience, by bombarding the subconscious mind with new internal images and experiences, it said that one could re-write one's internal mind script. As a consequence, ones' outward experiences are realigned to match with this new inward image of reality.

transpersonal counselling (New Age) Also, transpersonal psychology, transpersonal counselling psychology. An approach to healing and wellbeing, which combines JUNGIAN PSYCHOLOGY, PSYCHOSYNTHESIS, and EASTERN MYSTICISM. The approach emphasizes MEDITATION, PRAYER and self-transcendence. Stanislav Grof (b. 1931) a Czechoslavakia-born psychiatrist is a pioneer in transpersonal psychology and has researched into the use of altered states of CONSCIOUSNESS for healing, growth and insight.

transpersonal psychotherapy (New Age) Also, transpersonal therapy. A branch of PSYCHOTHERAPY which recognizes the interconnectedness of life in a mutually affecting web of experience. Viewing individual identity primarily as a Soul, the hallmark of transpersonal psychotherapy is integration, valuing wholeness of being and SELF-REALIZATION. The transpersonal perspective of psychotherapy attempts to see all symptoms as part of a larger picture of 'energy moving'. Transpersonal psychotherapy approaches healing and growth through recognition of the centrality of a Self in the therapeutic process. Transpersonal therapy, psychotherapy and counselling work towards the development of a whole life skill whereby the individual awakens from a limited personal identity to a widened universal knowledge of self.

trataka (Ind) Also, gazing. From the Sanskrit word, meaning to gaze. One of the SHAT KARMAS, trataka is an important practice in YOGA, of staring at an object intensely without blinking. Trataka is of two forms: the inner gaze (ANTARANGA TRATAKA) and the outer gaze (BAHIRANGA TRATAKA). The practice is said to develop concentration by stimulating the AJNA CHAKRA, and strengthening the eyes and eye-muscles. The practitioner fixes his or her attention on a symbol, dot, image of a deity or one's own image in a mirror, focussing his attention completely on each thought or feeling that arises. The idea is to absorb one's mind completely in the object. The practise is continued until the eyes become watery or he loses awareness of the body in which case the eyes are closed and relaxed, before the procedure is restarted. The second stage comprises staring at a candle flame and later an attempt is made to concentrate on the after-image by holding it for as long as possible. This practice is said to correct eye-related defects including nearsightedness, besides developing the power of concentration. It is also said to develop one's intuitive or psychic power.

> 'Tell me, I'll forget; show me I may remember; involve me and I'll understand.'
>
> —a Chinese proverb

trauma release therapy (New Age) A healing method, developed by Karl Nishimura, an orthodontist from California, which aims to remove all suppressed traumas. It is believed to remove by autogenic means, the body's natural healing capacity, a lifetime of accumulated, suppressed traumas that have been shielded from conscious awareness. It consists of a fourteen-step protocol to reactivate old traumas and remove individual injuries, layer by layer, until rejuvenation occurs.

trauma search therapy (New Age) Also, repressed memory therapy. A type of PSYCHOTHERAPY which assumes that problems such as bulimia, depression, sexual inhibition, insomnia and excessive anxiety occur due to unconsciously repressed memories of childhood sexual abuse and a healthy psychological state can be restored only by recovering and facing these repressed memories. However, there appears little scientific evidence supporting the notions that memories of childhood sexual abuse are *unconsciously* repressed or that recovering repressed memories of abuse leads to significant improvement in one's psychological health. See also TRAUMA TOUCH THERAPY.

trauma touch therapy (New Age) A certified programme aimed at addressing clients with trauma and abuse histories. Therapists encourage empowerment and choice, which assists clients in accessing a bodily experience in a safe, nurturing environment. See also TRAUMA SEARCH THERAPY.

treat-the-patient-not-the-disease concept (Hom.) A belief of HAHNEMANN and the basis of all holistic medical interventions which takes into account the uniqueness of the constitution of the individual as well as illness to be treated.

treat-the-whole-person concept (Hom.) Also, the concept of multifactorial nature of health and disease. Health and disease are taken as conditions of the whole organism, involving a complex interaction of physical, spiritual, mental, emotional, genetic, environmental, social, and other factors. According to this hypothesis, a physician must therefore treat the whole person by taking all of these factors into account.

treatment, the four pillars of (Ind.) The four pillars of an ideal or successful treatment setting as recognized in AYURVEDA include the physician, the drug, the attendant and the patient.

treatment principles in ayurveda (Ind.) Both diagnosis and treatment, in AYURVEDA are based on the doctrine of humours (DOSHAs). The following table shows the basic principles adopted while prescribing a schedule of treatment:

Nature of Affliction	The elements (in diet or drug) prescribed
KAPHA aggravation	Less of PRITHVI and JALA, but more of AGNI, VAYU and AKASHA
PITTA aggravation	Less of AGNI
VATA aggravation	Less of VAYU and AKASHA

tree remedies (Eur.) Remedies, considered 'subtle elixirs', made from flowers of certain trees such as birch, fir, hawthorn, beech, wild rose, pine, boxwood, broom and walnut. In folk usage, such remedies are believed to bring relief from unsettling moods and emotions such as anxiety, fear, guilt and anger.

trepanation (Afr.) Also, trepanning, trephination, trephining, burr hole. An ancient African medico-mystical practice, still an accepted medical practice, of drilling a hole in the skull to relieve 'pressure' on the brain, caused by a disease or trauma.

Evidence of trepanation has been found in prehistoric cave paintings from Neolithic times onwards, suggesting that the practice was used to cure epileptic seizures, migraines, and mental disorders.

tribhuvana kirti (Ind.) A compound preparation of AMLA, VIBHITAKI and other ingredients in AYURVEDA, often administered in conditions such as fevers and influenza.

tridhatu siddhanta (Ind.) A branch of AYURVEDA, dealing with human anatomy and physiology.

tridosha siddhanta (Ind.) A branch of AYURVEDA dealing with pathology.

triggers mind programming system (New Age) An approach to harness the hidden powers in one's personality for solving problems through reprogramming.

trigger point (Mod.) A knot or ropy band of muscle formed when a muscle fails to relax. The knot could be felt under the skin and may even twitch involuntarily when touched. The trigger point can trap or irritate surrounding nerves and cause referred pain—pain felt in another part of the body.

trigger point acupuncture (New Age) The application of ACUPUNCTURE needles to the TRIGGER POINTS, the sites of pain.

trigger point myotherapy (New Age) Also, myotherapy. A pain-relieving approach, developed by Bonnie Prudden in 1976, aimed at diffusing TRIGGER POINTS. The approach consists of a hands-on, drugless, non-invasive method of relieving muscle-related pain. To diffuse 'trigger points', pressure is applied to the muscle for several seconds by fingers, knuckles and elbows. It emphasizes speedy, cost effective recovery and active patient participation for long-term relief. Myotherapy relaxes muscles and alleviates pain, while increasing strength and flexibility. Myotherapy is said to be useful in the treatment of addictions, arthritis, backache, colic, Epstein-Barr, headaches, migraine, sinusitis, sports injuries and tendonitis.

trikatu (Ind.) Also, trikadugam. From the Sanskrit word, meaning three pungents. A formulation of GINGER, black pepper and long pepper (PIPPALI), to improve digestion and warm the system. The formulation is traditionally used to treat hay fever and colds and stimulate the respiratory organs. It is also used as a part of weight-loss regime.

trikon asana (Yoga). An asana, aimed at strengthening the calf and thigh muscles, and correcting a hunch back or flat foot.

trikon mudra (Yoga). A MUDRA formed by touching both the thumbs, index finger, middle finger and the ring finger, placed on the nail of the middle finger. This mudra is said to improve digestion.

trikuti (Yoga) The meeting point of the two nasal passages in the human body. See also IDA, PINGALA, SUSHUMNA.

triphala (Ind.). A popular herbal mixture in AYURVEDA, made of the three varieties of myrobalans including AMLAKI, HARITAKI and VIBHITAKI. The drug is regarded as an efficient colon cleanser which helps in the detoxification of the body without depleting the body's reserves.

triphala guggulu (Ind.) A compound preparation of TRIPHALA and GUGGULU. This mixture is said to be useful for detoxifying the body. It is also recommended for those who are conscious of their weight.

tripti mudra (Yoga) A MUDRA formed by folding the fingers of one hand in to the other hand, with the tips of both the thumbs touching each other. This mudra is recommended for those who suffer from paralysis and Parkinson's disease.

Tri Yoga (New Age) A modern version of the ancient system of YOGA, aimed at integrating Eastern traditions to suit Western needs. Tri Yoga exercises combine flowing and sustained postures following a spinal wavelike movement, economy of motion, and synchronized breath and MUDRA. The flows can be either gentle or challenging, according to what one prefers. Its regular practise is believed to increase flexibility, strength, endurance and knowledge of the practitioner.

tsubos (Jap./New Age) The electrically sensitive ACUPOINTS in the human body. The CHAKRAs in the body are referred to as giant tsubos, functioning over a broad range of frequencies and containing large quantities of neurotransmitters. Their malfunctioning is said to cause diseases in the body.

tsubo therapy (Jap./New Age) A form of ACUPRESSURE, that involves the application of MASSAGE, needles, or electricity to ACUPOINTS.

tuina (Chi.) (pronounced tway na) Also, Chinese massage therapy, push-grab massage, tuei-na, tui na an mo, tuina therapy. An ancient system of Chinese MASSAGE, aimed at regulating the flow of CHI and restoring the balance of YIN AND YANG. Fingers, fists, elbows, knees and arms are used on MERIDIAN lines to manipulate muscles to release tensions and enhance the healing process. An important component of TRADITIONAL CHINESE MEDICINE, tuina is easy to perform, convenient, inexpensive, safe and effective.

tulsi See HOLI BASIL.

turiya (Yoga) 1.The transcendental state beyond the waking (jagrat), dream (svapna) and deep sleep (susupti) states. This is the fourth state believed to reflect the true nature of reality, as many Indian philosophers consider the waking state as MAYA or illusion. 2. The state of deep meditation or SAMADHI.

'This state (turiya) is not that which is conscious of the subjective, nor that which is conscious of the objective, nor that which is conscious of both, nor that which is simple consciousness, nor that which is all-sentient mass, nor that which is all darkness. It is unseen, transcendent, the sole essence of the consciousness of self, the completion of the world.'

—*Mandukya Upanishad*

turmeric (Ind.) *Curcuma longa*. Also, haldi. A spice commonly used in Indian cuisine from ancient times and known for its antibacterial and therapeutic properties. It is also used to give a yellow colour to certain preparations. In AYURVEDIC medicine, turmeric is used as a cure for stomach-related problems. Curcumin, the active ingredient in turmeric, is believed to have benefits in Alzheimer's disease, pancreatic and colorectal cancers, and liver disorders. It is also used in the formulation of some sunscreens.

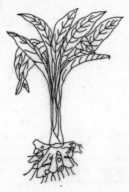

Turmeric

Turkish bath (Turk.) Also, hamam. A bath which comprises exposure to warm air, steam, massage and finally a cold water shower, with the bather moving from one chamber to another. This bath, originating in the Middle East, is said to be ideal for the weight-watchers. It is also known for its cleansing and relaxing effect.

turquoise (Gem.) A stone of protection. It is also believed to bring its wearer a strong willpower and effective communication when worn near thhe throat. It is also believed to slow ageing.

twelve stages in healing (New Age) An approach to healing, based on the concept of twelve stages of CONSCIOUSNESS corresponding to twelve basic rhythms. Developed by Donald M. Epstein, the approach includes QIGONG-like exercises and ASANA-like postures.

> 'The most appropriate response to suffering is to stop thinking about its causes.'
>
> —Donald M. Epstein

twelve steps (New Age) A system, consisting of twelve steps, aimed at recovery from addiction and compulsive behaviour. The steps include MEDITATION and PRAYER.

twenty-one day rejuvenation programme (New Age) A system of rejuvenation, as promoted by Joseph Kurian, including the use of a skin-care cream, said to be helpful in unblocking energy channels.

type (Hom.) A person's general personality and approach to life. Homoeopaths and Bach Flower therapists use it to refer to a constitutional picture, relating to a specific remedy. See also PRAKRITI.

typtology (Occ.) A method of communication with spirits. This is done by means of rapping with various codes being arranged for the purpose. One rap could thus signify the answer 'yes' while two could mean 'no'. See also PLANCHETTE, SEANCE.

udana (Yoga) From the Sanskrit word, meaning upward moving air. One of the five types of PRANA, known for its qualitative and transformative role in AYURVEDA, udana is said to be responsible for one's physical and spiritual development, besides the ability to express and effort.

udana mudra (Yoga) A MUDRA formed by touching the tips of the middle finger, index finger and ring finger with that of the thumb. This mudra is said to heal sore throats, coughs and thyroid problems.

udana vata (Ind.) A form of VATA, located in the chest and the throat, aiding functions connected to speech and singing, and enhancing confidence, enthusiasm and mental strength. Its derangement is believed to cause various diseases of the eyes, mouth, nose, ear, larynx and pharynx.

uddiyana bandha (Yoga) One of the three BANDHAs in YOGA the other two being JALANDHARA and MULADHARA BANDHAs. Uddiyana bandha is said to be helpful in reducing fat in the belly.

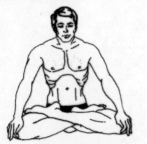

Uddiyana bandha

udvartana (Ind.) An exfoliating MASSAGE, using pastes of barley, chickpea and gram flours along with herbs that are tuned to the client's needs. The treatment is aimed at imparting mobility to joints, strengthening muscles, and rejuvenating the body. This massage balances VATA, removes fat, cleanses and nourishes the skin and increases circulation. It is best for Vata and KAPHA types. It works primarily on the lymphatic system, known as rasa dhatu and helps drain the lymph. It brings lightness and dryness in to the body.

ujjayi (Yoga) From the Sanskrit word, meaning victorious uprising. A form of BREATHING, characterized by (a) a distinctive sound and (b) a deliberate effort to maintain evenness of the flow of breath from the beginning to the end of each breath. The ujjayi sound is made by toning the throat and epiglottis as one would when whispering the sound 'haaa'—the breathy sound one makes when fogging a mirror. The purpose of sounding here is to maintain the quality and texture of one's breath throughout the exercise. It is also said to enhance one's ability to absorb the PRANA from the air, infusing energy into the body. With a subtle, relaxed practice of ujjayi breath, the soothing currents of energy moving through one's head, along the spine and passing throughout the body can be experienced. The practice is aimed at cleaning toxins accumulated in both the digestive and nerve passages.

Unani (Ind.) Derived from the Greek Ionia, a narrow coastal strip in Asia Minor. Unani is a system of healing influenced by HIPPOCRATES, the 'father of medicine', and dominated by the works of Greek physician, Galen. it owes much to the work of the tenth-century Persian physician, Ibn Sina who came to be known in the West as AVICENNA. The system which developed in India, recognizes that every individual has a unique constitution, combining a unique proportion of humours, blood (dam), phlegm (balgam), yellow bile (safra) and black bile (souda). It also recognizes that the body is composed of seven components, including elements, functions, humours, organs, powers, temperament and the vital spirit. Additional factors such as atmospheric air, food and beverages, physical and psychological movements and response of the body, sleep and alertness, evacuation or retention are believed to affect one's health directly or indirectly, along with factors such as geography of the nation, residence, occupation, habits, age and sex. Through pulse reading, the physician understands heart-rhythms and other factors such as blood circulation (i.e. volume, tension, condition of the blood vessels, duration and the rate of movement, tactus, rhythm, regularity and equilibrium). Diet restriction is an important component of treatment. Other methods include CUPPING, diaphoresis, exercise, MASSAGE, purging, TURKISH BATH and venesection. Unani uses honey as a base for its medicine, many of which comprise pearls and metals.

unconscious mind (New Age) The area of the psyche which is said to harbour unknown wishes and needs that influence conscious behaviour. According to Freud, mental states are essentially unconscious in nature and a store-house of socially unacceptable ideas, wishes and desires, traumatic memories and painful emotions put out of the mind by the mechanism of psychological regression. The part of the brain that regulates autonomic body functions, regulates the physical expression of emotions (e.g., shedding tears when one is sad) .

underwater massage (New Age) A form of HYDROTHERAPY in which a patient lying in the bathtub is massaged by a strong jet of water at a considerable pressure (35 lb per square inch). As a submerged body is weightless, an underwater massage is considered more vigorous than one above water. This treatment is found useful to people with chronic pain, like arthritis, since the water's buoyancy makes it easier to move without discomfort.

unicist homeopathy (Hom.) See CLASSICAL HOMOEOPATHY.

universe Based on the context in which the word occurs, it has a variety of meanings. In the physical sense, a universe is the summation of all matter that exists and the space in which all events occur or could occur.

> 'When I open my eyes to the outer world, I feel myself as a drop in the sea. But, when I close my eyes and look within. I see the whole universe as a bubble raised in the ocean of my heart!'
>
> —Inayat Khan

> 'The universe is not required to be in perfect harmony with human ambition.'
>
> —Carl Sagan

universal balm (New Age) A remedy considered practically for every ailment.

universal energy (Misc.) Energy-flow in the human body as well as in the UNIVERSE, variously referred to as CHI, PRANA, QI, SEFIROT, SHAKTI, spirit, vital energy, VITAL FORCE. Energy therapies presuppose that matter and energy are not exclusive opposites, but that matter is just a denser or condensed form of energy.

Universal Spirit of Oneness (New Age) Also para brahma. The mighty energy of the universe which creates, maintains and destroys through continuous transformation. This metaphysical principle of the universe is also referred to in ancient Indian philosophy as pure consciousness or pure bliss. It is formless and characterless (NIRGUNA) and is not bound by the laws of space, time or causation.

> 'I am the mist of morning, the wreath of evening... I am the spark in the stone, the gleam of gold in the metal...I am the chain of being, the circle of spheres, the scale of creation, the creation, the rise and the fall. I am what is and what is not.'
>
> —Rumi

upanaha svedana (Ind.) The application of warm, medicated poultices, often in the treatment of arthritis.

upanshu japa (Ind.) The mental repetition of a MANTRA. Silent japa is said to be more powerful than the one verbalized.

upaprana See MINOR PRANAS.

upgrades (New Age) The technique of merging a hypnotized person into a positive state (such as self esteem, acceptance, or inner peace) visually perceived by him or her.

urine analysis (Ind./Tib.) Urine is used in diagnosis in most systems of medicine. In TIBETAN MEDICINE, for example, urine is diagnosed by two ways: by 'listening' to the noisy bubbles while stirred in a jar and by smelling; a strong odour indicates an overheated body and lots of noisy bubbling in the urine when stirred, indicates that the patient is mentally stressed and restless. In SIDDHA MEDICINE, the colour of urine indicates the problem; straw-coloured urine indicates indigestion, reddish-yellow indicates excessive heat and a rosy tinge, blood pressure. The shape a drop of oil takes when placed on urine which is kept in a tray in sunlight is believed to determine vitiated humour: if it spreads like a snake, it indicates VATA, if it makes a ring it indicates PITTA, and if it floats like a pearl it indicates KAPHA.

urine therapy (Ind.) An ancient custom of use of urine for therapeutic purposes. See also, AUTO-URINE THERAPY, SHIVAMBU.

urobasti (Ind.) Also, hridbasti. A healing treatment for the chest or heart-area (ANAHATA CHAKRA), especially for patients with cardiac disorders. Medicated oil is filled in a dough dam, specially made to hold over the client's chest, and allowed to be there for thirty to forty minutes. The oil may be enriched with milk, ghee, arjuna, rose, hibiscus or herbs. The treatment is said to soothe and nourish the heart region and emotions. It is normally given in hospital under the care of a doctor.

ustrasana (Yoga) Derived from the Sanskrit ustra, meaning camel, as the shape assumed by the practitioner is that of a camel. The ASANA is considered beneficial for white-collar workers who do sedentary desk jobs. The practise of this asana is said to relieve stiffness in the ankles, back, neck and shoulders by toning up the muscles of the spine and enhancing the lung capacity and the blood circulation.

Usui, Mikao (1865–1926) (Jap.) Also, Usui Sensei. The re-discoverer of REIKI and founder of the Usui system of reiki.

utkatasana (Yoga) Also, the power posture. This ASANA comprises the following steps:

Step 1. Sit on the toes, positioning the thighs parallel to the ground.
Step 2. Place the fists on the shoulders.
Step 3. Do breathing exercise 10 times in the following way: Inhale slowly and gently, retain the breath and exhale softly and relax. This asana facilitates relaxation.

utkleshana basti (Ind.) The administration of medicated decoctions through the rectum. The treatment is said to promote secretions in the colon that liquefy and expel AMA.

utsaha (Yoga) Sanskrit, meaning zeal. One of the three essential qualities required for YOGA aspirants, the other two being cheerfulness (sahasa) and tenacity (dridhata).

uttama (Yoga) One of the three types of PRANAYAMA in which the duration for inhaling the breath (PURAKA) is fixed at 32 MATRAS. As a consequence, the duration of retaining (KUMBHAKA) and exhaling (RECHAKA) the breath would work out to be 128 and 64 MATRAS respectively. Adhama and Madhyama, the other two types of pranayama consist of twelve and twenty-four MATRAS respectively.

uttanasana (Yoga) Also, forward bend. A popular HATHA YOGA posture, this ASANA consists of standing with feet together, hinging

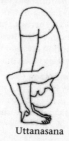

Uttanasana

forward from the hips, letting the head hang down, with palms placed flat on the floor. It provides a complete stretch to the back and is considered to be beneficial for depression and exhaustion. It is also said to rejuvenate the spinal nerves and the brain, besides lowering the heart rate.

uttar basti (Ind.) One of the eight BASTIs in AYURVEDA. Medicated oil is used for cleaning the urinary bladder by passing a catheter into the urethra in male patients and as a vaginal douche in women.

uttarabodhi mudra (Yoga) Also, gesture of supreme enlightenment. A MUDRA formed by touching the tip of the index fingers and thumbs of both the hands and interlocking other fingers. This mudra is said to strengthen the nervous system.

uzhichil (Ind.) AYURVEDIC oil-MASSAGE. The massage is done in two ways: with the help of one's hands (administered for children and seniors) and with legs (for others). Uzhichil is said to minimize the pressure on the heart while stimulating blood circulation. It is classified under the SVEDA system of PANCHA KARMA and is treated by the leading experts of kalari, the traditional martial art. UZHICHIL is said to be effective in treating of arthritis, breathing difficulties, rheumatism, slipped disc, spondylitis, and nervous weakness. Ancient texts such as *Ashtanga Hridayam* and *Yoga Ratnakaram* cite the supremacy of uzhichil over the various methods of treatment in AYURVEDA.

V

Vagabhatta (Ind.) (c.342 BC) A scholar and compiler of ancient texts on AYURVEDA, Vagabhatta is one of the main commentators of AYURVEDA. His *Ashtanga Hridaya* is regarded as the third major treatise on ayurveda, after the works of CHARAKA and SUSHRUTA. It contains information on the two schools of ayurveda—the school of surgery and the school of physicians. Vagabhatta is believed to be responsible for introducing a number of new herbs and surgical techniques to the system.

vaidya (Ind.) Also, vaid. A physician, a practitioner in AYURVEDA.

vaikhari (Yoga) An articulate form of sound, which refers to the sound spoken as the vehicle of thoughts.

vaikhari japa (Yoga). A JAPA repeated audibly.

vajikarana (Ind.) Sanskrit, meaning making or doing like a horse. 1. A procedure in AYURVEDA, aimed at promoting REJUVENATION 2. The source of strengthening the reproductive system. There is similarity in the procedures of RASAYANA and VAJIKARANA, though the former relates to the 'first' DHATU, called RASA (the body fluid), and the latter to the last, called SHUKRA (semen). See also APHRODISIAC.

vajra mudra (Yoga) A MUDRA which is considered the gesture of knowledge. It is made by making a fist with the right hand, index finger extending upward, and the left hand also making a fist and enclosing the index. The MUDRA is used along with MANTRA to enhance its effect.

vajrasana (Yoga) A popular ASANA considered ideal for meditation and for those who suffer from sciatica, stiff ankles and varicose veins.

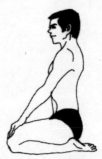

Vajrasana

vakrasana (Yoga) Also, twist posture. Derived from the Sanskrit for the crooked posture. An ASANA aimed at toning up the spinal nerves and considered ideal for diabetics and those who suffer from kidney ailments.

vamana (Ind.) Also, vamana karma. Induced vomiting; a technique in AYURVEDA to facilitate the expunging of toxins from the body by medicating with emetics. The technique is an important part of PANCHA KARMA and is considered the most effective treatment in vitiated conditions of KAPHA. In a disease having predominance of KAPHA DOSHA, Vamana can be performed at any time after performing SNEHANA and SVEDANA.

vamanopaga (Ind.) The natural substances used for stimulating vomiting. In AYURVEDA, several herbs are used for this purpose.

varma points (Ind.) The vital points as described in the ancient SIDDHA texts, akin to ACUPOINTS.

varma touch (Ind.) An ancient system of massage, prescribed in the SIDDHA texts, according to which a touch (thoduvarmam) or blow (paduvarmam) at the varma points, applied with a calculated force, frequency and pressure can prove to be life-saving. The basic features of the procedure include relaxation of varma points and their adjoining muscles through oil massage and fomentation.

varna dravyani (Cos.) Complexion-promoting substances.

varuna mudra (Yoga) A MUDRA formed by touching the tip of the thumb with that of the little finger. This mudra is considered ideal for controlling liquid outflows from the body such as mucous secretions and diarrhoea which cause dehydration.

vasaka (Ind.) *Adhatoda vasaka.* A medicinal shrub commonly found in the lower Himalayas. Vasaka is a popular drug known from ancient times. Its medicinal uses have been well-documented in several ancient texts. It is known for its therapeutic role in respiratory disorders like bronchial asthma and chronic bronchitis.

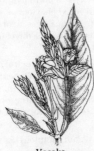

Vasaka

vastu (Ind.) Sanskrit, for physical environment. A traditional set of canons of Hindu architecture and town-planning as codified in ancient texts such as *Manasara* and *Mayamata*. The system is based on the belief that dwelling places should be built in harmony with the physical (e.g. gravitational, electro-magnetic) and metaphysical (e.g. supernatural) energies in the relevant area. Though vastu is conceptually similar to FENG SHUI, it differs from it in procedural details.

vata (Ind.) Sanskrit, meaning movement. One of the three humours (DOSHAs), recognized in the system of AYURVEDA, Vata represents a force created in nature by the dynamic interplay of ether (space) and air. It enables the other two DOSHAs, i.e. PITTA and KAPHA to be expressive. See also TRIDOSHA.

vata prakriti (Ind.) The overall predominance of VATA in the constitution of an individual. The dry quality of vata is manifested in the body in a dry skin and lean body, an appearance of dry hair, nails, teeth and eyes, and a low, weak crackling and hoarse voice. Vata prakriti people are hyperactive and require little sleep. Their movements, especially of the eyebrows, chin, lips, tongue and limbs, are quick and unsteady.

vata churna (Ind.) A combination of warming, calming, and slightly unctuous spices and herbs. Vata churna is eaten to counter constipation or flatulence and to promote the assimilation of nutrients.

vata shamaka oil (Ind.) A medicated oil used in AYURVEDA for countering the aggravating VATA. In Ayurveda, oils are prescribed according to the dosha of a person. For instance, calming oils like sesame, olive, almond, amla, bala, wheat germ or castor oil are used for vata dosha persons.

vaya (Ind.) The age of the patient; an important criterion for prescribing the course of treatment in AYURVEDA.

vayu (Ind.) Wind or air, one of the FIVE ELEMENTS (PANCHABHUTAS) regarded as the universal organizing principle of movement.

vayu mudra (Yoga) A MUDRA formed by touching the tip of the index finger at the base of the thumb. This mudra is believed to counter flatulence and wind disorders such as sciatica.

vayu surabhi mudra (Yoga) A variation of SURABHI MUDRA, this mudra is formed by touching the tip of the thumb with the base of the index finger. The mudra is considered a cure for gastric disorders.

Vedic therapy (Ind.) An approach to healing, with vibrations, contained especially in the Vedic chants.

veerya (Ind.) Power. According to the influence of nature a substance is believed to be either hot or cold in power. A drug is either ushna-veerya, or heating, or seeta-veerya, cooling. depending on its action.

veetrag mudra (Yoga) Also, dispassionate mudra. A common form of MUDRA, found in Jain art, especially in images of the Teerthankaras. The mudra is formed by placing the left palm near the navel, right palm over it and thumbs on each other. This mudra is aimed at developing dispassionate feelings and stability. It is also said to enhance the upward mobility of energy within the body.

vegan (New Age) An approach to healing and health through a plant-based diet, non-leather clothing, natural dwellings and a non-consumerist lifestyle in which compassion and contentment are intrinsic.

vegan diet (New Age) Uncooked or living-food diet, free from animal products, including meat, fish, seafood, eggs, and dairy. It provides significantly more dietary antioxidants than the cooked, omnivorous diet. As vegans eat no animal products, some dieticians emphasize the need for inclusion of vitamin B12 from fortified foods or supplements.

vegetarianism The dietary practice of subsisting on a diet composed primarily or wholly of vegetables, grains, nuts, flowers, leaves, fruits and seeds. It may or may not include dairy products.

velvet beans (Ind.) *Mucuna pruriens*. A popular Indian plant, velvet beans grow in the plains. Every part of the plant is used medicinally. According to recent research, the seeds contain L-dopa, an anti-Parkinson's disease drug. This discovery has created a new interest in the plant, motivating its commercial cultivation in various parts of India.

verbal therapy (New Age) An approach to healing, which relies upon IMAGINEERING, employing methods such as AUTO-SUGGESTION THERAPY, DIRECT COMMAND, FIVE-MINUTE FOCUS.

vessel organs (Tib.) The organs in the body, considered vessels in TIBETAN MEDICINE. There are five vessel organs, including the stomach, gall bladder, small intestine, large intestine, and the vesicle of regenerative organs.

vibhitaki (Ind.) *Terminalia bellirica*. Also, beleric myrobalan. The fruit of the vibhitaki constitutes one of the three ingredients of the ayurvedic preparation TRIPHALA. It is prescribed in a variety of diseases including anaemia, cough, fever, asthma, diarrhoea, dysentery, biliousness, diseases of the eyes, nose and throat. It is also believed to stimulate hair growth, cure leprosy and purify the blood.

vibrational medicine (Vib.) energy medicine; a healing system that treats the body on a vibrational or energy plane. The human body itself is believed to be made of denser forms of energy vibrations. Disease is considered a consequence of the depletion of energy, and the system attempts to select an exterior source of energy that can harmonize or synchronize energy pattern of the patient with the body.

Vietnamese traditional medicine The traditional system of medicine in Vietnam, which incorporates practices such as ACUPUNCTURE, CUPPING, MOXIBUSTION and SCARIFICATION.

vihara (Ind.) Sanskrit for practice. The activity or lifestyle of an individual. Vihara also refers to one's behaviour or conduct as influenced by the quality of his or her mind. It is considered to have a direct impact on one's health-profile.

vikruti (Ind.) The pathological condition as an indicator of health. There are numerous reasons for vikruti (or the imbalance of DOSHAS) to be manifest but the root cause of all disease is overindulgence of the senses or ignorance.

vilepi (Ind.) A soft, glutinous rice soup, prescribed in AYURVEDA for the second day after PANCHAKARMA.

Vini Yoga (New Age) A modern version of yoga, as popularized by T.K.V. Desikachar, an engineer-turned-yoga teacher. This form of yoga is performed one-on-one with an instructor, with poses and gentle flows performed at a slow pace.

Vini Yoga is based on the concept that by balancing the breath one balances the energy in the body and that improving breathing improves posture and develops a sense of being centred. It is also considered restorative and therapeutic. Postures are done with slightly bent knees and, as a result, Vini Yoga places little stress on the joints.

violet colour therapy (New Age) In COLOUR THERAPY, violet colour is believed to play a therapeutic role in several ailments including bladder problems, cramps, kidney diseases, mental illness, nervous disorders, neuralgia, rheumatism, sciatica, skin diseases and tumours. It is also believed that violet-coloured light, falling through a stained glass window, can increase the impact of meditation up to ten-fold.

vipaka (Ind.) The post-absorptive phase of digestion. It is the change which a drug undergoes in the organism under the influence of JATHARAGNI, the digestive fire. AYURVEDA believes that the post-digestive impact is an equally important criterion in the selection of a drug. According to ancient texts, three kinds of drug metabolism, namely, katu (pungent), amla (sour) and madhura (sweet), are responsible for an increase in vata, pitta and kapha respectively.

viparita karani (Yoga) A popular ASANA in which the body is inverted. It is believed that all the fluids in the body, viz. blood, lymph and hormones circulate more efficiently in the body, as a consequence of which the body is energized.

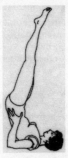

Viparita karani

vipassana (New Age) Also, vipashchana. A technique of self-observation and introspection, which has long been an integral part of Buddhism. The technique is considered useful in changing one's habit patterns and, as a consequence, brings freedom from aversion, craving and ignorance.

> 'The most basic requirement of the ten-day vipassana course is silence. Buddha was of the belief that nature does everything creative in silence. It is the basis for every process from degeneration to regeneration.'
>
> —Jayantilal Shah, vipassana teacher

virabhadrasana (Yoga) The warrior-pose. Named after Virabhadra, a legendary warrior who practised this ASANA, this posture is practised with the aim of enhancing breathing capacity.

virasana (Yoga) This ASANA, in which the chest is stretched, is said to help improve one's breathing capacity. It is also practised to alleviate or prevent backache, arthritis of the elbows, knee joints and fingers, stiff neck, frozen shoulders and the like.

virechana (Ind.) Purgation, one of the five methods of SHODHANA. A number of effective and safe herbs are used as laxatives in AYURVEDA. This includes bran, castor oil, cow's milk, dandelion root, flaxseed, mango juice, prune, psyllium, raisins and senna. Virechana is said to be beneficial to diabetes, skin ailments, chronic fevers and piles.

Vishuddhi (Yoga) Fifth Chakra, throat Chakra. One of the seven major CHAKRAS, vishuddhi is located in the spine behind the throat and connected with the cervical plexus, tonsils and thyroid glands.

Vis Medicatrix Naturae (Nat.) The healing power of nature. A fundamental principle in nature cure, which acknowledges the healing power in nature.

visualization (New Age) The process of creating MENTAL IMAGES. According to some psychologists, visualizing healing images may have a profound effect on the body and mind, strengthening the immune system of the body. In recent years Western writers notably, Norman Vincent Peale (*The Power of Positive Thinking*, 1952), Maxwall Maltz (*Psycho-Cybernetics*, 1960) and Shakti Gawain (*Creative Visualization*, 1979 have popularized the role of visualization.

vital force (New Age) Also, LIFE FORCE. A concept equivalent to the Chinese concept of QI and the Indian concept of PRANA. When the harmonious functions of a living system are threatened in any way, the vital force endeavours to restore the balance: the role of the vital force is to maintain a dynamic equilibrium in an organism.

vital organs (Tib.) According to TIBETAN MEDICINE, the five vital organs which sustain life processes are: heart, lungs, liver, spleen and kidneys.

vitala (Occ./Yoga) One of the fourteen CHAKRAS, representing raging anger. See CHAKRAS, LOWER.

Vodder massage (Mod./New Age) Also, lymphatic massage. A technique of MASSAGE, developed by Emil Vodder, a Danish physician, in the 1930s. The technique focusses on the lymphatic system. The procedure involves light repetitive strokes on a selected area, until a thin layer of lymphatic fluid appears on the skin. The therapist then moves onto another area to repeat the procedure. Through this methodical stimulation, the lymphatic liquid is directed towards the lymph nodes where the fluid can be filtered and the waste eliminated. The end result will be significantly decreased soreness or stiffness in the muscles. The technique is based on the concept that the proper flow of lymphatic fluid is vital for proper immune functioning through the elimination of wastes from the tissues and organs of the body.

voodoo (Afr.) The word comes from the West African word *vodun*, meaning spirit. It refers to a healing practice, derived from ancient African polytheism and was influenced by ancestor worship of Roman Catholicism. It is believed that God is manifest through the spirits of ancestors, which can bring good luck or bad days. To appease them, they are honoured through rites, rituals and ceremonies which include prayers, drumming, dancing, singing and animal sacrifice.

vowels (Misc.) One of the two elements in human speech (the other being consonants). Vowels are considered the most dynamic aspect of spoken sound, since without their involvement, no consonant can be sounded. Each vowel is said to affect a particular part of the body. This part of the body is visualized during the inhalation of the breath as the vowel is sounded silently. As one exhales, the vowel is sounded audibly with the outgoing breath. The breath penetrates deeply in to the concerned area as directed by our thought. As the breath infuses the area with PRANA, combining it with the vibrations in the vowel tone, it is said that the specific inner region is opened up with this practice. The purpose of toning is thus said to restore the vibrational pattern of the body (physical and subtle) to its perfect electromagnetic field, so as to enjoy good health. The following table indicates some vowel sounds which are believed to be healing:

Vowel	Area/limbs/organs activated or opened up
u	Pelvic region, i.e. hips, legs, feet and lower part of the body
o	Abdominal region, i.e., from the solar plexus to groin
a	Chest region, heart
e	Head region, above the upper chest including throat, forehead, crown and back of the skull

vyakta (Ind.) A stage of clinical manifestation of a disease. This stage is characterized by the manifestation of a conspicuous set of signs and symptoms.

vyana (Ind.) Literally outward-moving wind. One of the five forms of PRANA, located in the heart region, moving quickly in the body and attending to various activities relating to circulation. Vyana is said to move from the centre towards periphery and govern circulation. Apart from the circulation of oxygen, food and water in the body, it is also said to help in the circulation of information, thoughts and feelings.

'Vyana Vayu is the energy that envelops our body; it is often called an aura.'

—*Tathagata Abhidhamma*, Book I

vyana vata (Ind.) A form of VATA in the body, said to play a vital role in the transfer of elements (SAPTA DHATU). In derangement, this DOSHA produces aches and pains. It can also result in fever, diarrhoea and haemorrage.

vyayama (Ind.) From the Sanskrit vya meaning space, and yama, meaning restraint. A system of simple physical and movement exercises, comprising postures (ASANAS), body movements, breathing techniques and MUDRAS. HATHA YOGA postures, PRANAYAMA and SURYA NAMASKARA are examples of vyayama, which are energy-giving to the body, rather than energy-expending.

'Light, capacity for work, firmness, tolerance to hardship, subsidence of humoural discordance and stimulation of gastric fire are the (beneficial) results of practising vyayama.'

—an ancient Sanskrit text

vyayama shakti (Ind.) The capacity to work or physical exercises (VYAYAMA). It determines a patient's strength and morbidity.

vyayama vijnana (Yoga) A branch of AYURVEDA, dealing with the science of physical exercises (VYAYAMA). It covers the definition and concept of physical exercises, principles of the practice of exercises, the adverse impact of under- or over-exercising, appropriate diet for exercisers, therapeutic relevance of exercise, bodily strength physiology of strength, ideals for physical growth and development.

W

Wai Lana Yoga (New Age) A series of yogic exercises as developed by Wai Lana, a contemporary TV artist and musician from Hong Kong. It is based on the notion that yogic movements such as bending, pushing, squeezing, stretching and twisting 'bathe' the internal organs with vitality.

> 'The days you don't want to do Yoga are the days you need to do Yoga.'
>
> —Wai Lana

Waijia and Neijia (Jap.) External and internal martial arts (KUNGFU), respectively. Both these art forms have contributed significantly not only to Chinese culture but also to the world of health and fitness. The goal of Waijia practise is to increase the natural abilities (of speed, force, natural or normal movements and responses). All fighting skills combine these abilities. In Neijia practice, however, the goal is to change tactics rather than simply increasing one's natural abilities. Neijia practitioners achieve quickness and power by shifting their usual patterns of response. Though some Neijia training methods focus on increasing natural abilities, this goal has always been secondary to the goal of changing one's normal reactions. However the two systems are so conceived that both Waijia and Neijia students develop both external and internal skills. It is said that Waijia is practised from the outside (*wai*) to the inside (*nei*) and Neijia, from the inside to the outside.

waist–hip Ratio (Mod.) A ratio of the circumference of the waist at the umbilicus and of the hip around the fattest part of the buttocks. It is an indicator of body fat distribution. Values about 0.8 in women and 0.9 in men indicate a tendency towards central fat disposition and a possible increased health risk.

waitankung (Chi.) An ancient system of exercise of Taoist origin, said to allow CHI energy to fill up the body like an electric current. The system is said to be of help in strengthening the bones, joints and tendons of the legs besides improving the functions of the bladder, intestines and kidneys.

walking (Mod.) An ideal and simple exercise for the whole body, regular walking is recommended as a treatment for obesity, diabeties, heart and coronary diseases. The perfect means to weight loss and general fitness, regular walking strengthens one's heart, tones the muscles and instills a general feeling of wellbeing.

> 'Walk a mile, walk with smile!'
>
> —Anonymous

walking chi kung (Chi.) A special form of QIGONG that focusses on movement and walking. Each step in a move, requires one to stay in place till tension disipates. The exercise encompasses simple meditation, and more complex dance-like movements, controlled breathing, and guided imagery.

walking meditation (Jap.) KINHIN. A form of meditation, practised while walking. Walking meditation is essentially about being aware of one's movement, while concentrating on the component parts of the step. Walking meditation has been one of the most prevalent manifestations of Buddhist practice. It has the advantage of being able to be done anytime one is walking and is also used as a way to break up periods of sitting meditation.

> 'I walk on thorns but firmly as among flowers.'
>
> —Thich Nhat Hanh

walking pranayama (New Age) PRANAYAMA, practised while walking. Inhalation is done through both the nostrils chanting aum mentally for three times, one count for each step. The breath is retained for twelve counts of aum. Exhalation through both the nostrils is done for six counts. A respiratory pause or rest is taken after one pranayama for twelve counts of aum.

warm bath (Nat.) A simple, healing method, aimed at relaxing the mind and the body.

warm foot bath (Nat.) An alternative healing method in which the feet are kept in a warm water bath for a fixed duration, aimed at overcoming congestion and improving circulation.

water (Nat.) Known for its therapeutic value, water has the ability to store and transmit heat. It absorbs more heat for a given weight compared to any other substance. It has therefore been used in treatments in several medical systems. Its solvent properties find their application in HYDROTHERAPY. Increasing water intake when one feels sick or weak is the time-tested practice to regain one's vigour.

> 'There is no substitute for water.'
>
> —An old saying

water asceticism (New Age) A Japanese healing method, in which one douses oneself in buckets of icy water in mid-winter, or stands under a waterfall. This practice, like fasting, is said to help in the emergence of the super-conscious by slowing down the body's metabolism and calming the areas of consciousness related to bodily functions. Asceticism is the practice of austere self-discipline, voluntarily undertaken, in order to achieve a higher or spiritual ideal.

water birth (New Age) A natural birthing process, wherein child delivery takes place in a tub containing lukewarm water. By immersing the lower part of the body of the labouring mother in water, labour pains are said to reduce and delivery becomes gentle and smooth. The baby is offered the comfort of the warm and wet environment immediately after its arrival, and wallowing in warm water allows the mother relax.

water fast (New Age/Nat.) A method of FASTING, in which only water is consumed for a day or two with a view to cleansing and overhauling the digestive tract. It is believed that many diseases, such as asthma, cardiovascular disease, colitis, high blood pressure, psoriasis and various auto-immune disorders can be reversed through water fasting.

watsu (New Age) Also, water shiatsu. A healing massage treatment performed in a warm pool in which the therapist administers rhythmic movements, pressure-point massage and stretches to help clients achieve deep relaxation.

weight lifting work-out (New Age) Aerobic exercises that make use of the resistance offered by weights.

weight no more (New Age) An approach to weight reduction, as developed by Edgar Cayce. It is based on the concept that tapping into the life-force in a positive way, i.e. allowing it to flow without hindrance through the body, is the key for correcting physical deficiencies. The approach is based on the notion that the individual possesses three 'bodies': physical, mental and spiritual.

weight training (New Age) The use of free weights or weight machines in a structured and repetitive exercise programme, aimed both at toning the body and adding or replacing lean muscle mass.

wei qi (Chi.) A form of immune energy or force (QI) which protects the body against foreign pathogens.

wet-sock compress (Nat.) A simple healing method in which socks are drenched in ice water, squeezed, and then used. The application of wet socks is said to remove exhaustion and head congestion during a bad cold. It is also reportedly effective in insomnia and relaxes the body and mind.

whirlpool (Spa) A tub of hot water with jets of high-pressure water pumped from the sides and bottom. The regular use of whirlpools is prescribed for patients who experience chronic pain or who are to completely recover from injury. The treatment is also said to soothe muscle tension and induce relaxation.

whole health shiatsu (New Age) An approach to healing, combining SHIATSU and dietary treatment, as designed by Shizuko Yamamoto and Patrick McCarty in 1998. The system is oriented towards promoting the flow of QI energy in the body.

wicca (New Age) A religious movement popularized in 1954 by Gerald Gardner, a British civil servant. Considered a modern survivor of the ancient art of witchcraft, the movement aims at healing through beliefs, rituals and practices energizing the practitioner. In the US, it is reported that there were more than a million adult wiccans in 2001.

wisdom sheath (Occ.) See COGNITIVE BODY.

'By three methods we may learn wisdom; first by reflection, which is noblest; second, by initiation, which is easier; and third, by experience, which is the bitterest.'

—Confucius

wortcunning (Occ.) Also, herbal magick. An ancient art of tapping the 'power' of the HERBs, plants, trees and shrubs. Herbs are first 'enchanted', to ensure that their vibrations are attuned to the needs of an individual and oils, ointments and incense are made from such 'attuned' herbs. The simple method comprises rubbing herb-scent into a coloured candle, setting it in a holder and lighting it while visualizing one's magical needs. Ancient religions have incorporated such life-giving herbs into the realm of legends, mythology, rituals and worship. In Hinduism, gods and goddesses are associated with herbs and trees whose worship is believed to be as rewarding as worshipping the deity. The following table indicates beliefs concerning some a few healing herbs:

Herb	Properties	Uses
Angelica root (*Angelica officinalis*) ('The root of the Holy Ghost') (root)	Masculine, Sun, fire	For protection. Root is carried with as an amulet; dried leaves are burnt in EXORCISM rituals
Aloe (*Aloe Americana*) (leaves)	Feminine, Moon, water	For beauty, luck and success. Hung at doorways or in ceilings to attract luck and protection
Anise (*Pimpinella anisum*) (seeds)	Masculine, Jupiter, air	Burnt while meditating; worn in person; used in pillows for good sleep
Basil (*Ocimum basilicum*)	Masculine, Mars, fire	For courage, fertility, love, wealth and protection. Added to love sachets and incenses
Caraway (*Carum carvi*) (seeds)	Masculine, Mercury, air	Seeds used in sleep pillows to strengthen one's memory
Cinnamon (*Cinnmomum zeylanicum*) (bark)	Masculine, Sun, fire	For spirituality and success. When burnt as incense, it enhances one's spiritual and psychic powers
Cloves (*Syzigium aromaticum*) (dried flower buds)	Masculine, Jupiter, fire	For love, money and protection. Burning cloves is believed to attract riches
Garlic (*Allium sativum*) (Bulbs)	Masculine, Mars, fire	For healing and protection. Hung in kitchen, it is said to keep up one's will-power

Mugwort (*Artemesia vulgaris*)	Feminine, Venus, earth	For strength and psychic powers Stuffed in pillows for sweet dreams Infusion used in cleaning crystals and gems
Pine (*Pinus* spp.) (cones)	Masculine, Mars, air	For fertility, money and protection. Cones are carried to increase fertility for a productive old age
Rose (*Rosa* spp) (buds)	Feminine, Venus, water	For love, luck and psychic powers. Rose is traditionally associated with emotional health
Sandal wood (*Santalum album*)	Feminine, Moon; water	For spirituality and protection. Powdered sandalwood scattered to clear off negativities

wu ming qigong (Chi.) An ancient technique of self-healing, based on the notion that healing energy is transferred from teacher to student. The Chinese expression 'wu ming', literally means 'no name', and refers to the universal force or energy

wu xing (Chi.) Also, wu zhong liu xing zhi chi. From the Chinese *wu*, meaning five, it is the philosophy of the dynamic states of change. It refers to the five types of CHI dominating at different times in the body. According to this concept, water dominates in winter, wood in spring, fire in summer, and metal in autumn. At the intersection between two seasons, the transitional period is dominated by earth. The concept of wu xing is a central theme not only in TRADITIONAL CHINESE MEDICINE but also in all aspects of Chinese thought, including philosophy, astrology and FENG SHUI.

X

X (Hom.) The Roman numeral, which indicates the DECIMAL SCALE, the second potency scale, which has a dilution factor of 1:10 meaning that one part of the mother tincture or potency gets diluted in 9 parts of water-alochol mixture. As decimal potencies are 'low potency' remedies, they are easy to use and hence commonly sold in retail outlets. See also POTENCY; SUCCUSSION.

xi (Chi.) Inhalation; drawing in.

xi mai (Chi.) fine or thin pulsation.

xia qi (Chi.) Driving QI downwards.

xian (Chi.) Salt; salty taste. In Chinese medicine, a balanced diet is one which includes five tastes: spicy, sour, bitter, salty and sweet. Xian refers to the salty taste. As the herbs and foods with the salty taste tends to be warming and moistening, they are used in the treatment of cold and dryness and avoided or used cautiously for patients who are diagnosed as 'hot and damp'. As salty taste dries up the blood, it is avoided by those suffering from anaemia or blood deficiency.

xian mai (Chi.) Wiry pulsation.

xiang fu (Arab./Chi./Ind.) Also, cocograss; nut-grass. *Cyperus rotundus*. A troublesome weed, native to central Europe and south Asia, also known for its culinary and medicinal importance in folk medicine. In TRADITIONAL CHINESE MEDICINE, it is the primary QI-regulator.Charaka Samhita, the ancient ayurvedic text too recognizes it in the treatment of fevers, digestive disorders and dysmenorhoea. The roasted tubers are used in the treatments of bruises, carbuncles and wounds.

xie qi (Chi.) Pathogenic QI.

xin (Chi) Acrid.

xin ji (Chi.) Palpitations.

xing qi (Chi.) Facilitating the movement of QI.

xing ren (Chi.) *Prunus armenica*. Also, apricot kernel. The bitter seeds of this plant is used in TRADITIONAL CHINESE MEDICINE, to arrest coughs and help in stopping wheezing.

xing shui (Chi.) Facilitating the dissipation of pathogenic fluids.

xiong (Chi.) Virile and robust.

xu (Chi.) Deficiency.

xu mai (Chi.) Deficient pulsation.

xue xu (Chi.) Blood deficiency.

yama (Yoga) Restraint, a rule or code of conduct for living. The ancient scriptures of Hinduism list ten moral restraints, including non-violence and abstinence from injury (AHIMSA), truthfulness (SATYA), not stealing or coveting (ASTEYA), continence and celibacy (BRAHMACHARYA), patience (KSHAMA), steadfastness (DHRITI), compassion (daya), honesty (arjava), moderate appetite (MITAHARA), and purity of body, mind and speech (SHAUCHA). In the Yoga Sutras of Patanjali, the YAMAS which form the first 'limb' of the 'eight-limbed' ASHTANGA YOGA are dealt with as summarized:

The Moral Restraints	Brief Explanation
AHIMSA	Non-violence (freedom from violence in thoughts, words and action)
SATYA	Truthfulness (freedom from falsehood)
ASTEYA	Freedom from avarice
BRAHMACHARYA	Celibacy (living in harmony with creative principles)
APARIGRAHA	Freedom from desires

'What is moral is what you feel good after.'

—Ernest Hemingway

yang (Chi.) In traditional Chinese philosophy, one of the two opposing forces (the other is YIN) whose ceaseless interplay with each other is said to give rise to five elements including fire, water, earth, wood and metal. The yang characteristics include activity, brightness, daylight, happiness, hardness, horizon, lightness, masculinity, positive dispositions, summer, sunshine, southern directions, upward-seeking and wakefulness. See YIN.

yang environment (Chi.) According to the Chinese notion of YIN AND YANG, a yang environment is characterized by hot, arid zones, such as the Middle East.

yang food (Chi.) According to the Chinese concepts of YIN AND YANG, foods which are salty, sour and dry, which are grown in YIN ENVIRONMENT are yang food. See also YIN AND YANG FOOD, YIN FOOD.

yantra (Num./Occ.) From the Sanskrit word, meaning a loom, tool or machine. An abstract interlocking matrix of geometric figures, circles, triangles, floral or aesthetic patterns, a yantra is composed of an outer geometrical pattern enclosing an interior pattern symbolic of the link between the macrocosm (or the universe) and the microcosm (the human body). Although it is drawn in two dimensions, a yantra represents a three-dimensional view and is used as a tool for contemplation. Some basic components in a yantra are bindu or an infinite point, a hexagram, a lotus, upward and downward pointing triangles symbolizing female and male principles respectively.

A yantra serves as an image used to maintain a focussed state during MEDITATION.

Meditating through a bindu, and expanding into the designs around and returning to bindu repeatedly is believed to lend an integrative experience as one takes charge of outward disturbances in one's life, paving the way for overcoming the negativities and stress in life.

Yantra Yoga (Tib.) A healing technique which incorporates the use of YANTRA, microcosmic representation of the macrocosm and traditionally considered proactive to MEDITATION. The technique combines styles of HATHA YOGA and QIGONG. The exercises are based on breathing, postures, MUDRAs and movements.

yastikasana (Yoga) An ASANA, recommended for slimming and increasing height. The steps in brief are: (1) lie supine (2) inhale for three seconds, legs fully extended, arms stretched above the head (3) retain the breath for six seconds, stretch toes and fingers outwards (4) exhale returning to normal position.

yavagu (Ind.) A dietary preparation of cereals such as powdered rice, wheat, or barley boiled with water, making a gruel in a liquid (manda), semi-liquid (vilepi) or solid (peya) consistency. It is considered an ideal food while undergoing the treatment routine in AYURVEDA.

yellow colour therapy (New Age) Yellow is considered the colour of joy and merriment, capable of lifting despondency. In CHROMOTHERAPY, yellow is associated with cure of ailments such as arthritis, constipation, diabetes, eczema, exhaustion, flatulence, hemiplegia, indigestion, kidney and liver ailments, mental depression, paralysis and paraplegia. The colour is not, however, recommended for people who are already overexcited. Yellow-coloured foods are believed to be beneficial when a person is nervous or confused or unable to make decisions. Some yellow-coloured foods can be sourced from bananas, butter, cheese, corn, ghee from cow's milk, cucumber, eggs, lime and lemon, musk melon, pineapple and turmeric.

yellow saphire (Gem.) This gemstone is believed to be the best for promoting the overall health in its wearer. It is said to influence the endocrine glands and balance all the DOSHAs. It is said to be effective, more particularly in decreasing excessive VATA.

yi (Chi.) A focus or an intent, essential in the practice of QIGONG. Focussing one's mind on body movements is considered an art as the focus cannot be just hard and fixed but should facilitate smooth transitions by carrying awareness while remaining connected to changes in the body movements.

yin (Chi.) One of the two opposing forces in the scheme of the universe (the other being YANG), which is said to give rise to five elements, fire, water, earth, wood and metal, through a ceaseless interplay between them. Yin characteristics can be explained by the following qualities: darkness, dullness, earth, female, negative characteristics, night-time, northern direction, passivity, sleep, softness and winter.

yin and yang (Chi.) A popular concept, originating in ancient Chinese philosophy and metaphysics, describing two primal opposing but complementary forces in the universe as well as in the human body. Yin and yang are descriptions of complementary opposites, rather than absolutes. While the categorization is seen as one of convenience, the two are usually in a dynamic state of movement rather than held in absolute state. Thus, most forces in nature can be seen as having yin and yang states, though nothing is totally yin or yang. Western culture views yin and yang as corresponding to 'evil' and 'good' respectively, whereas in EASTERN MYSTICISM, they are complementary to each other.

yin environment Cold locations or climatic zones.

yin and yang in food (Chi/New Age) The culinary concept of yin and yang. Metabolic rate is believed to be increased by yang foods, whereas yin food decreases the body's heat and thereby decreases the metabolic rate as well. Foods dense in FOOD ENERGY, especially energy from fat, are categorized as yang. Foods with a high water content are considered as yin. The Chinese ideal is to eat both types of food to maintain the body's balance. There are neutral foods, which can neither be grouped as yin nor yang. The following table indicates yin, yang and neutral types of foods. See also, YANG FOOD, YIN FOOD

Yin-type foods	Yang-type foods	Neutral-type foods
Almonds, apple, asparagus, bamboo, banana, barley, bean curd, bean sprouts, beer, broccoli, cabbage, cantaloupe, celery, clams, corn, corn flour, crab, cucumber, duck, eels, fish, grapes, green tea, honey, ice cream, lemon, melon, mushroom, mussels, oranges, oysters, peppermint tea, pineapple, salt, shrimps, spinach, strawberries, soya beans, white sugar, tomatoes, water-melon, water.	Beef, black pepper, brown sugar, butter, cheese, chilli pepper, chicken liver and fat, chillies, chocolate, coffee, deep-fried foods, eggs, smoked fish, garlic, green peppers, goose, ham, kidney beans, lamb, leeks, onions, peanut butter, roasted peanuts, potato, rabbit, turkey, walnuts, whisky, wine.	Bread, carrots, cauliflower, cherries, lean chicken meat, dates, milk, peaches, peas, pigeon, plums, raisins, brown rice, steamed white rice.

yin and yang in medical theory (Chi.) The age-old concepts of yin and yang and the Five Agents (WU XING) provided the basic framework in biology and medicine. The organs of the body were seen to be interrelated and best understood by looking for correlations and correspondences. Illness was interpreted as a disturbance in the equilibrium of yin and yang or the Five Agents. The causes were identified as emotions, heat or cold, or other influences. Therapy thus depended on diagnosis of the exact source of the imbalance.

yin and yang symbol (Chi.) In the symbol of yin and yang, the outer circle represents 'all', while the black and white shapes represent yin and yang respectively. The shape of these two energies in the symbol gives the impression of the continuous movements and dynamism of these two energies, their expansion and contraction.

yin food (Chi.) Food materials, having aroma, flavour and sap, usually grown in hot and dry parts of the world, such as the Middle East. See also YIN AND YANG IN FOOD and YANG FOOD.

yin style bagua (Chi./New Age) A Chinese martial, medical and internal arts system, yin style bagua combines ACUPRESSURE and TUI NA forms of BODYWORK. The emphasis is more on QI than on strength. (i.e., 'qi-first-then-strength' approach). To achieve this, YSB has a DAO YIN practice, specially designed for the bodyworkers. It enables them to cultivate QI energy in them, besides enhancing their sensitivity.

ying qi (Chi.) Also, nutrient qi. The nutritional aspects of QI energy that nourishes the body. It refers to the essence of food nutrients, which are believed to be produced by a combination of fresh air, inhaled through the lungs, with the food nutrients absorbed and transported by the spleen. The nutrient qi is said to nourish the internal organs so as to maintain their physiological functions. See also, FOOD ENERGY.

Yoga (Yoga) From the Sanskrit yuj, meaning to unite. The union and integration of all human aspects, from the subtle and innermost force to external influences that create, grow, nurture and end them. Yoga has both a philosophical and a practical dimension. The union inferred by the name 'yoga' refers not only to the intra-harmonization (of body, mind and spirit) but also inter-harmonization between humans and their surroundings. By practising yoga, the mind is quietened and 'purified'. The ego is erased. The end result is the emergence of positive feelings, acceptance, pure love, joy and respect to every fellow-being and event in one's life.

The practise of yoga, on the other hand, can indicate the practise of any activity that brings the practitioner closer to the mystical union of the universe and human, a state called SELF-REALIZATION.

> 'Yoga is nothing but the evenness of mind.'
>
> —Bhagavad Gita

yoga basti (Ind.) A type BASTI, using medicated oil administered for eight days. The treatment is aimed at nourishing the colon and neutralizing the aggravation of diseases caused by the aggravation of VATA.

yoga blankets (Mod.) Blankets made especially to suit the convenience of those who practise YOGA and ASANAS. In ancient times, animal skins were used by yoga practitioners. These have been replaced by woollen or cotton blankets. They are also used as yoga props, such as bolsters.

yoga chikista (Mod.) An individual-based prescription of ASANAS and breathing practices, aimed at developing health and vitality. Some systems of YOGA, such as IYENGAR YOGA, PHOENIX-RISING YOGA and VINI YOGA, cater to the needs of an individual; based on the body alignment, an informed instructor can prescribe asanas to counter problems such as diabetes, obesity and stress. The five basic guidelines to be followed while undertaking any yoga exercise for healing are: 1. relaxing the body and developing relaxed feelings 2. proper exercise 3. proper breathing 4. proper diet and 5. positive thinking and meditation.

'The practice of yoga destroys the impurities of the body and mind, after which maturity in intelligence and wisdom radiate from the core of the being to function in unison with the body, senses, mind, intelligence and consciousness.'

—Patanjali

yoga clothing (Mod.) Light, loose and comfortable clothes, which facilitate the practice of various ASANAS. Simple, cotton clothes without hooks, buttons and zips are recommended.

yoga equipment (Mod.) Gadgets and equipment which facilitate the practice of ASANAS. Most yoga props are designed to provide extra support to help one get deeper into a pose, or hold a pose for longer. There are also yoga CDs and videos which train beginners.

'The yoga mat is a good place to turn, when talk therapy and anti-depressants aren't enough.'

—Amy Weintraub

yoga incense (Mod.) The use of traditional aroma aimed at activating the limbic system, triggering deep-seated emotional responses.

yoga nidra (New Age). 1. Psychic sleep 2. A type of MEDITATION practice 3. A relaxation method aimed at withdrawing one's awareness from external stimuli, while remaining aware of internal processes.

yoga nutrition (New Age) A dietary prescription, based on the belief that PRANA, vital energy, is the 'real nourishment' one derives from the food consumed. Several indigestible, rich and devitalized foods ingested, according to this theory, deplete energy levels in the body, mind and spirit. From the yoga perspective, consuming small quantities of high-quality foods is adequate. High-quality foods include fruits, vegetables, whole grains and nuts. Moderate eating is the cornerstone of yoga nutrition.

'Just as in earthly life lovers long for the moment when they are able to breathe forth their love for each other, to let their souls blend in a soft whisper, so the mystic longs for the moment when in prayer he can, as it were, creep into God.'

—Soren Kierkegaard

yoga of synthesis (Occ.) A type of YOGA, which integrates all spiritual and religious paths. It is an eclectic and universalistic path that garners the best from each path and integrates them into one cohesive unified whole.

'Believe those who are seeking the truth; doubt those who find it.'

—Andre Gide

Yoga Sutra (Yoga) Composed by the sage PATANJALI, some three millennia ago, these ancient texts on the system of Yoga contain four chapters and 191 aphorisms ('sutras'). Fifty-one aphorisms in the first chapter deal with techniques of concentration; fifty-one in the second deal with the technique of the three-fold KRIYA YOGA, (comprising austerity, study and prayer); fifty-six in the third, on SIDDHIs and thirty-three in the fourth on the causes of bondage and methods of liberation. In the final chapter, it is mentioned that physical ailments (vyadhi) create emotional upheaval and that the task of yoga is to tackle them together. The ideal and practise of concentration, its spiritual benefits and the siddhis that one encounters in the spiritual pathway are also discussed.

> 'The objective of yoga is to calm down the chaos behind the conflicting impulses.'
>
> —Patanjali

yoga synergy (Mod.) A dynamic style of HATHA YOGA, which represents a synthesis between ASHTANGA YOGA, IYENGAR YOGA and modern medicine.

yoga therapy (Mod.) The application of yoga to treat physical and psychological ailments; using yoga postures with obvious effects on pressure points, body systems and organs. See also YOGA CHIKITSA.

> 'Yoga teaches us to cure what need not be endured and endure what cannot be cured'
>
> —B.K.S. Iyengar

Yogassage (New Age) A healing method which combines YOGA and MASSAGE. Yogassage is said to invigorate the mind and body while, at the same time, relaxing them. It is said to be useful in relieving stress, aches and pains.

yogic neuromuscular therapy (New Age) A technique aimed at stabilizing mind–body connections. Yogic neuromuscular therapy is said to release stress, tension, pain and trauma on physical, energetic and emotional levels by unwinding the traumatized tissues.

yokibics (New Age) A holistic movement programme, based on AIKIDO and the EIGHT LIMBS OF YOGA, yokibics is said to bring balance and symmetry in one's behaviour.

yoni mudra (Yoga) From the Sanskrit word, meaning the seal of the vulva, yoni mudra is a gesture of the source. An exercise in PRATYAHARA or sense-withdrawal, comprising blocking one's ears, eyes, nose and mouth with the fingers. To form the yoni mudra, the ears are closed with thumbs, eyes with forefingers, nostrils with middle fingers, upper lips with ring fingers and lower lips with little fingers. The mudra also involves breath-retention (KUMBHAKA). It is believed to help the mind focus inwards, by increasing one's feminine (YIN) energies. Considered difficult for even devas ('devanampi durlabha'), yoni mudra is advised to be practised with caution.

yuan qi (Chi.) Also, congenital qi, heavenly qi, original qi, source qi, qi, inherited by all living things from their parents, which animate them. Though TRADITIONAL CHINESE MEDICINE recognizes a variety of QI having a profound effect on one's health and wellbeing, it is believed that yuan qi cannot be created by energy-building exercises, though it can be topped with 'acquired qi'.

yusha (Ind.) Also, mudga yusha. A regime of soup diet in AYURVEDA, combining green gram (mung dal), soaked for three hours and boiled in water with spices such as black pepper, coriander, cumin, ginger and long pepper. Rock salt is also added. Yusha is prescribed on the second day of PANCHAKARMA.

Yuthog Yonten Gonpo (1112–1203) (Tib.) The 'father of the Tibetan system of medicine', who was respected as the emanation of 'Medicine Buddha'. He codified Buddhist medical techniques and cultural beliefs in his Four Tantras which form an essential text in TIBETAN MEDICINE.

zangfu (Chi.) A term used to describe the main YIN AND YANG organs in the human body. A YIN organ is called a zang, while a YANG organ is called a fu. Although the organs are identified by their Western anatomical names, TRADITIONAL CHINESE MEDICINE views their function in relation to the ancient concepts of QI. The twelve organs of Traditional Chinese Medicine, which correspond to the twelve MERIDIANS or channels within the body are classified in accordance with their functions as yin (e.g. transformation) or yang (e.g. transportation) organs. The zang is thus made of the following six 'solid' organs: heart, pericardium (i.e., the sac surrounding the heart), lungs, spleen, liver and kidneys. The fu consists of the six 'hollow' organs including the small intestine, triple warmer (an organ function), stomach, large intestine, gall bladder and the urinary bladder.

zangfu zhi qi (Chi.) The energy that nourishes the internal organs of the human body. See also ZANGFU.

zazen (Chi./Jap.) From the Chinese, for seated meditation. Also, zuochan, tso-chan. A form of ZEN meditation, aimed at awakening meditative absorption directly wherein all dualistic distinctions are dissolved. The position for zazen is sitting with folded legs and hands, and an erect but settled spine. Breathing is done from HARA, the centre of gravity in the belly. The eyelids are half-lowered, the eyes being neither fully closed, nor open. The practitioner, though aware of his surroundings, remains undistracted. Zazen practices are said to pave the way for the cultivation of a focussed state of mind with a relaxed body.

> 'Research is to think what nobody else has thought'.
>
> —Albert Szent Gyorgi

zdorovye (Eur./New Age) Also, zdorovye nature's legacy. A centuries-old Slavic natural health system, incorporating bodywork or 'somatic engineering', which integrates respiratory enhancement, structural alignment, and bio-mechanical efficiency in the body.

Zen (Chi./Jap.) Also, Chan, a derivation from the Sanskrit word dhyana. A Japanese concept, which traces its origin to China and India, Zen believes in direct, intuitive insight by focussing exclusively on one's essential nature. The approach emphasizes the importance of moment-by-moment awareness. Japanese Zen teachers hold that Zen is a way of life and not solely a state of CONSCIOUSNESS.

Zen Alexander Technique (New Age) A technique of healing, combining ALEXANDER TECHNIQUE and TRADITIONAL CHINESE MEDICINE.

Zen gardens (Jap.) Also, Japanese rock gardens, karesansui. An enclosed shallow sandbox in which sand, gravel and rocks with occasional grass are arranged. While the sand symbolizes the ocean, the rocks, the islands of Japan. Plants may or may not be part of this garden. However, of late, the term refers to planted landscapes with rocks.

Zen shiatsu (New Age) A form of SHIATSU,

developed by Shizuto Masunaga (1925–81), a Japanese psychologist. Zen shiatsu is a form of BODYWORK, administered by the fingers, thumbs, palms and elbows, feet and knees with pressure applied to all parts of the body along the MERIDIANS. It includes the practice of MEDITATION.

zero-balancing (New Age) An approach to healing combining both Oriental and Western practises in healthcare. Developed in 1975 by Fritz Smith, an American acupuncturist, osteopath and physician, the technique stresses on achieving balance between bio-energy and the musculo-skeletal structure, using finger pressure and sustained stretching exercises to release tension, accumulated over years, deep inside the body.

zhang zhuang (Chi.) Also, stance training. A form of QI GONG. Known as 'standing meditation', the technique aims at enhancing one's energy levels.

zheng qi (Chi.) 'Upright' or normal QI; the energy that circulates through channels and organs in the body.

zinc An important nutrient, usually rare in the average diet. However, it is essential for the efficient functioning of the reproductive system, immune system and for healing. The table indicates zinc contents in some food sources:

Food items	Zinc (mg/100 gm)
Cheese	2-4
Eggs	1
Liver	6-8
Milk	0.4
Milk powder	4
Oysters	>7
Shrimps	2

zone diet (New Age) A recent approach to diet therapy propagated by Barry Sears (1940-). Called as a 'way of eating', it is said to help in maintaining the body's insulin levels within a particular 'zone'.

zone therapy (New Age) See REFLEXOLOGY.

zong qi (Chi.) QI that gathers in the chest area through the coming together of GU QI and KONG QI.

Zulu sangoma bones (Afr.) From *sangoma,* meaning healer. A South African DIVINATION method, which features herbal remedies and spirit healing.